Barbara I. Willinger, CSW, BCD
Alan Rice, CSW
Editors

A History of AIDS
Social Work in Hospitals
A Daring Response
to an Epidemic

D0022228

Pre-publication
REVIEWS,
COMMENTARIES,
EVALUATIONS . . .

"We are all living in the middle of AIDS history. This book is a necessary reference to what we have been through and what we will go through. It should be in every college library that teaches social work and on every desk of every social worker, regardless of whether they practice in HIV medicine. HIV touches all of our lives. When I read this book I cried for all of the friends I lost at the beginning of the AIDS epidemic when none of us knew what to do or what to say. Hopefully, this book will help everyone to get through that loss, until there is a cure."

Nancy "Buddy" Seaton, BA
AIDS Program Social Work Assistant,
St. Vincent's Hospital,
New York City

"Because of the emergent and unexpected appearance of HIV and AIDS, the history of the response to it has often been sacrificed in favor of doing the work. This book presents the recollections of social workers, their health professional colleagues, and their clients. The HIV/AIDS epidemic has 'grown up' with its own service networks, treatments, and recognition. We are all too often forgetful about how social workers first addressed the stigma and service voids surrounding the disease. Willinger and Rice have created a panel of front line experts who relate how social workers bridged medical staff, families, and communities, created or adapted support structures for families and community resources, and also created professional and personal support networks. These histories are vivid, evoking the personal and historical context and providing important lessons for the present and the future."

Nathan L. Linsk, PhD
Professor, Jane Addams
College of Social Work,
University of Illinois at Chicago

"**W**illinger and Rice have compiled a book that chronicles the historical and clinical aspects of the AIDS epidemic that had not previously been told. Many of the authors they bring together in this book were among the earliest heroes and heroines in the fight against AIDS as it struck the most disenfranchised segments of the American population. From the histories they tell, important lessons can still be learned that are immediately relevant to the challenges facing the current generation of social workers serving people living with HIV and AIDS in all segments of today's America. This book is immensely valuable to students preparing to enter the field as well as social workers currently on the front lines of working with clients and their families who are affected by the HIV/AIDS epidemic. *A History of AIDS Social Work in Hospitals* is also a valuable resource in terms of how it details public policy, administrative, organizational, and clinical issues all pertaining to the social work response to what has been called the most devastating epidemic of the twentieth and twenty-first centuries."

Michael Shernoff, MSW
Adjunct Faculty,
Columbia University
School of Social Work

"**T**his book is a powerful testament to the ability and desire of human beings to rise to the challenge to institute change during crises. It is a tribute to all individuals who struggled to make a difference from the beginning of the HIV/AIDS epidemic. These stories demonstrate the heroic feats of individual social workers and others who rose up to make a difference in the lives of those infected and affected by HIV/AIDS.

When you read this book you will feel sorrow, and then rejoice when you see how far things have progressed, then you will weep again. Reading it will take you on the roller-coaster ride of the epidemic, the twists and turns of the disease and social change. This book represents a torch to be passed to newcomers to AIDS social work."

L. Jeannine Bookhardt-Murray, MD
Medical Director of HIV Services,
Morris Heights Health Center,
Bronx, NY

The Haworth Press®
New York • London • Oxford

A History of AIDS Social Work in Hospitals

A Daring Response to an Epidemic

THE HAWORTH PRESS
Titles of Related Interest

A History of AIDS Social Work in Hospitals
A Daring Response to an Epidemic

Barbara I. Willinger, CSW, BCD
Alan Rice, CSW
Editors

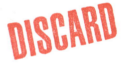

The Haworth Press®
New York • London • Oxford

TR: 8.9.04

The Haworth Press, Inc., 10 Alice Street, Binghamton, NY 13904-1580.

PUBLISHER'S NOTE
Identities and circumstances of individuals discussed in this book have been changed to protect confidentiality.

Cover design by Jennifer M. Gaska .

Library of Congress Cataloging-in-Publication Data

A history of AIDS social work in hospitals : a daring response to an epidemic / Barbara I. Willinger, Alan Rice, editors.
     p. cm.
Includes bibliographical references and index.
    ISBN 0-7890-1586-2 (hard cover : alk. paper)—ISBN 0-7890-1587-0 (soft cover : alk. paper)
    1. AIDS (Disease)—United States—History. 2. Medical social work—United States—History.
    [DNLM: 1. Acquired Immunodeficiency Syndrome—history—United States. 2. HIV Infections—history—United States. 3. Social Hospital—history—United States. 4. Social Work Department, Hospital—history—United States. WC 503.7 H673 2003] I. Willinger, Barbara I. II. Rice, Alan.

RA643.83 .H575 2003
362.1'969792'00973—dc21

2002015023

CONTENTS

ABOUT THE EDITORS

Barbara I. Willinger, CSW, BCD, maintains a psychotherapy practice and co-facilitates bereavement groups. She is currently an employee of the NYS Department of Health AIDS Institute in Manhattan. From 1989-2001, she was Social Work Manager and Clinical Supervisor for the Adult and later Pediatric HIV/AIDS Program at St. Luke's Hospital in New York City. She has also published clinical articles on social work practice, hemodialysis, and psychopharmacology. Over the years, she was asked to participate in various city and state committees and task forces. In the early 1990s, Ms. Willinger developed an innovative task force of hospital social workers and city administrators from the Division of AIDS Services to address the issues of HIV/AIDS patients accessing services/entitlements.

Alan Rice, MSW, is Director of Social Work at Highbridge WoodyCrest Center, an AIDS nursing home in the Bronx, New York. In 1983, he became one of the first hospital AIDS social workers in NYC at Beth Israel Medical Center. He has provided services to AIDS patients, their families, and the staff as a direct practice social worker, supervisor, and manager. Mr. Rice was the recipient of the first Rabbi Isaac N. Trainin award in 1986 "In Recognition of his Caring Spirit," and he received the Diego Lopez AIDS Service Award in 1995, presented by NASW-NYC Chapter HIV/AIDS Committee.

time in pursuit of a master's degree in health care administration. She has worked at Parkland Hospital with the HIV-infected population since 1996 and currently holds the position of HIV ER case manager. She feels blessed to be able to work with HIV-infected patients and their loved ones.

Holly H. Dando, MSW, CSW, is Senior Social Worker at the David E. Rogers unit of the Center for Special Studies of the New York Presbyterian Hospital. She graduated from Trinity College in Hartford, Connecticut, in 1986 with a BA in comparative literature. She has been a social worker in the HIV field since 1990 when she received her MSW from New York University.

Elaine Ehrlich, MSW, LSW, ACSW, has more than twenty years of experience in the not-for-profit and government sectors. Ehrlich has worked in the fields of HIV/AIDS, vocational rehabilitation, health care, social services, and developmental disabilities. She has served on boards in public education, mental health, and the arts. She provides consultation to boards, executive directors, senior management, and staff. Currently she is Director of Corporate and Foundation Relations at Saint Vincent Catholic Medical Centers of New York, a member of the board of directors of Gay Men's Health Crisis, and an editor for the *Journal of Gay and Lesbian Social Services.* She is also a member of the National Society of Fund Raising Executives.

Mera Eisen, MSW, ACSW, was formerly the assistant director for Community Services, Social Work Department, Montefiore Medical Center, Bronx, New York. She is a founding chairperson and current board member of Bronx AIDS Services, Inc. Eisen is newly retired from a professional career built upon the integration of community organization and clinical practice within the context of institutional and community-based service delivery.

Kevin Farrell, MSW, was Client Services Director at Face to Face and a member of the Sonoma County AIDS Commission during the process described in his article. Currently, he is employed by the University of California at San Francisco/AIDS Health Project on contract to the California State Office of AIDS, Department of Health Services. In that position, he is the consulting social worker for the Case Management program and the Medi-Cal Waiver program, which serves approximately 4,000 clients in forty-four sites around California.

Matthew Feldman, MSW, CSW, received his master's degree in social work from Columbia University in 1998. Until 2002, he worked at St. Luke's-Roosevelt Hospital in two positions: the outpatient division of child and adolescent psychiatry and the Center for Comprehensive Care's Morningside Clinic, which serves children and adults infected with and affected by HIV/AIDS.

Feldman is also an adjunct instructor at Columbia University as a social work field instructor. Currently he is pursuing a doctorate in social work, focusing on adolescents with HIV/AIDS.

Charles J. Finlon, MSW, CSW, is a clinical social worker at the Center for Special Studies of New York Presbyterian Hospital's Weill Cornell Medical Center. He has a post–master's certificate in end-of-life care from New York University and the Open Society's Project on Death in America and is a special features editor for the *Journal of Gay and Lesbian Social Services* (The Haworth Press, Inc.), in which he writes a regular column about Internet resources. He has been involved in HIV/AIDS organizations since the mid-1980s and currently maintains a private practice in New York City.

Dina Franchi, CSW, received an undergraduate degree in psychology from Hofstra University, New York. She received her master's degree in social work from Adelphi University, New York. Currently she is pursuing a PhD in social work at Fordham University, New York. Franchi began her AIDS work in 1987 and is currently the project manager of the Families in Transition Program at Beth Israel Medical Center in New York. She is also an adjunct professor at Molloy College.

Jay Freedman, BA, is Acting Director, Bureau of Community Support Services of the New York State Department of Health AIDS Institute. He is responsible for case management services in AIDS Institute contracts, Medicaid-funded initiatives including hospitals, primary care sites, and community-based organizations. Freedman has overseen the development of New York State's approach to both process and outcomes monitoring for case management services. He is responsible for the state's case management training initiatives, development of policy, fiscal and practice standards, and has designed methodologies for the evaluation of program effectiveness. Freedman has twenty years of experience with Medicaid-funded case management programs serving the geriatric and HIV communities. He has worked as a methadone maintenance treatment program case manager and holds a degree in counseling psychology.

Devin L. Griffith, MSW, is presently Community Programs Director for Randolph Hospital in Asheboro, North Carolina, where he directs the organization's home and community care services for older and disabled adults and manages the HIV/AIDS care services. Griffith has worked as a hospice social worker, HIV case manager, HIV support group facilitator, adult day health manager, and department director in a community-based hospital. Committed to increasing access to care for individuals infected with HIV/AIDS in rural areas, he has served on various state committees and task forces addressing pertinent health care issues. He began his work with HIV/AIDS clients in 1992 and continues the work today.

Susan W. Haikalis, ACSW, LCSW, has been a social work administrator in the field of HIV and AIDS for over twenty years. For the last seven years, she has been the director of the HIV Services and Treatment Support department of the San Francisco AIDS Foundation. She is responsible for planning, developing, and supervising all client services for over 2,000 clients seen annually. Services include client advocacy, financial benefits counseling, long-term subsidized housing, case management, treatment support/education, and publications. Haikalis is currently cochair of the NASW national HIV/AIDS Spectrum Project Advisory Committee, which provides workshops for social workers and allied health professionals on mental health, substance abuse, and ethics as well as HIV/AIDS. Haikalis is the past president of the Society of Social Work Leaders in Health Care and a recipient of the Ida Cannon Lifetime Achievement Award for her contributions to the field of health and social work.

John Kleinschmidt, MSW, CSW, graduated from New York University's Graduate School of Social Work in 1993. He has been active and involved in HIV/AIDS work since the late 1980s. He has been working as a clinical social worker with the HIV/AIDS program at St. Luke's Hospital in New York City since 1993. He is also a field work instructor for Columbia University School of Social Work since 1995. He maintains a small private psychotherapy practice and does per diem work for Visiting Nurse Service of New York in their Adult Care Services department.

Lorna Andria Lee, CSW, received her BA in 1986 from Mount Holyoke College and her MSW from Columbia University School of Social Work in 1990. She was a medical social worker at Beekman Downtown Hospital until 1992 when she began working with HIV/AIDS patients at St. Luke's Hospital, AIDS Center Program. She worked for eight years in the inpatient AIDS unit. Since then, she has worked at Jewish Home and Hospital Adult Geriatric Day Care Center and is currently employed by HIP Health Plan of New York in the Geriatric Case Management Department.

Vincent J. Lynch, MSW, PhD, is Director of Continuing Education and Adjunct Associate Professor at Boston College Graduate School of Social Work. In 1988 he founded, and continues to chair, the annual National Conference on Social Work and HIV/AIDS, which consistently draws over 500 people. Lynch has edited/co-edited four books that deal with social work and HIV/AIDS issues. His AIDS work has earned him awards from the Council on Social Work Education (1988), from the Harlem Community

AIDS Center, New York City (1998), and from the Massachusetts Chapter of NASW (2001). He also has an interest in ethical issues in research and serves as chair of the Boston College Institutional Review Board, which oversees the protection of human subjects who participate in research projects.

Sally Mason, PhD, LCSW, is Assistant Professor of Clinical Social Work at the Institute for Juvenile Research, Department of Psychiatry, University of Illinois at Chicago. She has over fifteen years' experience in the area of HIV/AIDS as a case manager, educator, therapist/group facilitator, program consultant, and researcher. Specializing in services to women, children, and families, she has played an active role in the development and evaluation of services for HIV-affected families in Chicago. In addition to HIV/AIDS, she has special interests in child welfare and kinship care. Her research includes the service and permanency planning needs of relatives who have taken on the care of HIV-affected children, custody planning with HIV-infected mothers, program evaluation of services for HIV-affected families, and community-based needs assessment of services for HIV-affected families.

Sister Rosemary Moynihan, SC, PhD, is a member of the general council of the Sisters of Charity of Saint Elizabeth, Convent Station, New Jersey. Prior to this, as Manager of Community Mental Health at St. Joseph's Regional Medical Center, Paterson, New Jersey, she developed the Ryan White-funded Mental Health Program for HIV-infected, multiply diagnosed individuals and family members. In addition, as Assistant Director of Social Work at Memorial Sloan-Kettering Cancer Center, she supervised the Social Work HIV/AIDS Program and collaborated in the establishment of the New York City Social Work AIDS Network. In conjunction with the New York City Department of Mental Health, Mental Retardation, and Alcoholism Services, she helped develop and clinically supervised the New York City AIDS Professional Education Program.

Nan O'Connor, LCSW, is a licensed clinical social worker in San Francisco. She is the project coordinator of the HIV Mental Health Case Management Program at the Center for Special Problems and is in private practice. She has been working with individuals with HIV for over fourteen years.

Daniel R. Ostrow, MSW, LCSW, is a licensed clinical social worker living and working in San Francisco. In 1992 he established the first publicly funded HIV primary care clinic at a private medical center in San Francisco. The program design later came to be the prototype of all San Francisco government-supported HIV primary care programs. He also designed and directed the first rehabilitation unit for people with severe AIDS-related dementia in the United States. He is currently the director of the medical clinic at San Francisco International Airport. He has maintained a psychotherapy practice since 1985.

Margaret E. Piazza, LCSW-C, RN, began her career in health care in 1967 as a registered nurse working in the areas of medicine and surgery. She received her BSN in 1983 and practiced in the areas of home care and community health. She graduated from the University of Maryland School of Social Work and Community Planning in 1989 and began her second career in social work and HIV/AIDS in 1988 while in her second year of social work school. She continues to be challenged and rewarded by her work.

Cynthia Cannon Poindexter, MSW, PhD, is currently an associate professor at Fordham University Graduate School of Social Sciences. Prior to that she held the position of assistant professor at the Boston University Graduate School of Social Work. She received her BA from Duke University, her MSW from the University of South Carolina, and her PhD from the Jane Addams College of Social Work at the University of Illinois at Chicago. She has been a social worker for twenty-five years, fifteen of which have been in the HIV field. Her current research concerns older HIV-related caregivers, HIV training evaluation, and participation of HIV-infected volunteers and employees in the AIDS service system.

Martha Powers, MSW, CSW, received her social work degree in 1992 and worked with HIV/AIDS patients at St. Luke's Hospital, AIDS Center Program until 1995. Currently she is the clinical social worker at the Miriam Hospital Immunology Center, working for Timothy Flanigan, Charles Carpenter, and Susan Cu-Uvin. Her work with HIV/AIDS clients includes individual and group counseling, crisis intervention, and case management.

Matthew Rofofsky, MSW, CSW, received his master's degree in social work from Columbia University in 1996. He began his work with HIV/AIDS clients in 1996 working for the Center for Urban Community Services as Assistant Team Leader at the Times Square Hotel, a model SRO serving a multitude of clients, and then as team leader at Flemister House, a fifty-bed congregate care facility for people with AIDS. Mr. Rofofsky gained his inpatient HIV/AIDS experience at St. Luke's Hospital (Center for Comprehensive Care Program). He also has supervised BSW students and is an adjunct instructor at Mercy College. Currently he is the program coordinator of the Mobile Mental Health Team at Harlem United Community AIDS Center.

Susan C. Rucker, CSW, came to social work after a twelve-year career in elementary education. She graduated from the University of Maryland School of Social Work and Community Planning in 1983. Except for eight weeks of temporary work at a state psychiatric facility, her social work career has been spent at Johns Hopkins Hospital and Johns Hopkins University AIDS Service. She began her work in HIV/AIDS in 1986 and has continued to the present time.

Patricia A. Stewart, MSS, ACSW, LSW, BCD, received her master of social service degree (MSS) from Bryn Mawr College Graduate School of Social Work and Social Research in 1981. She manages an independent psychotherapy and consulting practice in the Philadelphia area. She also works part-time supervising Widener University graduate social work students at a grant-funded program in Chester, Pennsylvania. Since the early 1990s, Stewart has been extensively involved in work with and on behalf of people living with HIV/AIDS. She has designed and facilitated more than fifty workshops both locally and nationally and has been involved in the planning of many conferences and institutes across the United States. She is the founder of a very successful conference by and about African Americans and HIV, held annually since 1996 in Philadelphia, Pennsylvania, and has also published a number of articles and book chapters.

Diane Pincus Strom, CSW, is the administrative director of the department of medicine and the AIDS program at Bronx Lebanon Hospital Center in the Bronx, New York. She received her BA from City College of New York and her MSW from New York University. Strom developed and supervised the AIDS case management program at Bronx Lebanon from 1986 through 1996, at which time she assumed the broader responsibilities of the overall AIDS program. Present interests include training and developing peers as case management extenders and educators concerning adherence to HIV treatments and the provision of care to mentally ill chemically addicted patients with HIV. Strom lives in the Bronx with her two children.

David Strug, MSW, PhD, MPH, obtained his PhD in anthropology from Columbia University in 1975, his MPH from the University of California at Berkeley in 1977, and his MSW from Hunter College in 1987. He is an associate professor at the Wurzweiler School of Social Work at Yeshiva University. He has been involved in HIV/AIDS research since the beginning of the AIDS epidemic. He began his clinical and supervisory work with HIV/AIDS clients in 1992 and continued until 1999.

Mary Tucker, MSW, CSW, is a social work supervisor at the Daniel Leicht Clinic (HIV/AIDS) attached to Gouveneur Hospital. She received a master's degree in social work at New York University in 1994 and has worked in the clinic since. Tucker lives in New York City.

Charlene Turner, LCSW, ACSW, graduated from Howard University's School of Social Work where her specialization was group work. She held the position of Director of Social Service at Grady Hospital for over twenty years. She is currently the administrative director of Care Management for the Grady Health System in Atlanta, Georgia.

Anita Vitale, BA, was born and raised in New York City. She graduated from Hunter College with a degree in history. Most of her working life has been spent in New York City government in a variety of direct service and administrative positions. In 1986, she was hired to be the director of the AIDS Case Management Unit, then a small program in the New York City Human Resources Administration. She became the citywide director of case management operations when the program expanded and became known as the Division of AIDS Services. She held that position until 1994. In recognition of her work with persons with AIDS, she was awarded the Samuel and May Rudin Award for Community Service in 1998. From 1994 to 2002 she was the director of AIDS services at the Visiting Nurse Service of New York.

Darrell P. Wheeler, PhD, MPH, ACSW, is currently an assistant professor at the Hunter College School of Social Work in New York City. He teaches community organizing and social administration methods. He has previously held faculty positions at the University of North Carolina–Greensboro, Columbia University, and the University of California, San Francisco. Wheeler is actively involved in HIV/AIDS prevention work and is the coprincipal investigator on a Centers for Disease Control and Prevention-funded seroprevalence study of African-American gay men. He began his HIV/AIDS work in Pittsburgh, Pennsylvania, as a peer outreach worker in 1989. Wheeler also holds national NASW board positions.

Lori Wiener, ACSW, PhD, has been working in the field of HIV/AIDS since 1982. Originally from New York, Wiener accepted a position at the National Institutes of Health in 1986 to help the chief of the pediatric branch of the National Cancer Institute incorporate pediatric HIV disease into the existing pediatric oncology program. To date, close to 600 HIV-infected children and their families have been cared for at the HIV/AIDS Malignancy Branch of the National Cancer Institute. Wiener has carried out numerous studies examining parental needs and coping, children and adolescent coping, as well as interventions designed to meet their needs. She also brings with her a wealth of information about the inner worlds of these children and their families, some of which has been published in a book titled *Be a Friend* (1994) and in *An Alphabet About Families Living with HIV/AIDS* (1998).

Acknowledgments

This book grew out of conversations between the editors reflecting on their conversations with and observations of social workers who have committed themselves to working with the thousands of men, women, and children infected with and affected by HIV/AIDS. We dedicate this book to the spirit and courage of all those social workers, as well as to the infected and affected men, women, and children.

When the editors originally conceptualized this book, we thought it would focus only on New York State, but our myopic outlook was quickly broadened, thanks to the suggestion of Michael Shernoff. This started us on an exciting journey. We wish to thank all the contributors across the country who participated in the writing of these chapters and who gave so freely of their time and experiences. A special acknowledgment to Marta Friedman who, without knowing either of us, provided the San Francisco "connection."

The co-editors wish to acknowledge the following people: Seth Parrish who provided Alan the supervision and guidance to help him obtain his MSW; Fred Nenner who provided Alan the opportunity to work with AIDS patients; Lu Czynski for giving Alan the time from work needed to complete this project; and Jeremy Willinger, a special acknowledgment for his invaluable technical skill and assistance.

A very special thanks to our spouses: Robert Willinger for his continued support, patience, and encouragement in moving this project forward, and Barbara Rice for having the courage to allow Alan to accept the AIDS social work position and always being by his side. And to both for being the people they are.

Introduction

Barbara Willinger
Alan Rice

There are moments in your personal and/or professional life that are defining and impossible to forget. Such moments occurred for us in the early 1980s at the beginning of the AIDS epidemic. We and other social workers, who were assessing patients' needs during hospitalizations, were confronted with colored signs on closed doors that gave the following instructions:

IF YOU ARE ENTERING THIS ROOM YOU MUST
    PUT ON A GOWN
    PUT ON A MASK
    PUT ON GLOVES

Some of us tried not to think of the implications of these signs. Many of us had internal dialogues about what we might be getting ourselves into. What if the information is wrong and casual contact leads to infection? Is it too late to tell my director this job is not for me? Most often, however, these were transitory thoughts, and we entered the patient's room.

Barbara's initial recollection of passing through that door was looking at an extremely cachetic Latino male, José, who was gasping for breath in spite of the oxygen mask covering his face. While Barbara could easily see José's frail body, covered by the white sheet, José could see nothing but Barbara's brown eyes peering from atop her mask. José repeated over and over, "What am I going to tell my wife?" He died soon after, never realizing his wife knew that he had AIDS and was only worried about what to tell their seven-year-old son.

Alan's first recollection is a Latino man named Joseph, who quickly understood the reason for Alan's precautions. For whatever the reason, Alan found himself sitting on the edge of the bed. What he thought would be a brief encounter turned into an hour's talk, a discussion of what could and could not be done for Joseph, but, most important, about who Joseph was. As Alan rose to leave, Joseph said to him, "In the last hour you were closer to me physically and emotionally than my wife has been since she found out I have AIDS—I can't thank you enough."

It is the thousands of José and Joseph interactions that have made this work so fulfilling and rewarding to all those social workers who were there during the early days, as well as now.

AIDS burst on the American scene in 1981, creating panic and fear in the American public. For some time no one knew what this disease was, where it came from, or how it was transmitted. For many it came as a relief when the disease was given a name—gay-related infectious disease. The relief of heterosexual men and women was short-lived, however, as more information became known.

For those of us working in hospitals, the early 1980s were a time of fear, challenge, and extreme caution. For some it was a period of denial and counterphobic behavior, thinking, "We could never catch this." Others acted like ostriches. Along with medical and nursing staffs, social workers were on the front lines. The social work profession found itself faced with the new challenge of helping young adults in their early twenties and thirties face the shock of a devastating illness that often quickly resulted in death or, for the more fortunate, the need to review and change their lifestyles. For some clients, the disease meant "outing" themselves to family; for others, it meant partial or total dependency on friends, family, or strangers and agencies.

The gay community in major cities such as New York and San Francisco quickly rallied, reacting to the multiple losses of friends and lovers that happened so quickly. Built-in support groups emerged, albeit oftentimes they were bereavement groups. Many others found little if any support, even though families and significant others existed. Many chose not to "burden" their loved ones in order to continue the status quo.

Social work values and ethics took on a new life in the midst of accumulated death. Confidentiality and patient rights took on new meanings as social workers grappled with "not telling," too often carrying the burden of hiding information from the patients' friends, families, and partners or spouses as we spoke with them about planning for their loved one's death. On-the-job training took on a new meaning as new resources were created and existing resources barred their doors. Social workers continued to advocate on behalf of their clients. The early AIDS social workers needed to be creative and patient.

Many hospital social work departments established task forces or specialized teams whose responsibility was not only to "work" with AIDS patients and their families but also to design programs and identify system issues within their respective sites that needed to be bridged. Among the earliest programs in New York City was the Social Work Department of Memorial Sloan-Kettering Hospital Center, which in 1982 "developed a psychosocial intervention program for patients, their friends and relatives, and the center's staff" (Christ, Wiener, and Moynihan, 1986, p. 176). In other hospitals executive committees were formed, chaired by top doctors, nurses, and administrative personnel. Social workers were asked to participate in these committees—not only the directors of social work but designated line staff as well. In San Francisco, the Social Work AIDS Network (SWAN) formed in 1985. For sixteen years it was a vehicle of peer support, education, and political activism.

In 1983, the governor of New York created a new state agency, the AIDS Institute, to deal with the multifaceted aspects of the new epidemic. Each discipline—medicine, nursing, social work, nutrition, to name a few—was to establish its own guidelines for patient care in hospitals. Social work drew on the model of case management, already utilized in the fields of mental health and long-term care, and adopted the model's core concepts for utilization with HIV/AIDS patients (Lambright and O'Gorman, 1992). It was a time of "cutting edge" care, program development, and resource building.

Until late 1986 there was no major influx of monies to provide increased services to AIDS patients within the New York health care system (Mantell et al., 1989). In the wake of the AIDS Institute's designation of hospital-based comprehensive AIDS program centers came increased funding streams that resulted in the expansion and provision of services to patients. Ryan White funds, the federal government's response to AIDS, soon provided additional monies through grant-funded programs.

Social work was often unable to utilize existing staff for newly created AIDS social work positions unless there were "personal reasons" that motivated the transfer; many staff members were too frightened. Alternatively, gay and lesbian social workers who once hid their identities more and more frequently gravitated to seeking work in the HIV/AIDS field in the late 1980s and early 1990s. Many felt a personal identification with the patients while others had been affected personally by the disease. New social workers, frequently recent graduates, were eager to learn and chose this area.

From the mid-1980s to the mid-1990s social workers in hospital-based AIDS care experienced a heyday—excitement, feeling renewed purpose and acting as agents of change. New and expanding roles that were not taught in the schools of social work emerged, such as arranging burials, assisting with wills, and learning how to discuss advanced directives long before the governor of New York signed the law making it a "patient right."

In the mid-1990s came a breakthrough: the introduction and widespread use of highly active antiretroviral therapy (HAART), which changed the face of HIV/AIDS from a crisis of dying to a situation with hope and chronicity. (In smaller cities and towns this phenomenon may be more recent because of expanding medications availability.) Separate and apart from the disease itself was the growing and encroaching impact of managed care and the phenomenon of hospital mergers in many parts of the country. These changes and the changes in the federal reimbursement guidelines to hospitals all collided in a trickle-down effect of reducing staff. In the social work world, particularly in New York City, the result was a dramatic change in organization and functions of departments of social work. For several hospitals it meant the decimation of HIV/AIDS social work programs that had existed.

Although patient longevity has increased and the numbers of admissions have decreased, does this necessarily mean that hospital social workers no longer need expertise in HIV/AIDS? We think not. Newly diagnosed patients continue to be seen, and the shock of acknowledging the existence of the virus is still powerful and "deadly" in the minds of many. Clients still need to be educated about prevention, particularly in light of the increase of unsafe sex practice among the young gay male population (AIDS Alliance for Children, Youth, and Families, 2001; Stolberg, 2001). Substance use, homelessness, and mental illnesses are again the pervue of social work interventions, but now social workers must consider the context of HIV/AIDS. Adherence to medications is crucial to reestablishing or maintaining a modicum of patient health that can result in a return to employment or educational training, or a resumption of homemaking activities. This often occurs in the context of social work support, referrals, interventions, and collaboration with multidisciplinary teams and/or outside agencies. Ultimately, patients are still sick and dying, even though diabetic and cardiac complications and lymphomas have replaced Kaposi's sarcoma, *Pneumocystis carinii* pneumonia, and toxoplasmosis. In general, however, the emphasis is on outpatient care and assisting patients to redefine their quality of life, their goals, and their medication management or adherence readiness.

This book presents an overview of some of the historical roles of hospital-based social workers from their personal and professional views—from the beginning of the epidemic to the present to the question of their future. This book is dedicated to all of us who were there with AIDS patients through the devastating times and to those who are still there in these changing times. Whether we live in New York City, San Francisco, Dallas, Atlanta, or somewhere in between, our responses and efforts have carried and continue to carry a common message: *we care.*

REFERENCES

AIDS Alliance for Children, Youth, and Families (2001). Press release, May 31.

Christ, Grace H., Wiener, Lori S., and Moynihan, Rosemary T. (1986). Psycho-social issues in AIDS. *Psychiatric Annals* 16(3): 173-179.

Lambright, W. Henry and O'Gorman, Mark J. 1992. New York State's response to AIDS: Evolution of an advocacy agency. *Journal of Public Administration, Research and Theory* 2: 174-198.

Mantell, Joanne E., Shulman, Lawrence C., Belmont, Mary F., and Spivak, Howard B. (1989). Social workers respond to the AIDS epidemic in an acute care hospital. *Health and Social Work* 14(1): 41-51.

Stolberg, Sheryl Gay (2001). In AIDS war, new weapons and new victims. *The New York Times,* June 3.

SECTION I:
MEDICAL OVERVIEW

Chapter 1

An Adult Infectious Disease Doctor's Encounter with HIV/AIDS

Alan Berkman

There is no straightforward history of the AIDS epidemic nor any way to achieve a coherent overview. HIV is a virus, a tiny particle that lacks the basic characteristics associated with life yet has the capacity to systematically destroy the 100 trillion cells that constitute a human being. It is transmitted through intimate acts—sex, birth, breast-feeding, needle sharing, and blood transfusions—and is responsible for a global pandemic that threatens to reverse decades of economic and political development in sizeable parts of the globe. The history of HIV in the United States is intertwined with the politics and popular perceptions and misconceptions that surround sexuality, gender, and race. HIV, the people infected with it, and those affected by it have challenged and changed how medicine is practiced, how medical research is done, and how personal rights and public health should be balanced.

In the beginning, it had no name. In 1977, I was an internist practicing community medicine on the Lower East Side of Manhattan. Most of my patients were women, struggling to make ends meet through low-paying jobs or welfare and doing everything they could to keep their children off the streets and off drugs. Carlton was an exception. He was a man in his late thirties who worked in a nearby hospital as a licensed practical nurse. He shaved his head before it was popular and had a wonderful sense of humor that could sometimes slide into maliciousness. He made no secret of his affinity for much younger men. One of the places—but certainly not the only one—where he met those younger men was Haiti, where he vacationed twice a year.

Carlton had been my patient for two years, coming regularly to have his blood pressure and diabetes checked and to engage in our ongoing discussion of how good it would be if he could lose twenty pounds. By the end of

1977, it seemed that he had finally succeeded in doing just that. He went from 200 pounds to 175, and his blood pressure and blood sugar both normalized. It was great to be able to take him off of the medications.

By January 1978, his weight had fallen to the low 160s. Further questioning revealed that he was having fevers and drenching night sweats. His appetite was good, but he was having diarrhea four to five times a day. On physical exam, he had markedly enlarged, nontender lymph nodes and an enlarged liver. Tuberculosis was a possibility, but he had no cough; parasites could be causing diarrhea and weight loss but wouldn't account for his swollen lymph nodes. The most likely diagnosis, I thought, was a lymphoma—a cancer of the lymph nodes. I arranged for an inpatient evaluation, including a lymph node biopsy.

The pathologist couldn't make a definitive diagnosis. The lymph node cells were definitely abnormal but not malignant. The pathologist from the well-known university hospital sent the slides to several colleagues, all of whom agreed with his description of the cells and none of whom could give a definitive diagnosis. All the other tests I ordered were also nondiagnostic, although they confirmed that he had an enlarged liver, no evidence of pulmonary tuberculosis, and no parasites in the stool.

He left the hospital with a clean bill of health and a progressive downhill course. It was not straight downhill, however. He would stabilize for a month or two and even regain some of his lost weight, but the diarrhea and fever inevitably returned and were unresponsive to any of the treatments I could prescribe. He became progressively weaker and more fatigued, and I had to work hard to come up with a diagnosis so that he could receive disability. Shortly before Thanksgiving in 1979, Carlton came to see me complaining of a cough and shortness of breath. He was skeletal, and walking down the hall made him breathe rapidly. I immediately arranged for hospitalization. His chest X ray showed pneumonia in both lungs, but he wasn't bringing up much sputum. Tests showed that his blood wasn't getting enough oxygen from his lungs. Intravenous antibiotics didn't help, and he was placed on a respirator. The oxygen in his blood continued to drop despite all our interventions, and he died just a few days after admission. Descriptively, he had experienced respiratory distress syndrome, but I had no idea what had brought it on.

By this time, I had another patient whose medical problems seemed equally mysterious. She was a nun in her late forties. Thin, with sparkling eyes and great energy, Sister Louise came to see me because she was losing weight and having fevers. In her lilting Irish brogue, she told me she thought that perhaps her malaria had returned. She had been a teaching missionary in West Africa for decades and had contracted malaria, tuberculosis, and a whole range of infections that would intrigue any tropical disease doctor.

She had needed blood transfusions because of anemia on a number of occasions.

Sister Louise had been in the United States for almost two years. Her order had sent her to St. John's University to study for a doctorate in American literature. She had finished her course work for a PhD and had just decided on the topic for her dissertation. She chose Saul Bellow, the quintessential Jewish writer. She hated to come to the doctor, but she was feeling weaker and knew she would need all her strength to complete her dissertation. It was my job to figure out what was wrong with her. I tried! A physical exam and routine blood tests revealed only enlarged lymph nodes and moderate anemia. She was twenty to thirty pounds below her ideal body weight.

I suggested a hospitalization that would enable a lymph node biopsy and several other studies, as well as a consultation from a physician more knowledgeable about tropical medicine. She outright refused, citing her upcoming oral exams as well as great distrust for doctors (no disrespect intended). We battled until we came up with a compromise that involved waiting until her orals were over and limiting the hospital stay to just a few days. We both kept to our word, but the only information that I got from all the tests and consultations was a lymph node biopsy that demonstrated pathology identical to Carlton's.

Sister Louise left the hospital and seemed to do better for a while. She attributed her improvement to twenty-four hours of continuous prayer by the sisters at the convent. It certainly seemed to work better than anything I had to offer. Sister Louise worked nonstop on her dissertation and came by the clinic every month or two to let me know how things were going.

She was stable for almost a year and rather miraculously completed the first draft of her dissertation. The fevers and weight loss resumed while she was doing revisions and preparing to defend her thesis. She worked hard and prayed hard and her body somehow sustained both, although she then weighed less than 100 pounds. She talked of returning to the convent in Ireland where she had entered the Church and where her blood sister still lived. Her admiration for a Jewish writer and her dreams of Ireland energized her while her physical being failed.

She invited my wife and me to her graduation, and we got to see her in her doctoral robes. After the ceremony, she was joyfully surrounded by the nuns from her adoptive American convent. We had a moment alone, and she told me she would write when she had settled in at the convent in Ireland. I never heard from her.

A gay man and a nun: Both had fever, sweats, diarrhea, marked weight loss, and enlarged lymph nodes. Neither could be diagnosed because we had no name for what they had—the first series of cases of what we now call AIDS would not be reported for another two years (Wolf, 2002). Yet, in retrospect, I am certain that each of them had AIDS. Carlton contracted HIV through sex and Sister Louise through blood transfusions in Africa. Or so I hypothesize. Epidemiologists categorize risk factors and even have a hierarchy of risk; for example, if a person who is an injection drug user and has unsafe sex gets infected with HIV and is reported to the Centers for Disease Control (CDC), his or her primary risk group will always be injection drug use. But like so many issues involved with HIV, the complexities of human behavior thoroughly muddle our categories.

A risk behavior history is only as good as the skills of the interviewer asking the questions and the honesty and memory of the patient. When behaviors are stigmatized or when an interviewer makes his or her own biases clear, the person being interviewed is unlikely to give an honest history. How many men have high-risk sexual encounters with other men but insist that they are exclusively heterosexual? How many women have had receptive anal intercourse but answer negatively when asked? One thread of the history of HIV has been a gradual awakening to the diversity of human sexual behaviors and the recognition that categories are merely abstractions that enable us to make neat tables to present data and perform statistical analyses but may say little about sexual safety and risk.

Twenty years after AIDS was first described (but not yet named), health care workers in the United States may have no direct knowledge or just lingering memories of the terrible suffering associated with it. As the immune system is progressively destroyed, every organ system can be affected. Early in the development of the illness, the patient may just notice mild weight loss and frequent bouts of diarrhea; a variety of sores, infections, and inflammatory changes involving the mucous membranes (mouth, vagina, and rectum) are frequent. As the T-cell count drops further, cytomegalovirus (CMV) disease can cause blindness in a matter of days. Toxoplasmosis, a minor problem in most healthy individuals, can cause seizures and destroy the brain. Cryptococcus, a rather common fungus in the environment, invades the membranes surrounding the brain and spinal cord and causes meningitis. CMV can cause excruciating ulcers in the esophagus that make eating almost impossible. Tuberculosis can cause disease in even healthy hosts but is much more likely to cause disease in those with impaired immune systems. A related organism, *Mycobacterium avium intracellulare* (MAI), can cause high fevers, profuse night sweats, and wasting in the advanced stages of HIV. HIV itself can cause painful nerve damage similar to that suffered by some diabetics and can destroy brain tissue, causing progressive dementia. A formerly rare skin cancer, Kaposi's sarcoma, can present as purplish lesions on the skin and can spread to the lungs and other internal organs. The list of HIV-related illnesses goes on and on.

HIV is not the only medical condition that causes suffering, but the number of combinations and permutations of diseases and symptoms is unmatched. For those caring for or about people with HIV, there seemed to be no way to comfort them. The patients were usually young and sometimes very articulate. Often, we could only empathize with them, and in that way extend our human solidarity in the face of suffering, disfigurement, and death. For social workers, the demand for help with benefits, home care services, end-of-life and guardianship planning, and counseling skyrocketed.

Fear accompanied the suffering. Many health care workers in the United States are now dismayed when they read about the stigma and fear that so often accompanies AIDS in Africa or other areas. Yet many of the earlier generation of American health care workers refused to touch infected people or even work on a floor that had AIDS patients. Some doctors and dentists would not accept people with HIV as patients; some nurses and social workers would not go into their hospital rooms. It was common knowledge among those of us working with HIV/AIDS patients that some prestigious hospitals in high seroprevalence areas such as San Francisco and New York tried to minimize the number of HIV patients admitted as inpatients or attending outpatient clinics.

Fortunately, many patients and their lovers, friends, and families refused to accept such treatment. They demanded that the health care system respond to their needs, and some of the finest doctors, dentists, nurses, and social workers finally did. The gay community in several large cities, particularly in New York and San Francisco, established and supported AIDS service organizations that became leading institutions for both care and prevention efforts. Advocacy groups such as ACT UP (AIDS Coalition to Unleash Power) broke the silence surrounding HIV (Silence = Death) and demanded that politicians and society as a whole respond to the AIDS epidemic. Social activism is one of the historical threads that makes up the story of HIV in the United States.

One of the demands raised by AIDS activists was for effective treatment. Part of what made HIV so frightening for patients and medical practitioners alike was the inability to effectively intervene. The progression of the illness seemed to be periods of acute illness followed by periods of recovery. But the patient never returned to baseline, and the next decompensation started from a lower level. HIV was like a roller coaster, with each infection resulting in a sharper drop for the patient.

Treatment for HIV has also developed in a step-wise fashion, but there has been movement both upward and downward. AZT was introduced in 1987 after a clinical trial showed that it decreased mortality and reduced new opportunistic infections in a group of patients with advanced HIV disease. Patients and their physicians were desperate for treatment, and soon tens of thousands of patients were setting their alarms and shaping their lives around a schedule of AZT every four hours around the clock. Many responded dramatically to AZT, but almost everyone experienced significant side effects as well. The improvement was short-lived, though, and after six months or so the downward progression usually resumed. AZT was followed by the "d" drugs: ddC (1993) and ddI (1991). Investigators and patients spent the next few years trying the three drugs in sequential order, hoping that a second drug would work when the first one failed.

Sequential monotherapy of HIV increased life expectancy in only small increments, but treatment of AIDS improved as doctors became more experienced in treating some of the common HIV-related diseases. Bactrim, a widely used sulfa-based antibiotic, was shown to both prevent and treat most cases of *Pneumocystis carinii* pneumonia (PCP), the most common cause of death in people who were severely immunocompromised. The average time from AIDS diagnosis to death stretched from one year to more than two.

HIV, the world's newest epidemic, brought with it one of the oldest epidemics known to humanity, tuberculosis. Tuberculosis flourishes when malnutrition, disease, or old age weakens the immune system; HIV made individuals extremely vulnerable to the disease. Most people with healthy immune systems who are exposed to the tuberculosis germ effectively fight the infection and never develop the disease. People infected with HIV, in contrast, are at great risk of developing tuberculosis either in their lungs or in a number of other organs.

New York City and other large urban areas began to experience a dramatic increase in tuberculosis during the late 1980s and early 1990s. HIV, linked initially in the public's mind with the gay community and people with hemophilia, had become epidemic among injection drug users. It was estimated that more than half of all injection drug users in New York City were HIV positive by the late 1980s (MacMaster and Womack, 2002). Injection drug use often accompanied poverty and poor living conditions, and tuberculosis has historically flourished under those conditions. Poverty and HIV were powerful and synergistic catalysts for a tuberculosis epidemic. Closed institutions, such as hospitals and prisons, accelerated its spread. A generation of health care workers that had seen only sporadic cases of TB now had to confront their own fears and get comfortable with masks, high-efficiency particulate air (HEPA), filters, and negative-pressure rooms.

Both the epidemiology and the management of HIV was changing dramatically by the early to mid-1990s. In large urban areas and in the rural South, the rate of infection was increasing rapidly among women. HIV infecting women was not new. Female sex workers, women who used injection drugs, and the sexual partners of bisexual men, hemophiliacs, and male injection drug users were all among the first impacted by the epidemic (CDC, 2001). In 1993, activists forced the CDC to recognize cancer of the cervix as an AIDS-defining malignancy. The growing number of women with HIV or who were AIDS activists compelled agencies such as the Federal Drug Administration and the National Institutes of Health to mandate that clinical and prevention research and new drug development include women in research studies (Project Inform, 2001).

The number of infants born with HIV began a dramatic decline in 1994 when the results of the 076 study were published. This clinical trial compared the percentage of infants born HIV infected to mothers and babies given AZT versus those who received no intervention. In the control (no intervention) group, approximately 25 percent of the infants were born infected. In the AZT group, this was reduced to approximately 8 percent. Adverse events among both mothers and babies were generally minor, and the 076 protocol was widely and aggressively adopted in the United States and Europe—both areas in which AZT was available (Connor et al., 1994).

Mortality due to AIDS declined in 1995 for the first time since the beginning of the epidemic (CDC, 1997). Many believe that one significant factor was that increased funding, particularly through Ryan White government grants, made it possible for a higher proportion of HIV-infected people to access care and treatment. Another factor was more effective care and treatment as health care practitioners in high prevalence areas became experienced in recognizing, preventing, and treating life-threatening complications of HIV. In addition to Bactrim, which was used for prophylaxis of both PCP and toxoplasmosis, protocols had been developed for prevention and treatment of MAI, a common cause of death in people with T-cell counts below fifty.

A third factor was that the treatments for HIV itself improved. Although sequential monotherapy had added little to people's life spans, therapy with two drugs simultaneously (dual therapy) did result in a modest clinical improvement and a rise in T-cell count. The introduction of two additional drugs, d4T (Zerit), and particularly 3TC (Epivir), increased the possibility of finding a two-drug combination that a patient could tolerate (Wolf, 2002).

The era of dual therapy came to an abrupt end with the introduction of a whole new class of antiretrovirals (ARVs) in late 1995 and early 1996. Unlike the five earlier drugs that were all of one class known as nucleoside reverse transcriptase inhibitors (NRTIs), protease inhibitors (PIs) attacked HIV replication at a different stage. Laboratory investigators, and subsequently clinical investigators, demonstrated that attacking HIV at two different enzymatic processes using NRTIs and PIs in combination could result in dramatic clinical improvement, improvement in immunological function, and reduction in the viral load (number of HIV particles) (Wolf, 2002). The use of three-drug combinations, usually targeting at least two different HIV enzymes, became known as highly active antiretroviral therapy (HAART).

We are now in the seventh year of HAART. A third class of drugs—N-NRTIs (non-NRTIs)—has been developed, and an additional variant of the NRTIs has just been introduced. There has been a marked reduction in deaths, in-patient hospital stays, and development of new opportunistic infections since HAART became widespread (Shernoff, 2002; THEORI, 2003). Initial hopes for a cure, or even for indefinite control of HIV replication, have disappeared as the limits of HAART have become apparent. Some of those limits are related to the drugs themselves and to the rapid replication and mutation of HIV. HAART is often (but definitely not always) able to slow HIV replication to a point at which the viral load cannot be measured, but the current regimens cannot totally eliminate HIV from the body.

We now understand that control over HIV replication comes at a considerable cost in terms of both short-term side effects and long-term complications from the therapy. Side effects, ranging from headache to nausea and vomiting to nerve damage to life-threatening pancreatitis and liver damage, have accompanied the introduction of newer and more effective ARVs. Fortunately, many of these side effects are temporary, and it is almost always possible to choose a regimen that a patient can tolerate. Unfortunately, long-term metabolic complications of HAART are now posing more of a challenge for both patients and practitioners as life spans are extended. Diabetes, high cholesterol and triglycerides, and dramatic changes in the fat distribution throughout a patient's body are all relatively common issues.

Medications are effective only if they are taken as prescribed. HAART therapy challenges human behavior. People may be willing to modify their schedules around dosing intervals and suffer from side effects when they are feeling ill and have been near death, but most find it hard to maintain that discipline when feeling better. Most studies (Meichenbaum and Turk, 1987; Sackett and Snow, 1979) have shown that less than half the people with a significant illness but without symptoms (such as people with high blood pressure) take medications correctly even when their pill burden is only one pill once or twice a day. HAART often requires several pills twice a day, and anything less than almost-perfect adherence will often lead to the emergence of drug-resistant HIV and failure of the therapy. Promoting and sustaining high levels of adherence has emerged as a critical aspect of treatment in the HAART era.

For people living with HIV, HAART has definitely offered hope and reasonable optimism for additional years of life. This comes at a cost—and not just the cost of rigorous drug adherence and side effects. There is also uncertainty about whether a particular regimen will continue to work and whether new medications will be available to try when and if it does fail. For people who might want to return to work, there is uncertainty about whether to give up important health benefits that come with disability. For women who want to have children, although there is much less uncertainty about whether a child will be born infected, there is great uncertainty about whether they will live long enough to raise their children.

What do these changes mean for those who care for people with HIV? In the early years of the epidemic, we had to find the place within ourselves that enabled us to relate to our clients' or patients' encounters with suffering and almost certain death. Now we are challenged to look inside ourselves to learn how to relate to patients and clients going through cycles of hope and despair, periods of good health and acute illness, and living day to day with profound uncertainty about long-term outcomes. Nevertheless, the one constant through the twenty years of changes brought about by the AIDS epidemic is that it continues to offer us the opportunity to learn more about what it means to be human.

REFERENCES

Centers for Disease Control and Prevention (CDC) (1997). 1996 HIV/AIDS trends provide evidence of success in HIV prevention and treatment: AIDS deaths decline for the first time. Press release, February 28.

Centers for Disease Control and Prevention (CDC) (2001). *HIV/AIDS Surveillance Report* 13(2).

Connor, E.M., Sperling, R.S., Gelber, R., Kiselev, P., Scott, G., O'Sullivan, M.J., Van Dyke, R., Bey, M., Shearer, J., Jacobson, R.L., et al. (1994). Reduction of maternal-infant transmission of human immunodeficiency virus type 1 with zidovudine treatment. *New England Journal of Medicine* 331: 1173-1180.

The Health, Economics, and Outcomes Research Institute (THEORI) (2003). SPARKS inpatient data, 1995-2002.

MacMaster, S.A. and Womack, B.G. (2002). HIV prevention for active injection drug users: A brief history of syringe exchange programs. *Journal of HIV/AIDS and Social Services* 1(1): 95-112.

Meichenbaum, D. and Turk, D. (1987). *Facilitating treatment adherence: A practitioner's guidebook.* New York: Plenum Press.

Project Inform (2001). Women and AIDS at twenty. *Perspective* 33: 9-10.

Sackett, D.L. and Snow, J.S. (1979). The magnitude of compliance and non-compliance. In R.B. Haynes, D.W. Taylor, and D.L. Sackett (Eds.), *Compliance in health care.* Baltimore, MD: Johns Hopkins University Press.

Shernoff, M. (2002). Uncertainty and quality of life: Psychosocial realities of combination antiretroviral therapy. *Journal of HIV/AIDS and Social Services* 1(1): 25-43.

Wolf, E. (2002). The HIV time line: 1980-2001. *Journal of HIV/AIDS and Social Services* 1(1): 11-23.

Chapter 2

A Pediatrician's Encounter with HIV/AIDS

Elaine J. Abrams

For me, the pediatric AIDS epidemic began in Central Harlem, New York City in 1982. I was a medical student learning about general pediatrics at Harlem Hospital Center, a municipal hospital serving the local community. A six-month-old boy was admitted to the pediatric wards with pneumonia. Despite routine treatment with antibiotics, he continued to worsen, requiring high levels of oxygen and respiratory support. His diagnosis eluded the team of medical providers, and he was eventually scheduled for an open lung biopsy. Under general anesthesia, a small piece of lung tissue was surgically removed and then examined under a microscope. Other pieces were sent to the laboratory to identify microbiologic pathogens. He was diagnosed with lymphoid interstitial pneumonia (LIP). No infectious agent was identified. With LIP, the white blood cells accumulate in an organized fashion in the lungs and cause limited oxygen exchange and difficulty breathing. Months later, we understood that this child also had what would eventually be identified as the human immunodeficiency virus (HIV) infection.

Twenty years later I continue to work at Harlem Hospital providing care to children with HIV infection. This young man is still alive, teetering on the boundary between adolescence and adulthood. His story, as well as those of many young people with HIV, chronicles the advances and changes that have characterized the pediatric HIV epidemic in the United States. The struggles of these young people as they enter their second and third decades highlight our successes and failures, as well as the challenges that lie ahead.

Throughout the 1980s thousands of children with HIV and AIDS were identified in major cities in the United States and Europe. More often than not, infants and young children arrived in emergency rooms with severe medical complications of the infection. Pneumonia, severe growth failure, brain disease, and overwhelming bacterial infections were increasingly common diagnoses on pediatric wards (Scott et al., 1989). Thousands of these children died, unable to withstand the immunologic devastation of the virus. Others, like the young man described previously, survived the early, severe illnesses and continue to battle the countless manifestations of the disease.

For each child diagnosed with HIV, there was always a mother with the infection. The vast majority of children with HIV acquired the infection "vertically" or "perinatally," during pregnancy or delivery. Surprisingly, HIV showed itself to be not just the "gay disease," but also very much a "family disease" (Abrams and Nicholas, 1990). In addition to the child and mother, the father almost always tested positive for the virus. Older and younger siblings were often infected as well. And those family members who weren't infected were clearly profoundly affected—grandparents, aunts, uncles, cousins, and neighbors were all drawn into the circle of AIDS.

By the mid-1980s pediatric wards in New York City were filled with children with HIV infection. Many were ill, suffering the devastating effects of the untreated virus. Others, however, were subject to the more subtle social complexities of the infection. HIV affected the most disenfranchised women and families, those with histories of substance abuse, living marginal lives in disorganized social settings. Medically fragile, these children could not be discharged to tenuous home environments. Women were at high risk for HIV infection because of behavioral and lifestyle choices, which also often left them unable to appropriately care for a child, especially one with intensified medical needs. Many mothers were actively using drugs, suffering from mental illness, homeless, or simply inadequately equipped to handle the complexity of caring for a child with a life-threatening illness.

For many years, few people stepped forward to take these children home. Fear of contagion was everywhere. Medical staffs were initially frightened of touching these children. Foster parents did not want to take them home. Everyone was afraid of contracting HIV. As we grew to know the children, however, barriers dissolved. The children, these "boarder babies," stayed for months, and sometimes years, on the pediatric wards of city hospitals, and they gradually became part of the hospital family (Hegarty et al., 1988). We threw away the gowns, masks, and gloves (except when handling blood). Over time, the children were lovingly cared for by nurses, physicians, social workers, and countless other members of the hospital community. Many first steps were taken while holding a nurse's hands, teetering down the pediatric corridor. Birthday parties were celebrated with great fanfare, and volunteers lined the children up in strollers at the elevator each afternoon, heading out for a walk to the park. Sadly, the staff at Harlem Hospital also buried many children who spent their short lives on the pediatric ward.

Social workers were at the forefront of the boarder baby struggle. They straddled the chasm between medical staff and family. The issues were complex and the dialogue inadequate. Medical staff did not want to see children discharged to parents who they perceived to be unable to care for a medically fragile child. Parents, despite a long list of social ills, very often wanted and struggled to take their children home. Social workers were left to communicate the difficult news that the child could not go home. They had few if any resources to offer parents who wanted to attend to their own problems. Drugs were much easier to come by than were openings in substance abuse treatment programs.

Social workers also had the primary task of finding alternative homes for the boarder babies at a time when few such homes existed. Foster families weren't prepared to take in children with AIDS, and foster care agencies had not recognized this new and pressing need in the pediatric community. Once again, the social workers had to bridge the chasm, this time between health care providers and social service agencies. "Why must the children remain in the hospital?" demanded the clinicians. But where were they to go? Ultimately, the social workers, like everyone else, rolled up their sleeves and played peekaboo and patty-cake with the new family of children boarding on the wards.

By the late 1980s the situation began to improve. The pediatricians at Harlem Hospital took the lead in publicizing the boarder baby crisis while actively seeking a solution (Nicholas and Abrams, 2002). In response, a unique collaboration between medical providers, social workers, city officials, the Catholic archdiocese, Columbia University, Harlem Hospital, and a private philanthropist was crafted, and Incarnation Children's Center (ICC) opened its doors in upper Manhattan (Nicholas and Abrams, 2002). ICC was a transitional care setting, where children with HIV could live in a nurturing, homelike environment until foster homes became available. It also offered medical rehabilitation for children with specialized medical needs who didn't warrant hospitalization. Many children from hospitals throughout the city were admitted to ICC, and they thrived there. Skinny children got fat. Shy, withdrawn children started to smile and laugh. Eventually most children were placed in wonderful foster homes. Simultaneously, foster care and social service agencies rallied to the needs of these children and began actively recruiting foster parents who would open their homes to children with HIV. Specialized training, enhanced stipends, and general goodwill resulted in a surge in available foster homes and the end of the boarder baby crisis.

Slow progress was made during the early 1990s as medical care for children with HIV infection improved. Zidovudine (also known as AZT or ZDV), the first antiretroviral agent, became available, and many children with symptomatic HIV disease received treatment. Clinicians also recognized the value of good supportive care. Enhanced nutrition, antibiotics to treat and prevent bacterial infections, and close surveillance of immune function resulted in improved health for many children. The pivotal moment in the pediatric HIV epidemic occurred in 1994, however. Researchers with the National Institute of Health announced the findings of a study that was conducted at many centers in the United States and Europe (Connor et al., 1994). These findings transformed the course of the epidemic for women and children.

When a woman with HIV infection has a baby, the child has a one in four chance of getting the infection. It was initially a mystery why some babies got sick and others escaped the infection. A great deal of research was focused on understanding this conundrum, and the risk factors for transmission were slowly identified (Mofenson et al., 1999; International Perinatal HIV Group, 1999). The study of greatest import is known as PACTG protocol 076 (Connor et al., 1994). The research was organized and conducted by the Pediatric AIDS Clinical Trials Group (PACTG) and studied whether zidovudine, if given to the mother during pregnancy and delivery and to the newborn, could decrease the likelihood of mother-to-child HIV transmission. Half of the women enrolled in the study received zidovudine during pregnancy (starting after the first trimester) and during labor and delivery. Their infants received oral treatment with zidovudine for six weeks as well. Half of the women and babies received a placebo treatment. The study was ended prematurely when researchers determined that the transmission rate in the treatment group was significantly reduced compared to the placebo recipients. While close to one in four of the untreated infants were infected, only one in twelve of the zidovudine-treated mothers transmitted the virus. The results were trumpeted throughout the corridors of HIV programs, and a door into the next phase of the epidemic was opened.

The results of PACTG protocol 076 transformed the dialogue concerning HIV. First, there was effective treatment to reduce the likelihood of mother-to-child transmission. Pregnant women with HIV could be offered medication to help protect their babies. Health care providers were relieved and delighted to have an efficacious treatment to offer their patients. Women were relieved and delighted that they could do something to help their babies. The bleak prospect of perinatal transmission suddenly brightened.

The study results also mobilized the programmatic philosophy of HIV testing during pregnancy. Although efforts had been made to encourage women to learn their HIV status during pregnancy, significant obstacles persisted. In the absence of preventive treatment, learning one's results offered limited benefits to the mother and child. The HIV-exposed child would be watched closely and prescribed antibiotics to prevent pneumonia until the child's true infection status was determined, but the mother and the health care provider could do nothing to protect the baby from becoming infected.

Learning one's infection status also held the risk of loss of confidentiality and potential associated problems. The ambivalence between knowing and not knowing was shared by patients and the health care system. Consent forms for HIV testing included long lists of the risks of learning one's status compared to only a few items of benefit. Protocol 076 shifted the balance clearly in favor of learning one's status during pregnancy.

The health care establishment and health care consumers responded quickly. New guidelines urged voluntary HIV counseling and testing for all pregnant women (Centers for Disease Control and Prevention, 1995). Those found to be HIV positive should be offered treatment with zidovudine according to the PACTG 076 regimen (Centers for Disease Control and Prevention, 1998a). The effect was profound. Counseling and testing programs were funded. Women agreed to testing and those identified with HIV infection agreed to zidovudine treatment. The road from clinical trial to widespread implementation was very short (Centers for Disease Control and Prevention, 1998b; Lindegreen et al., 1999). Remarkably, mother-to-child HIV transmission rates started to fall (New York City Department of Health, 2001). The number of HIV-infected pregnant women in care increased and significantly fewer sick babies were born. As new, more powerful, antiretroviral medications became available they were used in combination with zidovudine to enhance maternal health and to protect the baby. Many medical centers are now reporting mother-to-child transmission rates of 1 to 5 percent (Cooper et al., 2002).

Over the next several years more antiretroviral therapies became available, increasing the possibilities for treatment of children with established infection. The medications were relatively weak, however, and children continued to suffer disease manifestations. Multiple hospitalizations, frequent infections, poor growth, and delayed development continued to characterize the medical lives of many infected children. Some, however, despite having HIV, remained relatively healthy. The course of disease in children varies: 20 to 40 percent of children develop AIDS or die during the first years of life, while the majority appears healthier, manifesting fewer symptoms and remaining relatively well with the passage of time (Blanche et al., 1990).

The social issues evolved as well. HIV spread beyond the drug-using population to affect poor women of color living in inner-city communities. Unaware that they were at risk for HIV, many were identified during routine pregnancy counseling and testing. Social workers were the first in line to offer comfort and support while helping these women prepare for the future. Myriad issues needed to be addressed, including disclosure to partners and family members. Social workers provided counseling and support, both individual and group, to countless women living with HIV. Although most women did not use drugs, many were poor with enormous needs for tangible services. Quietly and effectively, social work staff identified resources and engaged women in the process of coping with this chronic illness.

The next scientific breakthrough made its way to the pediatric population in the winter of 1996. A new class of antiretroviral agents was developed, far more potent than the previously available medications such as zidovudine. These medications, protease inhibitors, could decrease the amount of virus in the blood to below the level of measurement. The medications were prescribed for adults with HIV and remarkable results were reported. Once a liquid formulation became available, pediatricians caring for children with HIV began to prescribe the only liquid protease inhibitor, ritonavir, and miracles occurred. Children on the brink of death, struggling with the most severe manifestations of the disease, improved dramatically (Abrams et al., 2001; Gortmaker et al., 2001). Expected deaths didn't occur. The skinniest kids started to gain weight. Children who hadn't been to school in months and years left their hospital beds for the classroom. The landscape of this disease was transformed.

Additional therapies were subsequently introduced, and most children with established infection were treated with these powerful new medications in combination with other antiretroviral agents. The widespread availability and use of these treatments resulted in a significant decrease in morbidity and mortality in the population of children with HIV infection (Gortmaker et al., 2001). Though the medical community quickly realized that these treatments didn't offer the hoped-for cure, pediatric HIV infection can now be considered a chronic disease of childhood. Rather than dying from HIV infection, most children are living with the disease. With relatively few new babies being born with HIV infection secondary to successful perinatal prevention efforts and few children dying from the disease, the average age of children with HIV infection has increased substantially (Abrams et al., 2001). More than half of the children with HIV disease in the United States are ten years of age or older. Many children, like the young man mentioned earlier, are well into their teens.

HIV, in addition to being a complicated and destructive virus, has always forced us to confront complex social and ethical issues. At the onset of the epidemic, society was obligated to examine its views on sex, homosexuality, and substance abuse. As the epidemic continued, questions of health care access and funding, especially for disenfranchised populations, were openly addressed. Now, as health care providers for children with HIV, we face a new series of social and psychological conundrums and challenges.

Adherence to antiretroviral regimens is presently the greatest challenge to the health and well-being of children with HIV infection (Watson and Farley, 1999). We have available a variety of powerful antiretroviral treatments that are able to completely suppress viral reproduction. Taken properly, these treatments can restore and maintain the immune system and prevent disease progression. The medications, however, are difficult to take. Because several medications must be taken together in order to be effective, many pills must be ingested each day. Most children require ten to twenty pills daily. Many of the pills are large and difficult to swallow. Some need to be taken on an empty stomach and others with food. Liquid formulations are not always available, and some simply taste terrible. Many children, who otherwise feel well, begin to feel sick after so many pills. It is often difficult to convince children and their caretakers that medicines which make children feel sick are "good for them." Given these limitations, children are often unable to adhere to prescribed medication regimens. Some children miss an occasional dose each week or month. Others actively conspire to hide their pills on a daily basis. More than one parent has reported finding a month's worth of the big blue pills (Viracept) hidden in the couch. Furthermore, not all families are able to provide the intense level of supervision necessary to assure complete adherence with antiretroviral regimens. Disorganized lifestyles, competing priorities, poverty, and ambivalence about the treatments and the side effects conspire to hinder therapy.

Incomplete adherence to treatment can result in the development of resistant virus that is no longer sensitive to the medications. After years of inadequate adherence, many children and teens with HIV harbor resistant viral strains that are increasingly difficult to treat. Treatment of resistant virus often requires more medications that further hinder adherence. While simple, easier regimens are needed to enable children to comply with treatment, their viruses, more often than not, require more and more pills to ensure efficacy. The young man in our clinic, having tried multiple complex therapeutic regimens, decided to stop treatment entirely. Despite advanced immunosuppression, he is more comfortable off therapy. Adherence has quietly moved to the forefront of issues concerning children with HIV infection, their families, and their health care providers.

Tied perhaps to the struggles with adherence, the mental health needs of children with HIV infection have emerged as especially pressing. A unique set of factors increases the vulnerability of children with HIV to mental illness and emotional disorders (Havens, Ryan, and Mellins, 1999). Many children, especially those now in their teens, were born to women with a history of substance abuse. It is not unlikely that many of these women had emotional and mental disorders which, in the context of poor access to treatment, they self-medicated with illicit drugs and alcohol. Many children have family histories replete with generations of substance abuse. Children with HIV infection were often exposed to drugs and alcohol in utero and many were treated for withdrawal symptoms at birth. The confluence of family predisposition and in utero environment likely increases the risk of emotional problems as these children age. In addition, HIV can affect the brain, and some children experienced severe, neurologic deficits during early childhood. Finally, consider the emotional milieu of a child with HIV infection. Most have experienced enormous losses throughout their lives. Many have lost parents, siblings, and friends to HIV infection, violence, or other social ills. Others never met their parents but instead spent significant parts of their lives in the foster care system. These children and young people let us know that HIV is on their minds. They grapple with their disease, its manifestations, and a variety of feelings generated by this chronic illness.

In clinics throughout the country, health care providers are struggling with the emotional and mental health needs of children with HIV infection. A wide variety of diagnoses ranging from attention deficit disorder to depression to psychosis fill the medical records. Many children receive treatment for behavioral disorders and psychiatric diagnoses as well as HIV infection and shoulder the burden of two chronic illnesses. In some cases, parents and caregivers find themselves poorly equipped to care for children, especially teens, with emotional problems. Having agreed to take home babies with AIDS more than a decade ago, many foster parents are surprised and overwhelmed to find themselves considering the emotional and psychological issues of their emerging teenagers. Social workers are once again at the forefront of the dilemma, trying to address limited resources and limited understanding of mental illness within the communities, which just a short time ago learned to openly embrace children with HIV.

The special needs of teens with perinatal HIV are slowly coming into focus. These young people have grown up with a chronic, ultimately fatal disease. They have learned, one way or another, to balance the demands and restrictions of their illness with the ordinary wants, needs, and fantasies of childhood and adolescence. As they enter their teens, most young people with HIV are confronting the same thorny issues as their uninfected peers: the highs and lows of puberty, sexual desires and fantasies, peer pressure, and limit testing. But they remain aware of their special risks, and they are quite emphatic that they do not want to further spread the virus that has so affected their lives. Yet few are prepared or willing to share their status with boyfriends and girlfriends, and fewer still are willing to practice safe sex. Despite being able to make the clear connection between parental drug use and their own HIV infection, many of the teens carry cigarettes in their backpacks, smoke marijuana in the school hallways, and have started to experiment with alcohol and a variety of drugs.

As the young man from my medical school days celebrates his twentieth birthday, we have many triumphs to celebrate. HIV perinatal prevention efforts have been enormously successful, and few babies are now born with

HIV infection in the United States. Children with established infection are living longer, healthier lives. Improvements in care and treatment have transformed pediatric HIV infection into another chronic disease of childhood. Many children are entering their teens and others are emerging into adulthood. The battle, however, is not over and challenges abound. First, we must find ways to help these children and families adhere to complex, lifelong medication regimens. Without improved adherence, we can expect many of the gains that we have witnessed to slip away as viral resistance increases and medication efficacy wanes. The development of simple, palatable regimens, consistent with the lifestyles of busy young people would be a large accomplishment, but short of this, ongoing support and education must suffice. We must also continue to mold health care programs to meet the needs of these children and young people. Emerging mental health and behavioral disorders require urgent attention and should be handled with the same urgency and empathy that went into the design and development of pediatric and adolescent HIV care centers during the 1990s. We must stay with these children. We must be there to hear about the triumphs and tribulations of adolescence, the dates, the fights, and the first kisses. We must continue the dialogue about safe sex, drugs, and alcohol. Finally, we must be there to sit at their bedsides and hold their hands when they are sick and when they are dying. For many of these children, doctors, nurses, and social workers have become family—and as family, we must continue the work.

REFERENCES

Abrams, E.J. and Nicholas, S.W. (1990). Pediatric HIV infection. *Pediatric Annals* 19: 482-487.

Abrams, E.J., Weedon, J., Bertolli, J., Bornschlegel, K., Cervia, J., Mendez, H., Lambert, G., Singh, T., and Thomas, P. (2001). Aging cohort of perinatally human immunodeficiency virus-infected children in New York City. *Pediatric Infectious Disease Journal* 20: 511-517.

Blanche, S., Tardieu, M., Duliege, A., Rouzioux, C., Le Deist, F., Fukunaga, K., Caniglia, M., Jacomet, C., Messiah, A., and Griscelli, C. (1990). Longitudinal study of 94 symptomatic infants with perinatally acquired human immunodeficiency virus infection. *American Journal of Diseases in Children* 144: 1210-1215.

Centers for Disease Control and Prevention (1995). U.S. Health Service recommendations for human immunodeficiency virus counseling and voluntary testing for pregnant women. *Morbidity and Mortality Weekly Report* 44(RR-7): 1-14.

Centers for Disease Control and Prevention (1998a). Public Health Service Task Force recommendations for the use of antiretroviral drugs in pregnant women infected with HIV-1 for maternal health and for reducing perinatal HIV-1 transmission in the United States. *Morbidity and Mortality Weekly Report* 44(RR-2): 1-30. Available at <http:www.hivatis.org>.

Centers for Disease Control and Prevention (1998b). Success in implementing Public Health Service guidelines to reduce perinatal transmission in HIV: Louisiana, Michigan, New Jersey and South Carolina, 1993, 1995 and 1996. *Morbidity and Mortality Weekly Report* 47: 688-691.

Connor, E.M., Sperling, R.S., Gelber, R., Kiselev, P., Scott, G., O'Sullivan, M.J., VanDyke, R., Bey, M., Shearer, W., Jacobson, R.L., et al. (1994). Reduction of maternal-infant transmission of human immunodeficiency virus type 1 with zidovudine treatment. *New England Journal of Medicine* 331: 1173-1180.

Cooper, E.R., Charurat, M., Mofenson, L., Hanson, I.C., Pitt, J., Diaz, C., Hayani, K., Handelsman, E., Smeriglio, V., Hoff, R., and Blattner, W. (2002). Combination antiretroviral strategies for the treatment of pregnant HIV-1 infected women and prevention of perinatal HIV-1 transmission. *Journal of the Acquired Immune Deficiency Syndrome* 29(5): 484-494.

Gortmaker, S.L., Hughes, M., Cervia, J., Brady, M., Johnson, G.M., Seage, G.R. III Song, L.Y., Dankner, W.M., and Oleske, J.M. (2001). Effect of combination therapy including protease inhibitors on mortality among children and adolescents infected with HIV-1. *New England Journal of Medicine* 345: 1522-1528.

Havens, J., Ryan, S., and Mellins, C.A. (1999). Child psychiatry: Areas of special interest, psychiatric sequelae of HIV and AIDS. In H. Kaplan and B. Sadock (Eds.), *Comprehensive Textbook of Psychiatry,* Seventh Edition (pp. 2897-2902). Baltimore, MD: Williams and Williams.

Hegarty, J.D., Abrams, E.J., Hutchinson, V.E., Nicholas, S.W, Suarez, M.S., and Heagarty, M.C. (1988). The medical care costs of human immunodeficiency virus–infected children in Harlem. *JAMA* 260: 1901-1905.

International Perinatal HIV Group, The (1999). The mode of delivery and the risk of vertical transmission of human immunodeficiency virus type 1. A meta-analysis of 15 prospective cohort studies. *New England Journal of Medicine* 340: 977-987.

Lindegreen, M.L., Byers, R.H. Jr. Thomas, R., Davis, S.F., Caldwell, B., Rogers, M., Gwinn, M., Ward, J.W., and Fleming, P.L. (1999). Trends in perinatal transmission of HIV/AIDS in the United States. *JAMA* 282: 531-538.

Mofenson, L.M., Lambert, J.S., Stiehm, R., Bethel, J., Meyer, W.A. III, Whitehouse, J., Moye, J. Jr., Reichelderfer, P., Harris, D.R., Fowler, M.G., et al. (1999). Risk factors for perinatal transmission of human immunodeficiency virus type 1 in women treated with zidovudine. *New England Journal of Medicine* 341: 385-393.

New York City Department of Health, Office of AIDS Surveillance (2001). Children perinatally exposed to HIV in New York City: Semiannual surveillance update, May.

Nicholas, S.W. and Abrams, E.J. (2002). Boarder babies with AIDS in Harlem: Lessons in applied public health. *American Journal of Public Health* H 92: 163-165.

Scott, G.B., Hutto, C, Makuch, R.W., Mastrucci, M.T., O'Connor, T., Mitchell, C.D., Trapido, E.J., and Parks, W.P. (1989). Survival in children with perinatally acquired human immunodeficiency virus type 1 infection. *New England Journal of Medicine* 321: 1791-1796.

Watson, D.C. and Farley, J.J. (1999). Efficacy of and adherence to highly active antiretroviral therapy in children infected with human immunodeficiency virus infection. *Pediatric Infectious Disease Journal* 18: 682-689.

SECTION II:
UNCHARTED TERRITORY

Chapter 3

Response to the AIDS Epidemic: Metropolitan New York

Esther Chachkes
Elaine Ehrlich
Mera Eisen
Sister Rosemary Moynihan

I remember attending one of the first scientific meetings on AIDS held in New York City initiated by Dr. Karen Cobell of Lenox Hill Hospital in 1982. The meeting was organized to discuss the new, rapidly spreading disease, and several social workers and public health professionals were invited. At the time this illness was found mainly in California among the male homosexual population, but now the number of cases in New York City was growing. The illness was called GRID (gay-related immune deficiency). There was a prediction that the illness could possibly become an epidemic, and the group at the meeting was polled about whether we thought this was possible. We were split almost evenly in response. Standing next to me was Sister

This chapter is based on conversations with Gaetena Manuele, Mera Eisen, and Elaine Ehrlich, and on task force and network meeting notes, memos, and announcements, 1983 to 1990.

Rosemary Moynihan, a social work supervisor at Memorial Sloan-Kettering Hospital. We looked at each other and concluded that we must put together a social work response—just in case. We were concerned about homophobia, the apparent youth of the persons infected, and how society would respond. We began to meet, at first informally and then later with Roger McFarlane who was the director of the newly formed organization Gay Men's Health Crisis (GMHC). Roger had helped with a female patient admitted to Montefiore Medical Center when there were no services organized and little was known about the illness. Roger was available, generous, and committed to helping anyone who was affected by the illness. His energy, intelligence, and "take charge" presentation were reassuring and calming.

The original network group included social workers from several hospitals that were beginning to admit patients diagnosed with HIV/AIDS including Montefiore Medical Center in the Bronx, St. Vincent's, St. Claire's Hospital, and Beth Israel Medical Center in Manhattan. As the number of cases began to increase in New York City, we recognized that we must extend beyond our small group and organize the greater New York City social work community to provide education and a better understanding of the important issues. In June 1983, we sent a letter to twelve hospital social work departments inviting social work staff working with AIDS patients to a meeting to discuss common concerns. That was the beginning of the Kaposi's Sarcoma (KS)/AIDS Social Work Network. By 1986, seventy-two social workers were members, representing a significant percentage of the voluntary and municipal hospitals in Manhattan and the Bronx, as well as faculty from the city's schools of social work. The group was a mix of direct practice social workers and department supervisors.

In any discussion of the social work response, it is important to acknowledge that social workers throughout the city were trying to identify professional approaches to service that would meet the needs of people infected with this new and unknown illness. This was complicated by the overlapping issues related to KS/AIDS—generally a hidden gay lifestyle, for some substance abuse, and the universally fatal nature of the illness at that time. For many infected people, the fear of contagion and infection led to rejection by family, friends, and even health care providers. The risk of being identified as a pariah, an "undesirable" patient, was real, and many people complained of poor treatment and of being turned away from services. Even funeral directors were raising concerns about handling the bodies of deceased patients. Prejudice and alienation marked the experience of many ill patients in these early days.

The social work mission, however, to provide service to vulnerable populations and to advocate and take social action influenced many social workers to seek venues for support and assistance in advocating for services. Social workers in hospitals, community agencies, and government agencies joined together but also worked as individuals in their own areas to push for home care, medical services, psychological counseling, legal protections, and prevention education. The list of social workers that contributed to the strong response of the profession is long; however, special mention must be made of George Getzel, Gaetena Manuele, Patrick Moriarity, Alan Rice, Susan Rosenthal, and Robert Schachter—social workers committed at the very beginning of these efforts. For social workers on the front lines working with dying patients, it was a time filled with grief but it was also a time when the immediacy of our help and assistance was especially rewarding. We felt we were in an important battle to help stigmatized people, at risk for rejection due to homophobia and attitudes about drug use, advocate for their needs.

The network met monthly at Memorial Sloan-Kettering Cancer Center (MSKCC). Esther Chachkes and Rosemary Moynihan rotated as chair; members took responsibility for identifying the important issues and for facilitating the discussion. This helped social workers dealing with this new illness and the profound concerns it stirred to identify problems, share information, and mobilize key resources, including housing, medical, and financial services. Almost no resources existed in the beginning, and those that did exist were reluctant to include AIDS patients. This was a very difficult situation as social workers tried to understand what resources were needed while trying to protect the rights of patients so that access to resources would not be limited.

The network served as a forum for advocacy on policy issues such as whether to disclose a diagnosis that could result in discrimination, rejection, and, for some, loss of employment and family support. The network also provided a place of emotional support for stressed social work staff working with young AIDS patients who were dying of the illness. The network also served to promote creative models of practice, as the psychosocial aspects of the illness became better understood. At meetings, experts presented on a range of issues that included information about homophobic reactions, mental health issues, legal and ethical issues in AIDS research and public health initiatives, drug abuse and AIDS, human rights issues, and antibody testing and current treatments.

Minutes of the early meetings in 1983 reflect the network's focus on learning about the medical aspect of the illness and the associated mental health and psychosocial issues, with particular attention given to the impact on the gay community. As patients began to return home for periods of time, focus on caregivers expanded and the American Red Cross was asked to give a presentation on home nursing for AIDS caregivers. Diego Lopez from GMHC talked about patient and partner counseling, John Arras and

Nancy Dubler from Montefiore's Department of Social Medicine provided discussion on ethical and legal issues including child custody issues and the increasing problem of the many orphans left because of a parent's illness. An important role for the network was to provide information to the New York City Departments of Health, Mental Health, and Human Resources about the impact of the epidemic and the needs of patients. Network members were surveyed several times and information was sent to the appropriate government agencies. Case examples were provided, and the responses of transportation companies, insurance companies, and hospitals were documented. We became an important conduit of information and provided witnesses who could offer professional testimony about abuses and violations of rights and the extensive unavailability of essential services.

In 1983 the network collaborated with the New York City Department of Health to prepare an AIDS referral and resources manual. We gave feedback on which agencies were useful or not useful and the strengths or limitations of resources.

In September 1985, the network developed guidelines for HTLV-III antibody testing. These guidelines enabled social workers to provide practice that was clear, consistent, and appropriate. They also were incorporated into the guidelines developed by New York City Department of Health for counseling and treatment. The guidelines included a discussion of whether to take the test and how the test results should be handled. Social workers were concerned that adequate counseling be available to people who tested positive and that confidentiality be protected.

In 1986, the network became a task force with full National Association of Social Workers (NASW) chapter status. This official connection with NASW provided updated information on AIDS and helped in the development and dissemination of policy statements on standards for implementing research and stimulating service delivery. The task force developed collaborative relationships with the Mayor's Forum on AIDS, the Greater New York Hospital Association AIDS Task Force, the AIDS Institute, and other organizations that were being formed to deal with this illness. These connections strengthened advocacy efforts when gaps in services were identified.

Minutes from the April 16, 1986, meeting of the task force delineated several ideas about the functions of the task force: to provide leadership for social work professionals in addressing service and policy needs; to suggest policy stances on AIDS for the chapter's action; and to develop relevant educational opportunities and resources for chapter members. A mission statement and progress report was presented to the board of directors of the NASW New York City chapter in the spring of 1986 and approved. Subsequently, the chapter developed a position paper on social work practice for people with AIDS and HIV infection. The NASW task force continued its work well into the 1990s and produced some very important policy and position papers. The task force also continued to influence the practice of social workers in this arena and helped to make the lives of so many affected by the illness better through advocacy and informed clinical practice.

Because the social work community had developed an extraordinary ability to identify and evolve clinical and advocacy interventions to address many of the complex issues related to the service and treatment of people with AIDS, their families, and their children, in 1986 the New York City Department of Mental Health, Mental Retardation, and Alcoholism Services, recognizing the social work contribution to the epidemic, granted a contract for an AIDS professional education program to the Department of Social Work at MSKCC.

While this program was housed at MSKCC, social workers from the NASW task force and mental health and health professionals from hospitals and voluntary agencies in New York City served as faculty. Under the direction of Grace H. Christ, director of social work at MSKCC, Roger McFarlane, and Sister Rosemary Moynihan, assistant director of social work at MSKCC, this program educated hundreds of professionals from all over New York City. Programs were provided from 1987 to the early 1990s addressing a broad spectrum of issues relating to AIDS treatment and services. The insights and firsthand experience of the faculty gave an unparalleled depth and richness to these programs. Topics such as neuropsychiatric problems and implications for behaviors, risk reduction in adults and adolescents, AIDS and addiction, family systems, and strategies for helping the terminally ill were all featured. Other topics involved the pros and cons of testing, emerging models for HIV counseling, harm and risk reduction, and, as patients began to survive for longer periods of time, living with AIDS and being HIV positive.

In addition to what was happening at MSKCC, the Montefiore Hospital and Medical Center also developed services related to women and children. The medical center began to identify HIV/AIDS patients as early as 1981 when eleven out of fourteen cases were women. Many of these early patients were intravenous drug users who were "street people" without residences, rejected by their families and presenting severe challenges to the discharge planning process, in addition to the emotional and concrete service supports needed to address a terminal illness that had no known treatment. These patients were poor and were often members of minority communities. Monnie Callen was appointed to this program as the direct service social worker, and her dedication and devotion were significant in designing a family-oriented approach. The social work department worked on custody issues, helping the new orphans of the illness to plan for future care and manage their psychosocial needs as their mothers were dying. In 1985 Dr. Rosa

Gil, deputy administrator of the Family Children Service Agency of New York City, brought attention to the growing number of children diagnosed with AIDS and the myriad social and medical issues relevant to this situation. A program directed by Anita Septimus was also organized at the Albert Einstein College of Medicine to address the needs of children with AIDS.

The department shared the strong social mission established by the hospital's past president Martin Cherkasky who gave the department an "open ticket" to engage in community leadership and service development efforts as interpreted by the professional staff. As a result, Gerald Beallor, the director of social work at that time, charged his administrative staff to develop programs and services for patients with HIV. The community was overwhelmed by the need to identify resources such as housing, financial assistance, medical insurance, support groups, meals on wheels, child care, and advocacy for public benefits and entitlements. Pressures mounted to advance administrative procedures to expedite public assistance and SSI applications for the newly disabled.

Along with the development of the NASW AIDS Task Force that was addressing the issues surfacing in the metropolitan New York City area, Mera Eisen, assistant director for community services at Montefiore Medical Center, was working with Bronx-based groups to address the needs of the growing number of patients in the Bronx. Mera had been involved with the NASW task force but recognized the need to organize a Bronx-specific response. She worked with an existing network of over sixty community health and social agencies, and the Association of Bronx Agencies, Inc., began to organize an AIDS response. The Bronx issues were similar to those identified throughout the metropolitan area such as gaps and barriers to entitlements and the need to develop appropriate services. Social workers from the various agencies became leaders in the efforts to design services and to advocate for patient needs. Social workers gained access to agency directors, elected officials, and New York City officials in Human Resource Administration, the Department of Health, and elsewhere. The Association of Bronx Agencies organized the first public forum addressing AIDS in the Bronx in 1983 with speakers from GMHC and the New York State AIDS Institute.

With the help of Elaine Ehrlich, then the program officer at the New York State AIDS Institute, the association was alerted to a New York State AIDS Institute grant proposal to establish community resources. Mera Eisen, after contacting several community agencies, was successful in eliciting the administrative and professional support of the South Bronx Development Office, a former antipoverty organization, to submit a proposal on behalf of the newly created Bronx AIDS Task Force, a committee of the Association of Bronx Agencies. The request for proposal was specific that community-based, not hospital-based, services were needed. Through the understanding gained from the social workers in the hospital and the work of the New York City AIDS Task Force, the wide range of services needed by HIV/AIDS patients and their families and the appropriate community-based programs were identified. At this time all service providers and hospital staff were hungry for information, community resources, and advocacy efforts. The Bronx AIDS Task Force became a key information sharing and educational forum for all. It also provided a venue for newly developing programs to present their plans and to obtain support, including the Highbridge Community Life Center, God's Love We Deliver, the American Red Cross, and others. The grant was received and used to hire staff, provide office space, and establish an infrastructure to begin the organization of an agency that became the Bronx AIDS Services Project. The organization was incorporated by 1987.

The Bronx AIDS Services Agency has become a vital resource in the Bronx, initially providing consultation and technical assistance to newly developing AIDS community services. Currently the agency's services include counseling, case management, HIV testing, peer education, support groups, outreach education and prevention, a food pantry, legal services, and nutritional education. New programs include an adolescent girls mentoring program, domestic violence counseling, and prevention education.

Elaine Ehrlich was serving as the community services program coordinator for the AIDS Institute in the New York State Department of Health when she came aboard in 1984. At that time the AIDS Institute had only been in existence for a year and a half, and she was the seventh person hired. She was responsible for overseeing grants given to community-based organizations and other organizations, such as Montefiore Hospital. These grants were to support provision of case management services for those who had HIV/AIDS and for prevention activities.

Soon thereafter, Elaine advocated within the AIDS Institute for expansion of comprehensive community-based services in each of the five boroughs of New York City. The primary comprehensive community-based prevention and case management services available in Manhattan were at Gay Men's Health Crisis. This organization, a national leader in providing AIDS services in the community, was able to meet the needs of the many men in Manhattan. They too recognized that other programs needed to be developed and offered to provide consultation to any services developed in the other counties. Elaine understood that people in Queens, Staten Island, Brooklyn, and the Bronx wanted to access services where they lived, and her advocacy within the health department resulted in the development and funding of six new community-based comprehensive HIV/AIDS organizations in Brooklyn, Queens, Staten Island, the Bronx, Upper Manhattan, and

Lower Manhattan. She provided guidance to the executive leadership for implementing their programs and strengthening their boards. Elaine will best be remembered for explaining to grantees why data collection was necessary. They all came to realize that providing data strengthened their cases for increased funding.

At the same time, Elaine, a resident of New Jersey, was actively involved with NASW, New Jersey. Sometime during 1986-1987, the New Jersey Department of Health AIDS Division invited social workers from around the state to a meeting to inform them of the activities of the AIDS Division. Elaine attended that meeting and afterward met with a few of her NASW colleagues to see how NASW could become involved. She and Barry Moore became the cochairs of the NASW-NJ AIDS Task Force and invited social workers from around the state to join in their activities. Their first efforts were to raise the consciousness of their colleagues about HIV/AIDS and to develop workshops at the annual meetings that covered aspects of HIV/AIDS treatment and counseling. The task force reviews the governor's proposed budget each year and prepares written testimony about funding of the New Jersey Department of Health's AIDS Division. Members of the task force were also engaged in drafting NASW's position on HIV/AIDS and the national NASW has recognized the work of this task force. Within NASW-NJ, the group has moved from being a task force to being a permanent committee of the chapter.

Elaine had to step down as cochair in 1989 when she became the director of grant monitoring and evaluation for the New Jersey AIDS Division. She brought to her new position four years of AIDS grantsmanship, management, and community-building skills. She initiated open meetings for community-based and grassroots organizations so they could learn how to respond to requests for proposals.

The social work profession can be proud of how it responded during the epidemic's early days. Social workers took leadership roles not only within their own professional organizations and workplaces, but also in government and community agencies. The social work perspective influenced advocacy efforts and promoted the establishment of appropriate services. Social workers were courageous, oriented to social action, and concerned with good clinical practice. The values and the mission of the profession, to alleviate suffering and to articulate the voices of those who must be heard, were upheld and well served. In the early 1980s, when working with a largely gay and drug-using population ran the risk of extending the stigmatization to social workers on the front lines, we did not shy away from service and commitment. Social workers continue today to provide services in AIDS organizations and to assist colleagues in other countries as the epidemic marches across Africa and Asia, producing thousands of victims.

Chapter 4

The Emergence of Social Workers in the AIDS Epidemic: SWAN— Social Work AIDS Network, San Francisco

Daniel R. Ostrow

Many of us in our forties have similar stories: We left our hometowns in the 1970s, resettling in great American cities, finding membership in diverse, gay urban tribes.

It was a Sunday afternoon in 1979 when I met Scott. I had never been picked up in a bar. The Rainbow Cattle Company, San Francisco's own gay country and western bar, was an unlikely venue for me. Scott possessed that rare trait among men: an unassuming bar demeanor. He melted through my usual reserve with his affable grin and a sparkle in his eyes. Hours later our pleasure was interrupted when we heard Scott's front door opening. In the hurry of sorting through and throwing on clothing, flushed with excitement and fear, I met Scott's partner of many years. Scott later explained that his relationship was ending, and he proceeded to romance me over the next year with sweet notes written on the back of vintage San Francisco postcards hand delivered to my doorstep. Although the romance never came to fruition, sweet sentiment pervaded.

My mind filled with these memories as I learned of Scott's death several years later while visiting friends in New York City. It was a frosty early spring morning in 1982. I was enjoying my last break before completing my graduate studies at the School of Social Welfare at UC Berkeley. Scott died of AIDS-related complications in a hospital bed after a brief, painful illness. This was how I faced the reality of AIDS. I did not know then that a year later I would be working in a hospital, St. Mary's Medical Center in San Francisco, and that my career in hospital-based social work would span the next two decades as a clinician, educator, organizer advocate, and administrator.

My professional life was relatively untouched by AIDS until 1987. In that year I was recruited to serve as the medical social worker for the hospital's growing number of AIDS patients, both on the inpatient units and in the outpatient clinic. My first patient, Bill, was a friend and colleague with whom I had worked on the adolescent psychiatric unit and dated on occasion. Bill declined the only rudimentary treatment then available, AZT, and died a week later in the arms of his friends.

Soon thereafter my partner Ed was given the soon to be outdated diagnosis of AIDS Related Complex (ARC). He had been ill for months, but his primary care physician was thick in denial or discomfort. Whatever innocence Ed and I were clinging to vaporized when his physician stiffly announced Ed's positive HIV antibody result. My world, not unlike that of many of my colleagues, had become professionally and personally centered on the reality of AIDS. I felt stunned.

The Reagan years (1981-1989) were a period of tremendous change in hospitals. Corporations formed with the purpose of acquiring and consolidating hundreds of freestanding community hospitals under vast holding companies to reduce expenses and leverage better rates under the emergence of managed care in the health industry. In tandem with these economic changes, hospital social work departments were quickly transforming. At St. Mary's, the psychiatric and medical social work departments were consolidated, with the attendant termination of one of the two social work department managers and numerous social work staff members. A year later the hospital gravitated to nurse case manager positions to facilitate shortened hospital stays under vastly restructured government and private health industry reimbursement strategies. Clinical social workers who provided treatment to patients and their family members were less relevant to hospital administrators who were working under mandates to cut costs by eliminating positions and moving patients out of beds at a faster pace. Most of the remaining social workers were limited to discharge planning functions. Eventually St. Mary's completely eliminated the social work department and formed a case management department. A few of us remained scattered in various departments reporting to nursing directors.

THE EMERGENCE OF SWAN

Against this backdrop of mounting illness, death, restructuring, and "down-sizing" of hospital social work departments, Suzanne Dumont and Ro Hanus, both medical social workers, convened the first San Francisco meeting of social workers to address the explosion of AIDS caseloads in local hospitals. Fifteen hospital-based social workers gathered in October 1985 and established SWAN, the Social Work AIDS Network. It was the beginning of sixteen years of monthly meetings of a nascent grassroots professional group, boasting a roster of 150 members representing multiple practice sites throughout the San Francisco Bay Area. SWAN's founding purpose remains relevant: the provision of professional peer support, education, and opportunities for networking and political advocacy. I joined in 1987.

SWAN's organizational development began with the basic need to connect with other social workers who shared common work, seeking relevant, accurate, and critical information and resources and learning approaches to work with our clients in an uncharted field. We were then able to find affirmation in one another and used our camaraderie, notwithstanding competition and rivalries that would occasionally arise, for our own well-being and on behalf of our clients. We were then able to successfully advocate for our clients. Finally, we assisted social workers in other cities such as Chicago, New York City, and Los Angeles who looked to SWAN as a model in building their own organizations.

One of our first political acts was to advocate for time to gather during the workday and preferably to be paid for this time by our agencies. Most of us were under increased pressure to be more productive with greater responsibilities. Initially many of us experienced relatively low levels of political clout in our hospitals. We felt isolated and stigmatized, mirroring what many of our patients experienced.

In the early years of the epidemic many of us carried mixed caseloads, undermining our ability to effectively serve our patients. At that time I was responsible for providing clinical services to children and their families on an acute psychiatric inpatient service, and to AIDS patients hospitalized on the medical-surgical and critical care units, as well as to the hospital's outpatient clinic.

SWAN's visible presence was in itself often influential. Before SWAN found a permanent venue to hold monthly meetings, members rotated the hosting of meetings at their home agencies. When I invited SWAN to hold a meeting at St. Mary's and arranged for one of the nursing administrators to give welcoming remarks, SWAN's visible presence contributed to leveraging the hospital administration to support a dedicated AIDS social work position despite regular rounds of budget cuts. Hospital and social work directors were increasingly incorporating our operational recommendations.

The group had a resounding need for fellowship and sharing of information and resources. The accumulated distress and sorrow we witnessed—the illness and death of partners, friends, clients, and colleagues—required our association. For many of us, holidays, birthdays, and anniversaries were now being replaced with new markers: the onset of symptoms, diagnoses, and hospitalizations of our clients, friends, partners, and our fellow social work colleagues. We realized that if we were emotionally unavailable or psychologically closed then we would not be able to listen and be empathic in our work. Therefore, time was made available to take our pulse and provide time for participants to "check in" with the group as needed. We also held several overnight membership retreats and half-day gatherings focused on self-care and renewal.

THE GROWTH OF SWAN

As SWAN grew from fifteen to 150 social workers with monthly meetings regularly attended by thirty to sixty people, a structure began to take shape to facilitate and organize our time and work. A permanent meeting site was adopted, officers were elected for six-month periods, and minimal dues were instituted to support the reproduction of minutes and mailings. Committees organized to address the needs of the membership, developing programs, inviting speakers to meetings, recommending policy development, and organizing political action.

Educational sessions were held during every other meeting and included local governmental policy leaders from the mayor's office, the Departments of Health, Human Services, and the Redevelopment Authority. The NASW California chapter president met with us. Other guests and speakers included hospice and home care directors, persons with HIV, and AIDS advocates representing groups serving persons of color, women, families, children, the homeless, and injection drug users. These sessions not only provided us with knowledge but also earned SWAN valuable credibility and political leverage as we advocated for policy measures such as anonymous HIV testing and low-income housing availability.

THE POLITICALIZATION OF SWAN

The need to engage in political activism emerged out of SWAN as a place for collegial support, education, and shared association. Later we developed into a professional group that formulated policy positions and joined with other allies. We sought and received representation on local and statewide governmental and professional bodies and task forces. SWAN members participated in the development of California's five-year AIDS plans and worked with legislative analysts on statewide AIDS legislation. We were also buoyed by the 1988 mayoral election of Art Agnos, a social worker and progressive political figure who appointed key progressive advisors, commissioners, and department heads. We now enjoyed increased access to the body politic. In 1988 SWAN affiliated with NASW as a recognized council to broaden our influence addressing issues of professional standards of social workers employed in HIV work, as well as working conditions and salaries. These alliances and affiliations increased our visibility and strengthened SWAN as a convincing force able to exert increased influence in public policy.

The need for personal affiliation with SWAN evolved over the years. In 1989 SWAN hosted a large contingent of members decked out in SWAN T-shirts to march in San Francisco's annual Gay, Lesbian, Bisexual, and Transgender Pride Parade. In 1990 Suzanne Dumont stood alone at the designated parade formation site, SWAN banner in hand, feeling abandoned when no other members arrived. She observed later that SWAN social workers were now marching with their respective agencies. She recognized this reflected an integration and identification with their organizations and was indeed a positive development that did not diminish the relevancy of SWAN's existence, but the expression of member affiliation with SWAN was changing.

Those of us who moved onto managerial roles were able to draw upon our experiences in SWAN to be sensitive to our agency staff as they in turn addressed issues of grief and burnout in their lives and work. This meant committing resources for staff training and professional development, including paid educational leave and reimbursement of conference registration fees. Agency staff retreats were also provided to address issues of team building and burnout.

I modeled SWAN when I developed new programs at St. Mary's; annual staff retreats and regular staff meetings were designed and budgeted for to address issues of team building and burnout. A staff support group was incorporated into the design of the innovative AIDS Dementia Unit at St. Mary's. The group was available to all staff on the unit and was conducted on site by an independent consultant. The group was ongoing, voluntary, confidential, and unconnected to management.

In an unpublished paper, Dunkel, Dumont, and O'Neill (1987), all early SWAN members and pioneers in their own right, noted that SWAN effectively integrated the therapeutic aspects of the support group with the goals of a professional organization, leading to the building of a professional group. Our individually honorable work in the epidemic and together in SWAN has brought meaning and purpose to many of us and to those clients we served. The opportunity to provide direct services and to design and implement new programs for individuals with AIDS along with our commitment to social activism compensated, in part, for the helplessness we often experienced in our work and with our loved ones.

SWAN San Francisco continues as a viable, if more informal, body today under the able leadership of Gail Splaver who has facilitated the group's monthly meetings over the past four years. Few original members are among the social workers that gather. It is a smaller group; with the decrease in AIDS funding and the subsequent consolidation of programs and agencies, fewer social workers are employed and mobilized. Many of the current issues taken up by SWAN remain the same, notably affordable housing for people with debilitating HIV and AIDS. SWAN continues to offer a vibrant forum of guest speakers, case presentations by social work graduate students, and discussion that continues to spark creativity, political activism, and community building.

REFERENCE

Dunkel, J., Dumont, S., and O'Neil, M. (1987). Social Work AIDS Network (SWAN), a professional group: A prescription for burnout in the HIV pandemic. Unpublished Paper.

Chapter 5

The South Carolina Experience

Cynthia Cannon Poindexter

I have been asked to remember and reflect upon my experience as a social worker in the early years of HIV disease. From May 1987 to August 1994, I worked for Palmetto AIDS Life Support Services (PALSS), the first community-based AIDS service organization (ASO) in South Carolina (the Palmetto State). I began volunteering for PALSS eighteen months after its formation. I later became the first full-time social work intern at PALSS, and upon graduation I became the first staff member there to have a social work degree. I had various paid and unpaid roles, including crisis line volunteer, grants and policy consultant, social work intern, district director, program director, assistant director, acting executive director, and finally executive director. I was recruited and trained by Bill Edens Jr., who was the founding executive director and who led the agency until his death from AIDS in November 1993. For more than six years Edens and I were both colleagues and close friends. The final four months of his life put a strain on my emotional equilibrium, as I was doing his job and mine, as well as providing him with case management and personal care. His death devastated me, and I immediately started making plans to leave to pursue a doctorate because I felt that PALSS needed a director who was not grief stricken. I never left the HIV field, however, and remain involved professionally as a university teacher, community-based trainer, clinical supervisor, grants writer, and researcher.

ORGANIZATIONAL GENESIS

In September 1984, a local member of Parents and Friends of Lesbians and Gays (PFLAG) attended a national meeting in Denver where she became alarmed about AIDS and AIDS-related stigma and began expressing her concerns to others. There had been no organized response to AIDS at all in South Carolina at that time, except for testing, counseling, and some pre-liminary prevention efforts by the state Department of Health. In August 1985 she met with eleven others in the first planning meeting for what was to become PALSS. Participants in that meeting included advocates from PFLAG and the gay community, as well as an older heterosexual couple whose son had died of AIDS two months earlier. By September, this group had chosen officers and a name and had contracted with Edens, who had been a local gay bar owner and supporter of the gay community, to become the sole staff member for no pay. The secretary of state incorporated PALSS as a nonprofit agency on October 22, 1985, making it the first nongovern-mental organizational response to AIDS in South Carolina.

ORGANIZATIONAL PRACTICE AND CULTURE

PALSS was a social movement agency, advocating for change while of-fering consumer-centered practical and emotional support. This generalist approach called for balancing an inward service delivery focus with a con-stant lookout for political, governmental, financial, and media dangers and opportunities. In the conservative rural South in the first decade of the HIV epidemic it was challenging but imperative to formulate and fund high-quality social services while being clear and consistent spokespersons for the rights of persons with HIV. Barriers to social service delivery in a rural state included serious concerns about confidentiality, health care profes-sionals inexperienced with the complexities of HIV, long travel distances to receive treatment or services, lack of public transportation and support sys-tems, and the fact that AIDS service models were developed in large urban areas such as New York City and San Francisco, which had sophisticated transit and medical infrastructures.

PALSS espoused and articulated a service delivery philosophy that was consumer driven, community based, culturally relevant, and focused on liv-ing with HIV as fully as possible. Imperative organizational values included support of informed choice, confidentiality, and consistent advocacy. The most important organizational practices were participation of HIV-positive persons as volunteers, staff, and planners; providing the bulk of services through volunteers; case management and interagency collaboration; cre-ativity and flexibility in program development and implementation; and fostering a nurturing, collective, organizational culture so that staff and vol-unteers would feel supported in doing heart-wrenching work.

Due to confidentiality and safety concerns regarding service applicants and recipients, volunteers, staff, and board, the physical location of the of-fice was not published or publicized during the agency's first decade. People who called or wrote for services or to volunteer were told the address and directions, but HIV stigma was so virulent and rampant that it was deemed hazardous to allow the public to know where the AIDS service organization was located.

Early services included posttest counseling, crisis intervention, safer sex education for the public and for persons with HIV, advocacy with other systems and institutions, professional education and capacity building, support groups, case management and referrals, a psychoeducational course for persons who had recently received an HIV diagnosis, peer support, and emergency financial assistance. Advocacy efforts included legislative testimony and behind-the-scenes lobbying for or against proposals; media interviews on controversial policies; taking stances against state laws or policies; and suing the state legislature over the exclusion of HIV from the health care risk pool. Thanks in large measure to Edens's skill and passion as an advocate, legislators and bureaucrats hated to hear from us, but they seemed to respect us and listen nonetheless. Those of us at PALSS had constant contact—for case management, advocacy, and education—with social workers and other professionals in formal service systems, such as hospitals, clinics, shelters, prisons, legal services, public health departments, mental health providers, home care agencies, hospices, the Social Security Administration, the Department of Social Services, and vocational rehabilitation. Volunteers, students, and case managers were well known in social work departments of all major hospitals in the state. In addition, we were often called in when someone was diagnosed or dying, in addition to providing ongoing visitation.

DAILY LIFE IN AN EARLY ASO

When I am asked to think about what it was like to be in the HIV field in the 1980s, what comes to mind immediately is how I checked the obituary list on the front page of the daily newspaper first thing every morning, looking for but hoping not to see names I knew. I took my paper into the office to have everyone else check this as well. Death was what we dreaded but what was also foremost on our minds. It was commonplace, but we never became accustomed to it. The shock, sadness, and pain did not lessen as the numbers of dead rose. If anything, grief was cumulative and grew heavier over the years. It may be counterintuitive to say, but each death felt to us like a surprise. We would shake our heads and mutter "How could this happen?" "She was so young!" "I just talked to him." "I thought she was getting better!" "I can't believe it." Sometimes I or others would enter a period of numbness over hospitalizations and deaths, being both grateful for the reprieve and worried that we were becoming jaded. Always that grace period would end and every loss and fear that occurred in the interim would feel raw and fresh. We lived and worked in a pervasive state of anticipatory grief and amassed sadness.

I see now that we did not fully recognize the profound stress, frustration, fear, and sadness that were woven into the fabric of our days. Even though at PALSS we did a wonderful job of watching out for one another, and we made recognition and mediation of stress a routine, in some ways the emotional intensity was closeted. Perhaps to fully stop and feel it would be immobilizing. In the midst of an emergency one does not have the luxury of thinking or feeling. It was easier to just keep going because the work was so important, necessary, and rewarding. We knew that whatever we were feeling was minuscule compared to what people who were ill with HIV were experiencing. However, I think that the persistent trauma of those days affects physical and mental health in subtle ways, both then and now.

Although death never became routine, it did become a typical and acceptable topic of conversation, no longer taboo or strange. Sex and drugs also became matter-of-fact subjects to us. Sometimes in situations not related to HIV we would have to monitor ourselves to make sure that we did not drift into these socially taboo subjects that might offend others. Furthermore, we somehow could and had to be able to laugh about the most horrible things. Humor in an early ASO was similar to what is probably found in medical schools; outsiders might wonder if we were being disrespectful when we were actually embracing irony and pain in a communal, loving, joyful way. The humor never put anyone down or pitted one group against another; it was inclusive and often originated from persons who were living with HIV. The humor, laughter, and sense of deep joy at PALSS went deeper than any I have witnessed before or since.

Usual professional boundaries were malleable and stretched because of the life-threatening nature of HIV and because service recipients wanted that level of community and support. One important characteristic of our days was the way that volunteers and service recipients would drop by just for a quick hug and enthusiastic encouragement. There was always spontaneous genuine happiness and gratitude at seeing a colleague or client walk in. It is amazing to me in retrospect that this was the case, given how frantically busy we always were.

In sum, the early days were characterized by paradoxes. Although the work could be frightening, overwhelming, and sad, there was always humor, energy, courage, camaraderie, and commitment. Tasks could be faced only in the short term and long term if one was armored with optimism, yet there was a constant underlying grief. Everyone was ambivalent about being there. It was hard to make sense of how meaningful and fun working at PALSS could be while we hated the reason we were needed.

ORGANIZATIONAL CHALLENGES

Trying to sustain an early ASO was a struggle. HIV was new to everyone, and no one knew what to do; we were all unprepared and untrained. We hungered for acceptance and legitimacy as expert service providers, even as we were proud of our marginal status as advocates. Given the constant and rapid rise in requests for services, board and staff saw no choice but to expand the response, even when the financial basis to do so was nonexistent. As PALSS's services grew, the structure quickly became too much to handle and fund. The agency suffered from poor fiscal health for years, which threatened survival of the organization as well as created inordinate tension among and between board and staff. Then, as state, federal, corporate, and foundation funds became available, there were hard ethical decisions to make concerning how we were to accommodate constraints and value conflicts. One example occurred in August 1990 at a public hearing about funds available as the Ryan White CARE Act became law, at which PALSS staff were informed by state employees that subcontracting agencies would be required to report names of service recipients to the state. Due to strict confidentiality policies, this pronouncement precluded us from applying for federal funds, even though the agency was plummeting into debt and in danger of closing its doors. For two years PALSS's unwillingness to compromise confidentiality of records made these federal funds inaccessible and greatly increased its financial distress, until the state Department of Public Health negotiated an acceptable reporting system that allowed us to accept pass-through funding without releasing names to the bureaucracy.

Gradual professionalization caused another type of tension in the agency. It is typical for a social movement to experience a transition from a completely grassroots effort, through a mostly volunteer and paraprofessional staff, to the addition of more formally trained persons. Edens was always clear that he wanted a hybrid organization, with community members, consumers, volunteers, paraprofessionals, and professionals working side by side, supplementing and sustaining one another. For the nine years that he was director, this model worked fairly well. Yet there was never enough money to attract and keep trained social workers, even though we wanted and needed that level of expertise. Ironically, as more social work students and social workers came on board, there was less immediate identification with and connection to the affected community groups because social work students were for the most part HIV-negative, straight, middle-class white women. The goal of combining professionals and students with indigenous employees and volunteers was always at the forefront for me (as a trained social worker) and Bill (as a community-based leader), but it was understandably difficult to balance at times.

THE PAST IS PRESENT

Writing and talking about the early days of the HIV pandemic is a paradox, because in some ways the early days never ended. Although everyone is enormously grateful that the AIDS death rate has recently slowed in developed countries, we are painfully aware that people with HIV are not universally having an easy time of it. From the very beginning of this epidemic we were challenged with treatment access, adherence, and failure, as well as the unpredictability and uncertainty of HIV disease. Those issues are extremely salient now, perhaps in broader and more intense ways than before, but they are not new to long-term HIV advocates. There is a pervasive "here we go again" group sigh heaved over the resurfacing and continuation of these concerns.

Our experiences in this country fifteen to twenty years ago are being repeated in underdeveloped countries now. I remember being called in 1989 to one of the local hospitals to speak with a family, all of whom had tested positive. The baby, almost one year old, had been frail and failing to thrive, and was tested for HIV when other diagnoses had been ruled out. This, of course, led to the mother and father being advised to take the test; they had both just received their positive results. I remember feeling as if the breath had been knocked out of me after I hung up from talking with the hospital social worker, wondering what on earth I could say to this couple. But necessity prevailed, as it always did, and I spent the five-minute drive to the hospital shifting my focus away from being overwhelmed to being open to whatever this family might say, do, feel, or need. I was reminded of this incident recently when a former student called to say that her relatives in Africa—her brother, his wife, and their children—had all tested positive while they were visiting her in the states. These scenarios may not be as common in the United States as they once were, but they are still happening all over the world.

As a long-term HIV social worker, I find that the old days are also very much alive inside me. The old triggers for worry and panic often resurface. I cannot always get emotional memory to mesh with cognitive knowledge. Because I experienced the illnesses and deaths of many people, the resulting pain, insight, and sadness does not easily dissipate, even with the passage of time. I still at times inexplicably become tearful when the weight of the old accumulated grief surprises me, at the sight of an ambulance, at a memorial service, or upon passing a person who reminds me of someone who died from AIDS years ago. There can be a seeping and creeping of old grief and fears into current relationships. When a colleague or friend now has a HIV-related symptom, infection, or cancer, I can easily slip into a panic that may seem uncalled for and overblown. Yet seen as a posttraumatic response, this reaction is perhaps more understandable. I suspect that many long-term

HIV workers find that if we do not mediate this posttraumatic fear with encouraging information and self-talk, we can become burdensome to our HIV-positive loved ones who wonder why they must constantly calm us down and take care of us when there is any news of concern to deliver.

Another reason that the old days are still vital and significant is that colleagues and friends from that time are still part of our lives. Some of those who have HIV are doing well on combination treatments and have regained health and functioning after years of disability. Others are debilitated from treatment failures or treatment side effects. Recently several people with HIV whom I met in the 1980s have died. The old days have not yet gone away, either inside us or around us.

FAMILY SECRETS

I think that there are family or community secrets which long-term HIV workers are only comfortable admitting to one another, and then only hesitantly. We keep these feelings close, in fear of being judged or stigmatized for them, because there are parts of these hidden perspectives of which we are not proud. In talking to colleagues individually and in focus groups, I have heard similar confessions. I ask the reader to suspend judgment for a bit and attempt to temporarily accept the worldview of a battle-fatigued long-term HIV worker and allow me this space to be open about these usually private musings.

First, veterans sometimes shake their heads over how the newer workers, especially those who started work after 1994, can have no idea what it was like in the early days. Although we are joyful about that, we feel isolated in our memories and sometimes suspect that these newcomers consider our stories and reflections more histrionic than historical. In the new and improved world of federal funding and professionally trained administrators, it is hard for new workers to fathom why and how a group of grassroots community advocates and paraprofessionals would continue to raise their own paychecks every week. Some of the newcomers to the field do not realize that HIV services were invented, initiated, and implemented by gay men who had no formal training in service provision, but who responded creatively and humanely to an unprecedented danger to their community. Many of those early advocates are disabled or dead and thus not visible as mentors. Recently I was invited to give a case management in-service presentation at PALSS. Most of the staff had been there two years or less. Before I began, I was asked to talk a little about what brought me to PALSS and what the early days were like. I found in these workers a burning curiosity about those urgent, tragic times and what bordered on awe at the barriers and challenges that we considered then to be routine. They remarked that they wanted to remember, when they were feeling overwhelmed and underfunded, that things were indeed much better now. As I was talking about the genesis of the agency they now worked for, I felt a strong thread of connection with them due to a shared history and commitment. Simultaneously, however, I felt a distance between us that was more significant than merely time and experience. I felt that these case managers and advocates could never really understand the first fifteen years of the HIV pandemic. No one who wasn't in the thick of it will be able to truly grasp the depth of grief, rage, and fatigue that gripped us daily. It is a blessing that the HIV picture has improved so dramatically for many people in this country, and I am glad for these workers that they do not have to struggle as we did. Nevertheless, I feel and acknowledge that despite our bond, as past and present PALSS case managers, we come from different worlds. The danger of this division is that we can lose some of the solidarity that must exist if we are to form a united front to provide support, push for results, and nurture one another.

Second, sometimes our spirits feel crushed and battered when we face the fact that there is still no vaccine, still no cure, and the pandemic has still not been conquered. We ask ourselves if we have been spinning our wheels all this time. Have we been wrong about the effectiveness of culturally relevant, community-based prevention messages? How could we have been so mistaken in our hope—perhaps conviction—that if we just fight like hell for a little while, then we could speed up medical research, government, and the public so that this virulent virus could get beaten back into submission? I imagine pouring heart and soul into a cause that you believe to be a temporary emergency, only to realize with increasing horror that it is much bigger and worse than you imagined in your worst nightmares. At best, the current state of HIV on the earth can make one feel intensely tired and bemused; at worst, one can feel devastated, deeply helpless, and resigned. The peril here is that we will give up and move on, accepting the plague as inevitable rather than increasing our efforts and energy.

Third, we harbor a secret anger that people seem to think that this epidemic is over, that HIV is controllable, and that AIDS is a chronic condition. We react with a passion that surprises even us: How dare people wane in their attention? In our best moments, we can acknowledge that this can be reframed as hope and relief and that it is a normal response. We know on some level that urgency cannot be sustained indefinitely, yet we rant and rage. I bet that others are already tired of our collective foot stamping and wish we would move on. I am guessing that it is easy to turn away from our message because we are too strident and hysterical. Yet like those who have witnessed the devastation of war or genocide, we cannot let it go. We are aware of what is happening in other parts of the world, and we can see on the horizon the next wave of treatment failures and deaths in this country. We try to be polite and silent, but we cannot always contain this terror that most people have forgotten what it was like and do not realize what it will be like again. Of course, we acknowledge that there have been some societal, community, personal, and medical gains in the HIV field. Yet it feels too dangerous to say this too often or to the wrong people, because we risk someone thinking that we are rejoicing and resting when we are desperate to put out a call to arms. We are afraid that people will think we are asking for personal praise or thanks when we really just want our anger and fear heard and validated so that complacency will not prevail.

Perhaps the most difficult piece of our burnout to admit is the rage into which we can erupt when we contemplate continued or resurgent unsafe sex and drug practices. We—who fought so mightily against victim blaming and stigma, who took solid political and professional stands on starting where people are and working with them instead of against them— can fly into fits of anger over barebacking, for example. Even though we know in our heads that there are only minorities of men who have sex with men who are seeking or having unsafe sexual activity, in our guts we take this personally. Yet now, sometimes we confess, perhaps only silently, that we want to shout from the rooftops: How dare you? How dare you discount our grief? How dare you run roughshod over our hearts? How dare you ask us to take care of you? We already took care of hundreds of alienated and marginalized people who were very sick and dying, and we did it over and over and over without resentment. We railed against those who said that people with HIV deserved what they had and what they were facing. Now we look at one another in fear and bafflement and ask: Do we have the responsibility to advocate and care for this new group of men who did not heed the warnings? Then we pull back in horror at what and whom we sound like. How did we, of all people, turn into victim blamers? We have never believed in the worthy and unworthy sick! We ask ourselves: Is this the price of sustained stress and grief? Have we become the people whom we previously fought against?

CONCLUSION

It is interesting to contemplate why long-term HIV workers have not left the HIV field, given the stress overload from the early days, the changing structure of HIV services, the overwhelming nature of the pandemic, and the impossibility of keeping up to date with new treatment developments. I have some ideas about this phenomenon, based on my own gratitude that I had these experiences and on conversations with colleagues who feel the same. One is that HIV work feels imperative to us. It often seems that we have little choice but to offer who we are and what we know. We know that not everyone chooses this work, and that if we have some ability to do it, we have an obligation to do so. Another part of the explanation is that HIV work is both challenging and rewarding. Long-term HIV workers do not stop learning, become complacent, or lose awe and respect for those with whom we work. It is probably that combination of feeling compelled and feeling fulfilled which keeps us doing this work. To plagiarize a military advertisement, it is the toughest job we have ever loved.

In the early years, serious illness, dying, and death in an atmosphere of prejudice, underfunding, and social conflict characterized the HIV field. Yet in that atmosphere, compassion and creativity thrived. It is useful for the current HIV field to remember the lessons and challenges from the early years. The demographics and treatment have changed drastically; however, the participatory traditions, flexible approach, and social justice values of the early ASOs are highly relevant today. If the HIV field becomes too complacent in its traditional approach, turning more to the bureaucratic, professional end of the continuum than to the raw, angry, activist end, we will lose effectiveness and vision. Is it possible for HIV social workers to be both professional and to be partners with communities and persons with HIV? Absolutely. The HIV work pioneers have already shown us the way.

Chapter 6

Social Work in HIV Care:
A Labor of Love in Philadelphia

Patricia A. Stewart

It was 1992. I had determined that I wanted to do the kind of social work that allowed me to draw on my administrative skills and experience but would also offer the opportunity to work directly with consumers. That opportunity presented itself when I began work as Coordinator of Family Services in a family program in the Special Immunology Section at a children's hospital in Philadelphia, Pennsylvania. Medical, social work, nutrition, and a range of other services were provided to infants, children, adolescents, and adults who were living with HIV and AIDS. The program was large, with 350 families served in total and an average of fifty to sixty visits per week. This outpatient program was designed to serve mothers who were HIV positive and who had children who were diagnosed with or who were at risk for HIV.

The statistic time line illustrates that the number of reported cases of AIDS was at an all-time high in Philadelphia in 1992 and 1993. I may not have been aware of that at the time, but I did know that we were in the throes of an epidemic that called for a wide scope and depth of response unparalleled in the twenty years of experience I brought to the setting. For over a year, we routinely received two to four new referrals per week of HIV-positive women with children who were diagnosed with or at risk of HIV. The numbers alone were astounding and at that time, with limited drugs to combat the disease, a diagnosis was essentially a death sentence. Reinforcing the horror of the disease was the large number of men, women, and children who were dying in horrible physical ways due to complications of AIDS. We knew of people, many of whom were gay men, who had lost friends, lovers, and associates. HIV and AIDS hit the gay community very hard. As horrible as all of this was, it only begins to tell the story.

In this family program in an inner-city community, we witnessed and experienced many losses. At that time, there were no models of care and treatment for those who were being newly diagnosed in large numbers. Therefore, we extrapolated from models that were designed for a very different population—primarily white gay men, many of whom were accustomed to societal privilege. We did our best to adapt those models to the clients we were seeing: poor and African-American and Latino women and children and the men who were the women's partners and the fathers of their children. I must also say that we served others—including a nearly invisible population of men and women who had same-sex partners. They were "invisible" for a number of reasons, including the profound stigma arising from the fear of homosexuality that is rampant in the African-American and Latino communities we served.

Because of the poverty and disenfranchisement of our clientele, my colleagues in the program used to say that HIV was "tenth on a list" of social problems that poor people who are infected and affected may face. As grave as the disease was, it was telling that the effects of the medical illness, especially for the asymptomatic and/or the newly diagnosed, could sometimes feel incidental to the problems that people already were facing as black and Latino people living in poverty in America. For example, there were times that we were shocked to learn that we were stressing refrigeration of a medication for a patient who did not even own a refrigerator—in Philadelphia! In the twentieth century!

Some of the better-known issues of poverty were compounded to levels nearly intolerable when people were diagnosed. After perhaps a lifetime of struggling to live, they were then faced with having HIV and coping with issues such as living with the fear of getting sick and dying, trying to have hope while feeling hopeless, fears about sexual desirability on the one hand and transmission to loved ones on the other, guilt about past or present use of drugs, the fear of being exposed as a homosexual, children facing death and/or loss of siblings and parents, and child placement and custody issues involved in permanency planning.

I had been in the social work field for twenty years, seven of which had been providing social work services in an intensive care unit of a general hospital, yet at times I felt unprepared to address the magnitude of the suffering. We addressed the myriad psychosocial issues, yet more issues continued to emerge. It quickly became apparent that care for people living with HIV is largely social. One of the rewards of working in HIV care at that time was that physicians and other medical personnel who worked in the field were able to recognize this. Many considered the social worker an integral part of the team. This differed greatly from the regard for social work that was generally held in health care in my previous experience.

The high regard for social work values, skills, and perspectives was gratifying and, for me, tended to offset somewhat the immense sorrow inherent in the work. Social work with people living with HIV was (and is) cutting edge. There was always something new to learn as knowledge about the disease, derived from both clinical observation/experience and research efforts, became more and more available. There was usually money available and time given to attend seminars and conferences where we not only learned information to sharpen and develop our skills, but also had the opportunity to listen, to be heard, and to give and receive support in meetings with other social workers. Often during this networking I would identify others with whom I could have ongoing contact for mutual technical and emotional support.

This was especially important, because in the early days of the epidemic few people outside of the circle of those who did the work could be of substantive support. Even other social workers in different areas of practice and friends in the field would stop me short as I began to talk about the work. I didn't blame them; it was very difficult for those not doing this work to comprehend the gravity and intensity of it. In addition, I think ignorance and fear about the disease tapped into people's homophobia, disdain for drug addicts, and fears for their own safety. This then constituted a loss of connection with some colleagues with whom I had previously been able to share experiences and had the effect of compounding the many losses I experienced in doing the work. I was in the unique position of being a supervisor with a caseload, so I was giving in that arena as well. Many days I felt totally spent, with nothing left to give. I was fortunate, however, that the medical director recognized these feelings and readily agreed to pay for a supervisory consultant for me, which proved helpful. Yet the need for support grew beyond the sources of it, particularly because of the cumulative effects of all the loss. Learning how to help men, women, children, and babies die without having that affect the general emotional well-being of the practitioner is, to say the least, a challenge. I learned how to take good, frequent, low-cost Caribbean vacations as one way to nourish myself.

Let me pause here to say again that there were very few treatments then available to HIV-positive people. Even with the most conscientious medical care, numbers of opportunistic infections and deaths were still high. We knew our patients well and relationships developed as we helped them face yet another manifestation of the disease, which would surely mean loss of some function and more physical pain. The medical personnel on our team addressed the new findings with them, often requesting a social worker's presence to do so, and then the social worker would be with the patients as they processed the emotional and psychological pain—the fears, the hurt, the loneliness. Being there—allowing them to dissolve into tears, holding them, comforting them made the work at once so special and meaningful and yet at the same time so sad. Feelings of helplessness because there was no more to be offered medically were experienced at the same time as the profound reality of being in that very personal space with individuals facing their own mortality. I grew as a social worker and, more important, as a spiritual being as they allowed me to experience with them their attempts to somehow find the courage to live while facing death.

It was at times a surreal experience to be a part of a team of such caring human beings and competent health care professionals. Although I have mentioned there were not social work supports sometimes, there were, nonetheless, those on the team who were also experiencing the vicissitudes of mood and complexity of feelings in this very tender work. We devoted much time to being a working team. Weekly meetings lasted for hours—until each consumer and family was discussed and each team member had the opportunity to give input from his or her professional and personal perspective. It was intense, and I did not appreciate it as much then as I do in retrospect. It provided us with as good a model of a team approach as I have had in any of my professional experiences. That is not to say we did not have differences, including different training and different values, and different backgrounds and professions. The common thread, though, was that we all cared deeply about our work and about the people whom we served. Of that I am certain.

We also went to great lengths to communicate that care and concern to our patients. I can recall one case in which we had much involvement with an infected baby boy who was cared for excellently by nuns who operated a program for such babies. Our team, however, repeatedly felt concerned that the baby's mother had dropped out of care. She was addicted to crack cocaine and, therefore, was not able to function very well. She had little connection with her son since her visits were sporadic. Our concern for her, however, remained. I will never forget how it felt when the medical director suggested that he and I, the assigned social worker, make a home visit to encourage her to come in for her own treatment. When we arrived, she was disheveled and groggy, and we appealed to her as an equal human being. The doctor, at one point, was on his knee in front of her while I sat beside her on the sofa. Her mother was also present, and we connected with her as well. I think that the visit made an indelible impression. This young woman began coming regularly for her treatment. When she relapsed we would miss her and when she returned we would tell her so and welcome her with open arms, no matter how long it had been since she had last come. I remember her saying to a friend who accompanied her one time when we enthusiastically greeted her in the clinic, "See, I told you they cared about me here." As I write this, I feel the emotion of that, and I wonder where she is today.

In the early to mid-1990s, the social worker as integral team member was pretty much the norm in HIV work. There was something about the physicians and the nurses that was also different than other medical settings in which I had worked. They were more likely to allow their humanity and vulnerability to be seen. They also had a clear sense of the limitations of their training when it came to psychosocial issues and took great pains to select social workers with abilities in the areas of casework, advocacy, and counseling who could also work well on an interdisciplinary team. Knowledge of HIV medical issues was not as important because the information was ever changing, and they took responsibility for providing the medical training in ongoing formal and informal collaboration and education sessions. Professionals had numerous opportunities for formal training in those days, since monies for such programs were often included in funding proposals.

In our clinic, the social worker was the first person to have substantial contact with a new or prospective patient, after the client spoke with the very competent and personable front office staff. In the first clinic appointment, the patient met with the social worker for a complete psychosocial assessment. The social worker would then share relevant information with the team. The first medical appointment would be set for the second visit, unless there was a medical emergency. Social work follow-up was based on need, which at the very least coincided with each regularly scheduled medical clinic visit and sometimes was more frequent. Joining the team, at one point, was a grant-funded drug and alcohol counselor, with whom we interfaced for referrals and collaboration. If the client needed social work support at a meeting or a hearing, we were able to attend. When children were hospitalized, we provided services. Parents who were hospitalized in a nearby adult hospital were also visited, and we continued to provide services for them. Visits to patients in the community were difficult because of the caseload size but were done when necessary. In addition, when it came to giving parents the information that their hospitalized child was newly diagnosed with HIV, the social worker was there at the critical juncture to provide support and to begin the relationship. These are just some of the actions that demonstrate how highly we regarded the families. We went to great lengths to assure a meaningful connection and ongoing emotional support which increased the likelihood that they would remain in treatment, learning about the disease and getting support to make decisions for healthy lifestyles and activities.

After several months of doing the work, I decided that a way to foster more opportunities for nourishment was to develop a group of social workers who would meet periodically. That became a reality as the group, Social Workers in AIDS Care, was formed. Those who worked in other hospitals, outpatient clinics, and the community were welcome. We found it helpful to share information about everything from new entitlement programs to financial resources to the latest legislative initiatives. I had an interest in sharing difficult case material with some focus on the impact on the social worker.

We also had a few guest speakers. These meetings were held every two weeks for several months and were well attended with an average of fifteen to twenty people. As demands on our time grew, we had to meet less frequently—every three to four weeks—but we maintained the connection and called on one another for strength and support in the interim on an individual basis. These groups served a significant need, since many of the participants were practicing without social work supervision and some had no regular opportunity for such dialogues —not even with a superior from another discipline. The work we did together addressed some important needs and served to minimize the frustration, sense of "aloneness," and burnout. In those days, I did not know about the term *compassion fatigue,* but looking back, we were all familiar with the concept. We attended to people whom we had grown to respect and care about at bedside and on their "death-beds" and comforted their significant others at those times and at the funerals, which seemed endless. Did I mention how much I love doing this work? I think that is why many of us stayed in it for so long. There is something profoundly gratifying in working with people living with HIV/AIDS.

The other initiative that I developed was training providers about the nuances of working with African Americans with HIV. At the time, my anger about the ignorance and errors of omission propelled me to do something on behalf of people in my community. I was very aware of my commitment—and my responsibility—to offer the cultural perspective on an ongoing basis in patient care overall. I was also painfully aware of the proliferation of the disease in the African-American community. I was burying large numbers of my people and seeing astounding numbers of the newly infected, yet the models of care, the focus of training sessions, and sometimes the information presented were all too often devoid of content that felt relevant or meaningful to my work with African Americans. To that end, I approached a local agency with experience training health care professionals to assist me in the development of a conference by and about African Americans, open to all providers and, of course, consumers. That was 1995. In 2001, we held the fifth annual conference, "Breaking the Silence, Breaking Through the Fear: HIV/AIDS . . . African-American Perspectives." A group of ten constitutes the planning committee, six of whom are charter members—African-American professionals from varied disciplines and consumers who come together on a regular basis throughout the year and plan a unique, Afrocentric conference. The mission is to educate, in a nonthreatening, inspiring way, about the experience of being black in America and what that can teach us about providing culturally relevant services for African Americans—services that are caring, competent, and respectful. It is seen as a very meaningful conference with 100 to 200 participants in attendance each year.

I have worked with people from many racial and ethnic backgrounds who live with HIV/AIDS. For a number of reasons, my specialty with African Americans has evolved and opportunities to broaden that work have presented themselves. On a national level, from 1993 to 2000, I was privileged to be a member of a group of social workers, mostly educators with some practitioners, who met several times each year to plan national and regional conferences. During that time, with the growing numbers of new infections and cases of AIDS among African Americans, much of the focus (and the funding for) these planned conferences was on African Americans. That group of social work leaders from all parts of the country was in itself an inspiration to me as a social worker. Our activities served to keep me on the cutting edge of work that I dearly loved, long after my full-time direct service in HIV care ended. In part, because of that group, I continued to learn a great deal about HIV and social work in all its areas of practice and research, and I believe that I contributed to others with my areas of expertise as well.

In closing, the practice of social work in HIV care is without a doubt the most rewarding work of my career. It requires that we give much to others and, to be successful, to ourselves. That happens in a variety of ways, which I have described here. Having this opportunity to put that kind of meaningful giving and receiving of ourselves into words is both nostalgic and inspiring as I continue this labor of love.

NATIONAL, STATE, AND CITY MODEL INTERVENTIONS

Chapter 7

The New York State Response: Case Management for Persons Living with HIV and AIDS

Jay Freedman

The AIDS Institute (AI) of the New York State Department of Health was established in 1983 by the New York State legislature to coordinate the state's policies with respect to the growing AIDS epidemic. The mission of the AIDS Institute is "to promote, protect and advocate for health through science, prevention, and assurance of access to a coordinated system of quality health care and supportive services for people with HIV and AIDS" (New York State Session Laws, 1983). The institute undertakes its broad mission guided by the following principles: (1) science-based decision making, (2) prioritizing HIV/AIDS prevention, and (3) assuring a continuum of care and services. It is within this context that the AIDS Institute embarked on developing case management as a major focus of many of its programs.

In 1983, the AI was a unique, innovative organization within state government. Staffed from its initiation by advocates as well as professionals from within the state health department, the AI challenged those within government to move more rapidly and urgently than ever before. It also challenged those outside of government to work with it to remove barriers to the development of HIV services and programs. By the end of the decade, the AI had established itself as a leader in the development of HIV/AIDS services in New York State and the rest of the United States.

The AIDS Institute grew from a small staff of three individuals in 1983 to its current workforce of 417 individuals dispersed geographically (primarily in New York City and Albany) but united in dedication and commitment to working for the public good. Under the leadership of its early directors and most notably its third executive director, Nicholas A. Rango, MD, appointed in 1987, the institute began to develop a broad array of services and a continuum of care for persons with HIV/AIDS. Prior to joining the AIDS Institute, Dr. Rango, a geriatric physician, was the executive director of Village Nursing Home located in lower Manhattan. From his experiences as a physician and social scientist, Dr. Rango understood that case management and social work needed to be key components of AIDS Institute programs and services. He believed that case management was the thread that held the continuum of services together.

Case management had been a service developed and deployed early in the epidemic by organizations involved in the early battle against AIDS. However, there was no central coordinated effort to define, develop, or standardize case management throughout the state. Case management development in the early years of the epidemic was guided by the essential and well-intended efforts of the many AIDS organizations that offered and experimented with case management as a way of providing supportive services and counseling to clients who faced gross discrimination, fear, ignorance, and a devastating terminal illness. What resulted, in place of a planned and thoughtful approach to case management and systems development, was what Dr. Rango often referred to as "the Tower of Babel," a confusing and uncoordinated scenario of many case managers working on behalf of one client. It was not unusual for a case manager to learn of the involvement of other case managers working with the same client. At a time when people were living only twelve to eighteen months after diagnosis, a sense of urgency grew for the development of a full spectrum of health care and support services for infected individuals. As people lived longer, the need for a comprehensive statewide effort to coordinate the growth of case management also grew.

Case management was a natural but unplanned development in the evolution of the AIDS epidemic. Our medical and social service systems were often fragmented, with multiple barriers to access and delivery of care. From early in the epidemic to today, AIDS is a complex and evolving disease, and there was an obvious need for intervention with clients to provide them with assistance to increase access to and negotiate continuity of care. It was evident to service providers that a comprehensive approach to care and services was required; case management was the logical solution to managing a complicated service delivery system.

Case management had previously been deployed by New York State in times of crisis. In the 1970s, case management was utilized within various New York State programs for the aging under the Medicaid program. Thus, there was experience with case management by the time the AIDS Institute was ready to develop its AIDS case management system.

The mission of the Case Management Section (CMS) of the AIDS Institute, formed in 1989, was to better understand the structure that had developed within New York's continuum of AIDS case management. The institute began by undertaking several projects. The first was to adopt a common definition and develop guiding principles for case management. The AI then focused efforts on defining the models of case management practice that had evolved and developing standards and a financing strategy to promote the continued development of case management in the continuum of AIDS services in New York State.

The benefits of such an approach were obvious. The institute's goals were to promote uniformity in case management practices and to provide clear expectations for providers in the AIDS care system so that they understood their role and the roles of other agencies in case managing clients. A carefully planned systems development approach also helped to measure the success of case management efforts, promote quality, and foster the effective and efficient delivery of case management services.

The AIDS Institute adopted the following definition for case management:

> Case management is a multi-step process which ensures coordination and expedient access to a range of appropriate medical and social services for the client and his or her family and support system. The goal of case management is to promote and support the independent functioning of the client and family. Case management is a method of placing responsibility for service planning, service acquisition, service delivery, and systems coordination onto a person or a team. It is a client-centered service that links and ensures timely coordinated access to medically appropriate levels of care and support services. (AIDS Institute, 1994)

These guiding principles were developed in 1994:

1. Case management should be available statewide to all HIV-positive persons.
2. Case management should be integrated into a comprehensive service package.

3. The intensity of case management provided should be consistent with the needs of the clients.
4. The empowerment model should guide all case management efforts.
5. Developmental grant funding followed by enhanced Medicaid funding should lead an agency through developmental stages and provide for growth in order for it to become an experienced and mature provider of case management services.
6. The Ryan White HIV Care Networks in New York State should assume an active role in case management development for their regions.
7. Case management should be the process that assures continuity of care. Every client should have access to at least one primary care case management provider who coordinates and assures communication among other involved case managers. The institute recognized early on that it was essential for multiple case managers to be involved given New York's diverse service delivery system and the complex needs of persons with HIV/AIDS. It was not uncommon for a client to have both a medical and a psychosocial case manager. The two were not necessarily duplicative—one guided the medical care coordination effort, the other the entitlement-based and psychosocial needs of the client.
8. Case management should be a full-time effort whenever possible. Too many case management efforts were of poor quality because individuals who had another full-time role carried them out. Case management should not be an ancillary role; if case management is to succeed, it needs to be fully funded and a full-time effort. Case management should be proactive and empowering and include visits to clients in their home setting. (AIDS Institute, 1994)

Many of the activities of the Case Management Section in the early years included development of standards for already existing programs such as those within the designated AIDS centers (DACs), hospitals established as centers of HIV expertise with beds and units identified for AIDS patients. DACs received a higher Medicaid payment for enhanced services, including case management. From 1987 through 1989, the institute worked with committees of DAC social workers to promote best practices for case management in inpatient and outpatient settings and to build this continuum beyond the hospital setting.

As the epidemic shifted from an acute and terminal illness to a long-term chronic illness, the institute's approach shifted to expanding the availability of case management to serve people from their entry into the HIV prevention, counseling, and testing environment on into chronic care settings. The

AIDS Institute developed and made available case management components for primary care settings, substance use treatment, day treatment, community-based agency, home care, and housing settings. Financial support for case management was established through federal and state-funded grants as well as Medicaid reimbursement. Through the Medicaid rate structure, access to case management funding was provided to DACs, clinics, and community-based organizations.

DEVELOPMENT OF COBRA COMMUNITY FOLLOW-UP

In 1989, the institute began development of its intensive case management program through Medicaid's Comprehensive Medicaid Case Management (CMCM) program (under the COBRA legislation of 1985) by amending New York State's Medicaid plan to recognize case management as an optional Medicaid service for the HIV-infected population. This program, called the Community Follow-Up Program (CFP), was designed to be a comprehensive, family-centered intensive case management program utilizing a service delivery team of three dedicated full-time staff members consisting of a case manager, a case management technician, and a community follow-up worker. These three worked together as a team to provide an empowerment-oriented full-time intensive case management program whose defining mission was to leave the office and follow the client into the community. Small caseloads were encouraged, and frequent contact with a significant amount of home visitation was characteristic of the program.

The program was designed to incorporate a career ladder for case management personnel. Community follow-up workers, modeled after the community health worker concept, could be promoted after work experience to the next level—the case management technician position requiring one year of experience plus training. The team leaders were the case managers, whose qualifications were established at a minimum of an associate degree with experience up to and including bachelor of arts, master of social work, and nursing degrees. A unique and enhanced Medicaid case management rate was developed that allowed each agency to be reimbursed on an hourly basis for its direct and indirect costs associated with the program, including administrative and overhead costs not normally reimbursed in efforts of this nature.

From its early implementation in 1990 with just three or four providers and a handful of clients, the COBRA CFP has grown steadily through the years to encompass fifty agencies and over eighty sites statewide and has served more than 40,000 clients. The program has become a significant source of case management funding for New York State, currently bringing into the case management effort more than $40 million annually and more than $186 million in revenue since its implementation in 1990.

The COBRA CFP has been successful largely because of the dedication, commitment, and partnership of its provider staff and the staff of the AIDS institute, who work together to monitor, administer, and oversee the training for and development of these programs. COBRA program staff are required to undergo regular staff supervision, case record reviews, and peer review and are monitored on a frequent basis by AI staff of the Case Management Section. An extensive training program was also developed, funded by the institute, to offer both introductory and advanced-level case management training. In recent years this training has been made available to the wider case management community.

The Case Management Section also provides support to the sixteen federally funded Ryan White HIV Care Networks located throughout the state. Each network is required to have a case management committee that works at the provider level to promote communication and coordination between case management agencies, hold monthly case management meetings in their localities, and develop case management and HIV service directories for their communities.

MEASURING CASE MANAGEMENT OUTCOMES

The Case Management Section has been involved in conducting a number of evaluations over the years that have demonstrated the effectiveness of case management in a variety of different settings. Working with Union College of Schenectady, New York, evaluation studies have demonstrated the programmatic and cost effectiveness of New York's case management programs (Lehrman and Gentry, 1998; Lehrman, 2000; Chestnut et al., 2002). The CMS has promoted quality assurance and continuous quality improvement within case management agencies and has worked over the years to identify case management outcomes and indicators and help providers measure their efforts in moving clients along an outcome-based path.

By 1994 the Case Management Section recognized the importance of measuring HIV case management outcomes and identifying areas and processes that need attention to improve the quality of case management services. Outcomes analysis also assists in identifying training needs and improving case management processes within agencies. Measuring outcomes helps attract and sustain funding through government, third-party, and other sources, such as newly emerging managed care organizations which have a financial interest in ensuring that there is effective case management of their populations. Measuring outcomes assists in identifying areas of excellence, highlighting successes, attracting new clients, and increasing public recognition of the work being done by HIV case managers. In 1995, the Case Management Section began to work toward transitioning AI-funded agencies from traditional quality assurance review of case management processes to measurement of outcomes and quality improvement activities that would sustain and achieve better client outcomes.

To begin this effort, New York State assembled twenty-five of its most experienced case management directors and engaged them in a consensus-building exercise to identify case management activities, benchmarks, and outcomes. Through continued discussion and refinement, a number of broad outcome areas were identified. Over a two-year period, monthly quality subcommittee meetings debated the measurement indicators that could be used to actually monitor case management outcomes within the COBRA CFP. Consensus was reached on twenty-three indicators based on their measurability, applicability to the case manager's job, relevance, importance to the case management function, and finally the degree to which the case manager actually produced this particular outcome. Union College of Schenectady was hired to perform annual reviews of each COBRA CFP agency over a two-week period. Twenty-five case management records were randomly selected and exhaustively reviewed by research assistants in order to determine progress on these twenty-three measurement indicators. The eight broad outcome areas include

1. entitlements,
2. independent living,
3. adult education and employment,
4. family stability,
5. optimal health,
6. mental health,
7. substance use, and
8. use of legal services.

Measurement of outcome indicators in human services agencies is a new and emerging field. The results achieved by New York State's efforts have been heartening. Measurable improvement and better documentation have been demonstrated over the first two successive years. For example, within the optimal health area (outcome area number 5), a review of the indicators shows that the percentage of clients in the COBRA program enrolled with an identified primary care provider increased 3 percent between the initial round of reviews and the second year of reviews. The number of clients that kept primary care provider appointments increased 7 percent in the second year. A 15 percent increase was achieved in the number of clients that followed their medication regimen, and an even more impressive 37 percent increase in documented communication between the case manager and the primary care provider was demonstrated in the second year of the review. New York State is committed to continuing its work to evaluate case management outcomes and has broadened its efforts to train agencies to develop internal continuous quality improvement approaches, measure their own success, and initiate quality improvement projects designed to strengthen identified weaknesses.

Recent case management evaluation findings in other states also support the importance and value of case management for HIV populations. For example, a recent study of Florida's Medicaid Home and Community-Based Waiver for people with HIV/AIDS (July 2000) shows that people living with HIV and AIDS (PLWHAs) not enrolled in case management (when compared to case management enrollees) incurred significantly higher costs across the board, including higher inpatient and outpatient costs (Mitchell and Anderson, 2000). A study of South Carolina's HIV/AIDS Long-Term Medicaid Waiver demonstrated that noncase-managed HIV patients had higher costs (as much as 161 percent higher annual inpatient costs and 74 percent total annual spending costs) (Stoskopf and Richter, 1996). New Jersey's study of Medicaid case-managed individuals showed that case management was associated with a more appropriate pattern of protease and non-nucleoside reverse transcriptase inhibitor use and that case management also assisted in reducing interracial group differences between white and minority use of drug therapies, specifically increasing minority access to these therapies (Sambamoorthi et al., 2001).

A Health Resources and Services Administration (HRSA) study of case management showed that in New York City, clients were nine times more likely to enter medical care and three times more likely to enter appropriate medical care than those not receiving case management. In New Orleans, clients with case management were 2.6 times more likely to remain in medical care. In Boston, 80 percent of case-managed clients remained in care while only 66 percent of those not case managed remained in care. In Chicago, 13 percent of case-managed clients remained in care. These studies document that case management can be effective in helping clients remain in care (HRSA Publication, 1998).

New York State's recent study (Chestnut et al., 2002) of the cost effects of COBRA case-managed populations reveals that while statistically case management is cost neutral (i.e., the cost of providing case management is balanced by lower utilization of other services), there was a modest savings for the case-managed population. Regression analysis reveals that for those who are AIDS diagnosed, the savings are impressive, especially for those who utilize hospital-based care on a frequent basis. Case management helps to shorten the length of hospital stays and return clients to their home settings. This produces significant savings for the Medicaid program. (Approximately $10,000 per client per year or nine days of inpatient care per year were saved with case management.) COBRA case-managed individuals had better access to antiretroviral therapies than non-COBRA case-managed persons (57 percent versus 29 percent), were more likely to be cared for in a designated AIDS center (51 percent versus 34 percent), and were more likely to stay in primary care for the entire year of the study (45 percent versus 34 percent).

THE NEW ERA OF MANAGED CARE

Case management has been shown to promote timely access to crucially needed services in an effective and efficient manner. Thus, it is no surprise that when New York State began to develop its managed care approach for HIV populations in 1995, case management was seen as having a central and crucial role in special needs plans (SNPs, pronounced "snips"). SNPs are managed care Medicaid plans specifically for persons with HIV infection. SNPs will receive special capped rates to support the medical, case management, and psychosocial needs of their patients. In particular, HIV SNPs will be responsible for providing both client-centered and systems-centered case management services.

Clinical coordination and medical case management will be direct responsibilities of the newly formed SNPs. Each SNP patient must receive medical case management, but the manner in which this will be accomplished will vary in each SNP. Some have elected to utilize the primary care provider as the case manager; some have hired nursing care coordinators to provide medical case management; and others have delegated medical case management to networked providers such as the DACS.

SNP-based medical case managers will be expected to engage in utilization management, quality assurance, and continuous quality improvement efforts, as well as coordinate with two different levels of psychosocial case management provision. Each SNP will be required to assess the need for and refer clients to providers of either intensive or nonintensive psychosocial case management. During their first year of operations, SNPs must only ensure access to psychosocial case management, but in the second year of operation, each SNP will assume direct responsibility for providing needed psychosocial case management. Intensive case management, funded under Medicaid's COBRA CFP program, remains a carved-out service, which means these providers may bill directly to Medicaid for their services and the SNP does not have to pay for these services. Case management standards will require

SNPs to collaborate with other existing community case management providers to increase the effectiveness of case management for clients.

Implementation of SNPs will probably result in an increased demand for case management. As many as 30,000 to 40,000 clients could be brought into the case management system as a result of voluntary and eventually mandatory SNP enrollment of Medicaid recipients, which will undoubtedly have a dramatic effect on current case management capacity and the ability of the system to meet the new demand. The new case management system emerging after the SNPs become operational must unite the entitlement, clinical, and psychosocial case management community in one coordinated case management system that can successfully serve this expanded population.

Caseloads within the various SNP case management entities will vary. The SNP medical case manager is limited to a caseload of no more than 150 clients. This differs significantly from what is found in commercial managed care programs that often have ratios of one case manager to 10,000 to 14,000 enrollees. Our goal is to make SNP case management a viable proactive medical case management effort that does not solely target utilization management and high-cost catastrophic cases but provides realistic and effective medical care coordination. Caseloads for psychosocial case management are limited to sixty clients per manager for nonintensive case management and twenty clients per manager for intensive case management.

By designing their own case management structure, SNPs have been given flexibility as to how to provide and arrange for psychosocial case management. This flexibility will allow different models to emerge among the approved SNP entities. SNPs may elect to do all case management internally, taking responsibility for the medical and psychosocial case management with direct staff. Conversely, they may elect to refer all psychosocial case management to external providers, or they may triage populations and manage some internally and some externally based on the best fit for each patient. The efficiency and effectiveness of the various arrangements that arise over the next few years will be evaluated to determine which organizational structure of case management services provides the most effective approach. Evaluation findings will guide future decisions about case management models for SNPs.

THE FUTURE OF CASE MANAGEMENT IN NEW YORK STATE

Case management has come a long way since the mid-1980s and Dr. Rango's "Tower of Babel." A tremendous amount of effort has been put forth to define and guide the development of case management within New York State. The next few years will be a very interesting time with new challenges. After the September 11, 2001, disaster in New York State, we have witnessed a dramatic downturn in the economy, disturbing trends in HIV and STD seroprevalence, and a likelihood of increased demand for HIV case management. HIV funding has leveled, and there may be no further ability to expand case management against this backdrop of increased demands. The case management system of the future will have to do more and serve more, with fewer resources. It will be incumbent on all of us to demand greater efficiency and effectiveness from case management providers and service delivery systems. The impact of managed care may require evolved thinking about how case management services should be provided in these new settings. Case managers will be the key to identifying appropriate solutions to problems that arise. There is no doubt that the case management community will rise to the challenge and solve the complexities of the "Tower of Babel."

REFERENCES

AIDS Institute (1994). Unpublished memo.

Chestnut, T., Gimbel, R., Lehrman, S., Manna, V., Schnee, J., Freedman, J., Savicki, K., and Tackley, L. (2002). Effect of COBRA HIV/AIDS case management on Medicaid expenditures. Unpublished paper.

HRSA HIV/AIDS Bureau (1998). *Evaluating HIV case management: Invited research and evaluation papers.* HRSA Publication No. HAB00018.

Lehrman, S. (2000). *An evaluation of AIDS Institute HIV case management services in upstate New York and on Long Island.* New York: New York State Department of Health AIDS Institute.

Lehrman, S. and Gentry, D. (1998) *An evaluation of AIDS Institute HIV case management services in New York City.* New York: New York State Department of Health AIDS Institute.

Mitchell, J.M. and Anderson, K.H. (2000). Effects of case management and new drugs on Medicaid AIDS spending. *Health Affairs* 19: 233-243.

New York State Session Laws (1983). Chapter 822.

Sambamoorthi, U., Moynihan, P.J., McSpiritt, E., and Crystal, S. (2001). Use of protease inhibitors among Medicaid beneficiaries with AIDS. *American Journal of Public Health* 91: 1474-1481.

Stoskopf, C.H. and Richter, D.L. (1996). Evaluation of South Carolina's HIV/AIDS community long-term care Medicaid waiver: Cost comparison and patient satisfaction. *Journal of Health and Human Services Administration* 19: 79-98.

Chapter 8

The New York City Division of AIDS Services

Anita Vitale

BACKGROUND

It was 1985, and the New York City Human Resources Administration (HRA), the vast, sprawling bureaucracy responsible for the delivery of social and support services to millions of New Yorkers, including child welfare, public assistance, Medicaid, home care, and emergency homeless services, was experiencing a new and extremely troubling problem. It was the AIDS epidemic, and fear was rampant in the city over this new and apparently terminal disease. Caseworkers, who were responsible for interviewing clients to determine eligibility for entitlements and other services, were not immune to this fear. People with AIDS (PWAs), many of them gay men, no longer able to work, facing eviction, unable to buy food, and without health insurance, were coming to welfare centers to apply for public assistance and were being turned away. Some workers would not touch the paperwork of people who identified as having AIDS and even refused to be in the same room with them due to fear of transmission. These fears could not be allayed. Therefore, very sick and dying individuals were denied the basic help they needed by the very agency whose responsibility it was to provide it.

Equally terrible, the few clients who were actually able to get through the system and file applications for public assistance were dying before they received any benefits. The documentation requirements and an eligibility process that could take thirty to sixty days or longer were the major stumbling blocks. Moreover, the fragmented nature of HRA meant that individuals had to apply to separate agencies to receive different services including public assistance, Medicaid, and food stamps—tasks that are difficult enough when one is well but insurmountable when one is dying. It was finally becoming clear to city officials that the usual bureaucratic response would not suffice.

Pressure was also being placed upon the city by the hospitals for immediate action and from Gay Men's Health Crisis (GMHC), a new organization formed in response to AIDS. The hospitals had their own problems in handling the growing epidemic, including AIDS patients with no health insurance, no Medicaid, and no place to discharge them to if they became well enough to leave. Hospitals became substitute permanent housing for these people, and the alternate level of care days (ALOC) soared, placing the hospitals at great financial risk. At last Mayor Ed Koch took action.

It should be noted that there were some early heroes in HRA who single-handedly took on the cause of PWAs. Chuck Wallrich, a caseworker in Crisis Intervention Services, the agency that dealt with all kinds of disasters and emergencies (natural and otherwise), began learning of people losing their housing not only because they could not pay rent but also because of their AIDS diagnosis. With the approval of his supervisor Susan Urban, the director of Crisis and Disaster Services, he began to use the emergency financial services available to the agency to help provide food money and to avert evictions. These two people helped to shape the philosophy and the program that was established in mid-1985.

THE MODEL

Representatives from the New York State Department of Social Services (NYSDSS) and the city hammered out special agreements for this new initiative. A specialized program would act as the single entry point for PWAs to apply for and receive financial assistance and services—a one-stop shopping approach. Each client would be assigned to a case manager who would be responsible for coordinating and providing all that was needed. The services included:

- income maintenance (public assistance)
- rental assistance
- home care
- Medicaid
- food stamps
- Social Security referrals

NYSDSS agreed to allow the city to provide an enhanced public assistance rental allowance of $480 a month for a single person (the previous allowance was $215). Due to the wasting nature of the disease, representatives agreed that the food allowance be increased so that dietary supplements such as Ensure could be purchased (the prior approval process in place with Medicaid was too cumbersome to meet immediate needs). The eligibility criteria was CDC (Centers for Disease Control)-defined AIDS; those with ARC (AIDS related complex) qualified only if they needed home care.

A form already used by the HRA Home Care Program, the M11q, "Request for Home Care Services," which needed to be signed by a physician, would be utilized as the referral form and confirmation of diagnosis. These agreements constituted the basis of the program, along with an HRA official's stated but unwritten directive to Income Support and other HRA agencies: "Give them what they want." This directive lasted only a short period, as the official left and was replaced by someone with other ideas, but we ran with it for as long as we could. The reality of so many young people sick and dying, as well as their individual stories, touched even the most hardened of HRA bureaucrats and enabled us to get requests approved that would have been unthinkable under ordinary circumstances.

THE PROGRAM

The AIDS Case Management Unit (CMU) was established in Crisis Intervention Services in June 1985. CMU consisted of city workers who volunteered for the position. Joyce Gee was the supervisor; Dennis Velez, Sam Arus, Arthur McLean, and Kenny Long were the first caseworkers. They operated out of a small room at the agency's central office at 250 Church Street and were immediately flooded with referrals. There were few, if any, procedures. The staff members made it up as they went along, utterly committed to serving the needs of this population no matter what it took. On their own, they found housing for homeless clients, got them money, brought them food and other necessities, provided personal care in some instances, and helped them to die with dignity. They were able to get checks for food and rent to clients within a day, sometimes within hours, feats virtually unheard of in this bureaucracy. However, there was a backlog of referrals from day one, reduced only by the deaths of those on the waiting list.

In January 1986, I was hired as the director of Case Management to oversee the program's day-to-day operations. Additional supervisory and casework staff members were hired as well. In order to accommodate the increased staffing, the program moved to the Waverly Income Maintenance Center in Manhattan. It was clear that bureaucratic fear still existed. We had our own separate entrance, separate bathrooms for the clients, a separate ventilation system, and a wall that had been extended to the ceiling to keep us apart from the other programs in the building. The Serviceline was established as the intake section to handle all referrals, verify eligibility, and assign the cases to caseworkers. A special unit of Income Support workers was established to handle the public assistance applications submitted by caseworkers on behalf of the clients. The Income Support workers would not have to actually see the clients but would only review the paperwork and produce the checks. These workers were not part of the CMU and reported to a separate structure. This arrangement later created tensions and conflict, as Income Support took a strict interpretation of policies and procedures and sought to apply them to our requests. We, on the other hand, sought to make the system respond to the needs of our clients and attempted to bend the rules whenever possible.

Operating out of Manhattan, staff members began servicing all the boroughs. Each case manager had a caseload of thirty clients at any given time, and clients remained with the program throughout the course of their illness until they died (an average of two to three months).

Since only a handful of AIDS organizations existed, and the hospitals were bearing the brunt of the epidemic, the program was hailed and immediately utilized. The growth and need was phenomenal and beyond anyone's planning or expectations. Establishing communication and collaboration between the program and the other service providers was extremely important. This enabled the new program to gain credibility and become an integral part of the AIDS service delivery system.

In 1987, the program was shifted to the Medical Assistance Program and was given its new name, the Division of AIDS Services (DAS); according to the new administrator, Gordon Campbell, it was no longer a "mom and pop" operation but a program. We had started with one office and a caseload of approximately 200 cases; by September 1988, the program had expanded to include three borough offices; the staff had increased from sixty-five to 100 and the client caseload had increased to over 2,000. From 300 to 500 referrals were received each month. They came from everywhere: hospitals, correctional facilities, physicians, drug treatment programs, other community organizations, families and friends of those infected—each with their own needs and desperations. People with AIDS walked in off the streets to apply. In order to inform the public about our services a pamphlet titled "Who Cares? HRA Does" was printed and distributed throughout the city. However, it was the staff that made this program special.

THE STAFF

In the beginning and for several years, all of the DAS staff, including clerical and casework, volunteered for the unit; some were HRA veterans who were looking for a new challenge, and some were gay men looking for a way to help their community. Many believed it their mission to work with the disadvantaged and the stigmatized in society. Whatever their personal reasons, the staff was willing to take on the risk of working at the forefront of the epidemic, because there was an opportunity to actually help people without being encumbered by bureaucratic policies and rules. We saw ourselves as cutting through the red tape and making a difference in people's lives. All level supervisors, including the director of DAS Case Management Operations and the site directors also handled one or two clients so that they would have an understanding of what the staff was experiencing. During the times (and there were many) when hiring was frozen and our backlog was growing, the supervisors took on more clients to at least get them financial assistance. We visited clients in homes and in hospitals, often after work and on weekends. We accompanied them to appointments and listened to their fears. We were there when they died, sometimes as part of a group of friends and loved ones, sometimes all alone. We made burial arrangements and attended funerals. In some instances, families were so estranged from our clients that we not only made the arrangements but also kept the ashes. None of this was in the job description, but it became the standard.

However, the constant, unrelenting deaths of our clients eventually took its toll on all of us. In those first years, we knew that when we met a client for the first time, he or she would be dead within days or weeks. One was helpless against the disease, and it was almost too much to bear to witness the inexorable disintegration of a person's mind and body. For several years, until budget cuts struck, we were able to have a counselor who provided support for the staff. DAS also had its own psychiatrist who was hired to assess clients, but who often spent more time with the workers. However, budgetary problems, shifting priorities in HRA, and the normalization of AIDS in New York City changed our recruitment and support of staff. By 1990, workers were coming off civil service lists or even being involuntarily transferred from other programs. Although many proved to be good workers, the intense dedication and commitment of the original staff was no longer there.

THE CLIENTS

Each caseload was quite diverse and reflected the ever-changing face of the epidemic; the clients came from all walks of life and social strata. The common denominator was that they were all young and were all going to die. Many clients came in telling us they were going to beat "this" AIDS, and they fought to the end, demonstrating enormous courage and inspiring others. Some were able to give up drugs because they did not want to die with needles in their arms and wanted their families to be proud of them at the end; others became activists, fighting the stigma and the acts of hate with the skills they possessed. They included artists, musicians, performers, transvestites, sex workers, doctors, and lawyers. Some were people who, despite living on the edge, had been able to scrape together a way to survive without turning to public agencies; only AIDS brought them to us now.

They had no knowledge of the entitlement system and often could not produce the proper documentation or satisfactorily account for how they had supported themselves; DAS ensured that this barrier was overcome so that they could receive public assistance and Medicaid. Many were poor to begin with and familiar with a public assistance process that often denied them benefits; AIDS made the system more responsive to them.

When the CDC expanded the definition of AIDS to include a T-cell count of 200 or less, more people became eligible for DAS services. We had extraordinary scenes at the Serviceline of people who after literally weeks of bringing in M11q's to try to qualify for DAS services were finally eligible. James M. waved his M11q like a winning lottery ticket: "I now have AIDS; you have to give me a caseworker and a room." Clients brought in their siblings who had just been diagnosed and proudly told them that DAS would take care of them. We had to implement a stricter eligibility review process as a "black market" arose for the sale of forged M11qs. People were desperate to qualify for services.

At a time when most of the city viewed AIDS as an epidemic among gay men, we were also seeing substance abusers, women, and families. This required us to develop strategies on our own to handle and serve these populations and, in doing so, to push the system to respond in ways it had never considered or envisioned. The plight of women and children with AIDS was especially heartbreaking and demanded a special response. These women were often the sex partners of men with AIDS, and they were typically not diagnosed until they were either near death or had given birth to an HIV-infected child. Many were the sole caretakers of uninfected children who were now becoming orphans. Grandparents who were losing their children to AIDS were now being called upon to care for their grandchildren. They needed emotional support, emergency financial assistance for food and rent, and in some instances rehousing, but there was no one to help. Again, the traditional social service providers for families, both within HRA and the community, were not prepared and equipped to respond, so the referrals came to DAS.

Since DAS had been set up as a program for single adults, the staff and system were overwhelmed with handling the financial and psychosocial needs of these families. We decided to convince the administration that families needed a more specialized approach, and in 1988 were able to establish a pilot program with one family unit in the Bronx. Our goal was to keep the family intact during the course of the illness and plan for the future of the surviving family members. This included the provision of home care and homemaker services, permanency planning, and family counseling, as well as financial and housing services. The caseload was limited to fifteen cases per worker to enable the provision of intensive services. This model proved to be so successful that we were able to expand the program through a federal grant in 1989. At that time, over 400 families were receiving services through DAS and this number continued to grow.

Shawn came to us when she was seventeen, newly diagnosed with HIV and forced to leave the group home where she was living because the other girls had attacked her when they learned of her diagnosis. DAS was her safety net. Shawn had a child in foster care and was on her own. We housed her and linked her to some community-based services; however, as she was healthy and did not have AIDS, we were unable to keep her case open and lost track of her for several years. Then we received a telephone call from Bellevue Hospital. Shawn, now diagnosed with AIDS, had another child and was pregnant with a third. Her boyfriend had been murdered in their apartment, and she was forced to flee, leaving all of her possessions behind. She needed help, and we at DAS, who had never forgotten her, took her back into the program. We cared for Shawn and her children until her death several months later. She was able to plan for them, designate caretakers, and die peacefully.

HOUSING

Housing was another major issue—for us and for clients who were facing homelessness due to inability to pay rent, for those with precarious housing arrangements (e.g., subletting, sleeping on a friend's couch), and for those who were homeless. Although the public assistance rental allowance had been increased to $480 a month, this proved to be totally inadequate as our clients who had been working were paying significantly higher rents. Also, due to the rental market in New York City, it was extremely difficult to find apartments at the allowable rent for those who needed to move. Each situation involving excess rent had to be reviewed and considered on a case-by-case basis by an Income Support administrator for an "exception to policy." We became adept at these requests, fighting hard to get rents approved and working closely with GMHC, the hospitals, and other groups to get the needed information and advocacy. The staff worked out agreements with clients' friends and relatives to pay a portion of the rent, even at times convincing sympathetic landlords to lower the rent requested.

The homeless were even more challenging, as many were substance abusers who lived on and off in shelters or on the streets. Before AIDS, hospitals could discharge them to shelters, but the New York City Department of Health issued a memorandum stating that no person with AIDS could be discharged to a shelter. The question was where would they go? Nursing homes would not take them and with the exception of a few apartments operated by the AIDS Resource Center, a community agency, and plans for a residential facility (Bailey House) to be opened some time in the near future, there was no housing stock available. Although HRA was involved with providing emergency housing for homeless families, these resources were not extended to individuals with AIDS or to DAS caseworkers. So although homeless people with AIDS were waiting in our offices and hospitals were sending them to us by ambulette, the HRA commissioner was telling us that HRA did not belong in the business of housing people. As a result, DAS was on its own to find emergency housing, and the caseworkers found it in single-room occupancy hotels (SROs). It was not the best answer; the rates were expensive (often running $1,000 a month or more). Most were run-down with inadequate facilities, but it was better than leaving someone to die on the streets. We had no other options, and it was extremely frustrating. Often we would arrange for a room at one of these SROs yet when our client arrived he or she would be turned away for looking too sick or seeming gay or looking like a drug user. We coached our clients on how to speak to the hotel manager and helped them look as clean and as well dressed as possible. When absolutely necessary or when all else failed, we used subterfuge. When a client looked too ill, one of the DAS staff went to the hotel and made a reservation, and then we brought the client to the room. One of our better and safer housing placements was the McBurney YMCA, but they took only men. Late one day, we received a call from St. Clare's Hospital seeking housing for Crystal, a transsexual. "Can she act like a man?" we asked, because if she could, we would get her a room at the McBurney. The social worker came back on the phone and told us she would. So we were able to house Crystal for the night and many others in this way.

With no real housing policy (the development of housing programs did not begin until the late 1980s), we grew dependent on the SROs as the first resort and soon set up an internal housing unit to handle the placements as the numbers of people needing emergency housing increased. Often we all worked late into the night to ensure that everyone with a need for emergency housing had a place at least for that night; then we could begin again tomorrow. However, we were not able to house everyone sent to us. There were instances when extremely sick and disabled clients, some in wheelchairs, were brought from hospitals by ambulette to Waverly and deposited at the Serviceline for housing. We sent them back to emergency rooms, as there was no appropriate housing to meet their needs. We experienced the same problems with the state and city prisons who released sick, and now homeless, inmates with no planning and with only the address of the DAS Serviceline. We worked with the New York Division of Parole to develop discharge-planning procedures so that the needs of parolees with AIDS could be met immediately upon their discharge from prisons.

CHANGE

In 1989, DAS was transferred back to the oversight of the Adult Services Administration. This marked the program's third transfer in three years. Each different agency meant a shift in focus and priorities, as well as the necessity of convincing yet another group of administrators that DAS needed resources to meet its mission and to function on a level that met people's needs. The arguments often fell on deaf ears as other programs and issues took precedence. While the internal politics of HRA were being played out, more pressure was put on DAS to respond, and the system was breaking down under the strain. It was now taking weeks, not days, to assign a client to a caseworker. This meant that a client's receipt of financial and medical benefits was also delayed. Hospitals were unable to discharge patients who were homeless, because DAS could not assign them quickly enough or find housing for them. There were several reasons for this. The advent of AZT and other medical advances meant that clients were beginning to live longer, thus remaining on the DAS caseload for a longer period of time. The CDC's expansion of the definition of AIDS to include those with T-cell counts of 200 or less meant that more people were now eligible for DAS services. The city, in order to alleviate pressure on its shelter system for homeless individuals, also decided to go further in expanding the eligibility criteria for DAS services to include not only people with AIDS but also those with related HIV illness (as defined by the New York State AIDS Institute) who also needed assistance with the activities of daily living. Almost immediately, DAS was inundated with homeless clients who met these new criteria. There were not enough caseworkers or housing resources to meet the increased demand. As one GMHC advocate put it, "It's [DAS] been an enormous lifesaver for many clients. But as the program has fallen behind, it's become a nightmare."

Newly hired caseworkers were without desks or telephones and demonstrated at the HRA commissioner's office. The commissioner conceded that the city had miscalculated the number of clients who would be coming to DAS and the number of caseworkers needed but that the situation would improve. AIDS organizations became more militant and, with the establishment of ACT UP, more adversarial. ACT UP demanded that DAS expand its admission criteria even further to include all homeless persons living with HIV-related illness and to provide medically appropriate housing for them as well. ACT UP issued a "Wanted for Murder" poster against the deputy commissioner of adult services for failing to act and for restricting eligibility. It was a difficult atmosphere to work in, with pressure and criticism coming from all sides.

With the city facing fiscal problems in the early 1990s, the administration of Mayor David Dinkins began to look at programs to cut or eliminate. Since DAS was not a mandated program, its position had never been secure, and it always had to justify its reason to exist. Now the question was raised: What differences exist in AIDS clients that require a specialized case management approach to service delivery compared to other clients? To state it more bluntly, as one senior HRA administrator did, when people with AIDS were dying quickly, usually within two to three months, the city could afford to be generous in its approach as the investment of money was short term. Now that people were living longer, that changed everything.

DAS administration was given the difficult task to develop a restructuring plan that would better manage the caseload, which was approaching 16,000 clients, with 800 new applicants each month, without increasing staff or resources. Several plans were considered. A plan was finally decided upon in which there would be a two-tier system. DAS would provide intake and stabilization for all clients for the first ninety days, at which time a decision would be made as to how to handle the case. Those clients meeting specific criteria, e.g., those permanently housed and those that had entitlements in place, would be transferred to a holding unit in DAS and/or referred to other community-based organizations or HRA programs for continuing case management. There would be limited access to a DAS case manager until a problem arose needing intervention. At that point a caseworker would be assigned to resolve the problem and make appropriate referrals. Clients with unresolved housing and/or other issues after ninety days would continue to receive intensive case management services from DAS. This plan was loudly and severely criticized by the AIDS community, which viewed it as DAS seeking to shift its responsibilities to community-based organizations that were not funded to handle these issues. Due to the inability to work out the problems, the plan was not implemented at that time. Also, a new mayor would soon be elected to grapple with the problem.

In 1984, the new Giuliani administration took a different approach to the unrelenting and severe criticism of DAS by the AIDS advocates. DAS should not be reorganized; it should be completely disbanded. His administration believed that AIDS clients would be better served by being mainstreamed into existing city programs. However, when confronted with the possible loss of DAS, the AIDS advocates denounced Giuliani's plan and mounted demonstrations and lobbying to keep the flawed but necessary program. As a result of their efforts, DAS was saved. However, DAS was reorganized somewhat along the lines of the original restructuring plan with an important addition. With the goal to make the public assistance process more efficient, the Income Support staff and their functions were merged with DAS under one umbrella. This new structure was named the Division of AIDS

Services and Income Support (DASIS). Despite the restructuring and the new name, the old problems persisted. DASIS was unable to provide emergency and permanent housing to meet the need. In line with the harsher homeless policies of the Giuliani administration, homeless clients were sometimes instructed to make their own temporary arrangements as best they could, even if this meant staying on the streets. Delays continued in the processing of public assistance applications for food and rent, and tighter rules were implemented. Where were the advocates now?

The restructuring came at a time when there were significant changes in the treatment of HIV/AIDS due to the successful introduction of HAART therapy in 1996. People were becoming healthier and less subject to the debilitating and often life-ending opportunistic infections. This resulted in a dramatic decrease in the number and length of hospitalizations. Therefore, less pressure came from the hospitals to discharge patients. Many of the original AIDS activists had died and the advocacy organizations were no longer as militant; in fact, many of them now held contracts with the city for housing, case management, and other services. With the exception of Housing Works, a community-based organization with a militant advocacy component, dissent was muted. A system of community-based organizations, funded through Ryan White grants and other sources including Medicaid, was now in place to support the needs of persons living with HIV/AIDS. However, the role and importance of DASIS in providing housing and benefits was recognized and supported by all organizations. In order to protect the existence of DASIS from future problems, as well as to make it more accountable to PWAs, the advocates requested that the city council make DASIS a mandated program. After much debate, DASIS was mandated by the city council, so it became a permanent program that could not be dismantled at the whim of current and future mayors. The city council also mandated that DASIS establish and meet standards for the timeliness of processing housing requests and entitlements. The city council would monitor these on a regular basis.

Another name change occurred in 2001, when DASIS expanded to include a division for employment and rehabilitative services along with the original case management program. It was now known as the HIV/AIDS Services Administration (HASA). The small, almost "outlaw" program developed in 1985 to cut through the bureaucratic red tape was now a full-fledged member of the bureaucracy. Although the program continues to serve thousands of AIDS- and HIV-infected New Yorkers, it does so through systematic rules and regulations that are now harder to cut through, both for the staff and the advocates.

Chapter 9

A Case of Serendipity:
A Brief History of the Early Years
of the Annual National Conference
on Social Work and HIV/AIDS

Vincent J. Lynch

INTRODUCTION

In writing this chapter, I had many thoughts as to how I should organize it. First, I thought it should be a lengthy academic discourse that would focus on the history of HIV/AIDS in this country and the accompanying need for an AIDS conference for social workers. Or perhaps it might be an outline of the key topics that this conference has addressed over the years. However, what I have decided would be most useful is a simple reflection during which I informally discuss how I literally "stumbled" on the idea of an AIDS conference for social workers. I must confess at the outset that the decision to establish this conference was not the result of many extensive needs assessments, focus groups, or other sophisticated formal evaluation strategies. In all honesty, the decision to establish this conference was the result of (as the chapter title indicates) a fair amount of serendipity related to several events that converged at various points in time. Please indulge me as I discuss a number of events that led up to the founding of what we now refer to as the annual National Conference on Social Work and HIV/AIDS. I also will briefly discuss some key events in years two and three of the conference, as well as provide some brief information about more recent developments that have been important and that have enabled the conference to continue over these many years.

Since December 1986, I have served as Director of Continuing Education at Boston College Graduate School of Social Work. During the first few years in that position, I established a number of typical continuing education offerings for social workers in the Boston area. I enjoyed the work that I was doing and thought my work would probably remain the same in the years that lay ahead. In June 1988, however, I experienced a rather transforming event that impacted my personal and professional life. One early evening that June, I was casually listening to the National Public Radio news program *All Things Considered.* A segment reported on some of the political and logistical problems happening in Stockholm during the convening of the annual International AIDS Conference. Being a conference planner myself, some of these issues caught my attention.

Following that segment of the program was an interview with a young gay American man who was dying of AIDS. For the first time I learned of the issues of oppression and marginalization experienced by those who were living (and dying) with AIDS. I found his testimony extremely moving and troubling in a way that I could not fully describe. At the conclusion of the interview, I learned from the commentator that additional segments from the interview with this man would be broadcast over the next three days. I found myself compelled to listen to those additional programs, and each time I did, I learned more about this man's tragic suffering and increasing abandonment by his friends, by family members, and by the medical establishment as his illness progressed. When this radio series concluded at the end of the week, we learned that this young man had recently died.

In the days and weeks that followed, I continued to think about what I heard in this man's testimony. I also came to learn that his story was typical of so many of those who were living with and dying from AIDS at that time. This was the first time in my life that I had confronted AIDS as a reality, despite the fact that AIDS had been with us for at least seven or more years by that time. I began to wonder how it was that I, a social worker, knew so little about the reality of AIDS—a reality that contained issues supposedly so important to me as a social worker, issues such as oppression, marginalization, and social injustice. For several days I told no one of these internal struggles. I thought, perhaps on some level, that this discomfort would somehow just go away. It did not.

I first spoke of this discomfort to my wife, Mary T. (now deceased), explaining to her how troubled I felt. Although I believed that I strongly adhered to social work values, such as seeking social justice for others and fighting oppression, when it came to the AIDS epidemic I did nothing that put these values into action. I knew nothing about AIDS and contributed nothing to fighting this battle. Mary T., also a social worker, appreciated the values conflict in which I found myself. From these early discussions with her I decided, at a minimum, to try to become better informed.

I sought out information from fellow social workers in the Boston area who were working at AIDS Action, a major AIDS service organization.

These social workers included David Aronstein, David Brennan, Patricia Giulino, Dennis James, Rick Miller, Dianne Perlmutter, and Bruce Thompson. These colleagues opened my eyes to the realities of AIDS. I came to learn about their important AIDS work in great detail as well as their frustration with our profession. Specifically, they had described to me several efforts to communicate to various professional associations and organizations the need for social workers to learn about AIDS. Their perception was that although more and more social workers were dealing with AIDS in their practice settings, very few opportunities existed for them to learn in depth about the psychosocial aspects of AIDS. To the best of their knowledge, at that time there had not been any social work educational efforts either locally, nationally, or internationally that specifically focused on the growing AIDS crisis.

I also learned that they were not the only ones concerned about this issue. Indeed, they reported that social work colleagues in other cities who were doing AIDS work had similar frustrations and a similar lack of opportunities for social training and continuing education on AIDS topics. AIDS conferences that focused on medical issues abounded in 1988, but those that addressed psychosocial perspectives were scant. As my friends conveyed these concerns, it occurred to me one day that perhaps there was a way I could try to make a contribution—to make some difference in the AIDS battle they were waging. Although I possessed little knowledge about AIDS, I did have some expertise in organizing conferences. It occurred to me that perhaps I could explore the possibility of organizing a major AIDS social work conference in my role as Director of Continuing Education at Boston College Graduate School of Social Work.

CAN THIS IDEA WORK?

After some weeks of internal debate on the matter, I decided to approach my dean, June Gary Hopps. As I look back, I think I presented my idea in a way that was perhaps guaranteed to fail. After all, a part of me was frightened to undertake this venture and wanted to sabotage my efforts. For example, AIDS was a seriously controversial topic, especially at that time; it dealt with isssues such as sex, drugs, blood, homosexuality, and the deaths of young adults. On top of that, I was working at a Catholic university, and I frankly was nervous that such a conference would make "the powers that be" quite uncomfortable. Therefore, I presented a "sabotaging strategy" to Dean Hopps, proposing that we organize this major conference on a sensitive topic which we knew little about and that we commit significant human and financial resources of our school to this venture, having no guarantee that anyone would even come! To my "surprise" (i.e., read, dismay) Dean

Hopps thought it was a powerful idea and wholeheartedly gave it her approval. Within a few days of our discussion Dean Hopps was traveling to Stockholm for an international social work conference. She suggested I quickly develop a flyer to announce the conference, and she would distribute the flyer at this international social work conference. My initial thought was that the conference would be a regional one, targeting AIDS social workers in New England, perhaps. However, my dean had other plans. We were going international with this conference, like it or not. In the space of a twenty-four-hour period I needed to decide the dates, theme, venue, and other preliminary conference information that would be included in the flyer, as well as have 2,000 of these flyers printed and shipped to the dean at the conference hotel in Sweden. This flyer also had to describe procedures involved in submitting a presentation abstract for those who wished to give a workshop at the conference. This was a formidable task, to say the least!

Nonetheless, the venue for the conference was arranged, "procedures" were established, dates were set, and flyers were printed and shipped. This was moving much too quickly, I thought. As the famous proverb states: "Be careful what you wish for; you just might get it."

When Dean Hopps returned from Europe she reported that there was great enthusiasm about our proposed AIDS conference. I had selected June 12-15, 1989, as the dates for this conference, and we would hold it on the campus of Boston College. These dates were selected because they were dates when adequate meeting room space was available on campus and adequate on-campus university housing would also be available at that time for those conference attendees who wished that low-cost option. Dean Hopps reported that many people she spoke to at the conference indicated that they were planning to be in Montreal during June 1989 to attend the annual International AIDS Conference there (largely a medical conference) that was to conclude just three days before our Boston social work AIDS conference opened. Many individuals expressed an interest in coming to our conference directly from the Montreal conference. In addition, two major international social work organizations, the International Federation of Social Workers and the International Association of Schools of Social Work, generously offered to promote our conference and provide some very helpful in-kind services. Meanwhile, back in Boston, Carol Brill, the executive director of the Massachusetts chapter of the National Association of Social Workers, also generously committed support to the conference in many useful ways. At that time I sought out assistance from our New England AIDS Education and Training Center, and through the helpfulness of Donna Gallagher, its director, was able to secure a grant for the conference that supplemented the budget resources available at Boston College. All of these events took place during the late summer and early fall of 1988.

THE CONFERENCE BECOMES A REALITY

In late fall of 1988 I asked my friends at AIDS Action if they would work with me to form a planning committee for the conference and invited David Aronstein to join me as cochair of the committee and of the Boston conference. He graciously accepted. This committee shaped the program of the conference, evaluated submitted abstracts, and helped me develop strategies to promote this conference more extensively in the United States.

In an effort to broaden our planning committee beyond Boston, I invited three distinguished social work educators to join our effort. Two of these were American men who have been social work pioneers in AIDS care. Professor Gary Lloyd from Tulane University School of Social Work in New Orleans joined our planning efforts in the fall of 1988. At that time Gary was spending a fair amount of time in many African countries conducting trainings on AIDS prevention and treatment to health care professionals. He had also just developed an important manual on psychosocial issues and AIDS, which was used largely in developing nations. These activities were conducted as part of Gary's role as consultant to the World Health Organization's Global Programme on AIDS. Also, Professor Manuel Fimbres, another AIDS social work pioneer, joined our efforts. Manuel was on the faculty of San Jose State University College of Social Work in San Jose, California. He was co-author (along with Carl Leukefeld) of one of the first books that dealt with the psychosocial dimensions of AIDS, *Responding to AIDS: Psychosocial Initiatives* (1988). Manuel also held many important posts in the National Association of Social Workers, both in the California chapter and on the national level. As will be described in greater detail, after our first conference Gary and Manuel continued to work closely in planning future conferences until their respective retirements (Gary's in 1996 and Manuel's in 2000). The third social work educator who was of great help to me at that time was Professor Elaine Belanger from McGill University School of Social Work in Montreal. Elaine was involved in many international social activities, and she agreed to facilitate the "pilgrimage" of our many social work colleagues from the Montreal conference to the Boston conference.

Thus, by late October 1988, we had our planning activities in place and completed extensive mailings of a conference brochure nationally and internationally. However, we still had no clue whether anyone would actually attend this event. By Thanksgiving we had received only twelve presentation abstracts—quite discouraging. I remember meeting with Elaine Belanger in November 1988 and considering whether we should "pull the plug" on this venture before we utilized any more of our scarce resources. She encouraged me to wait and see what the next month would bring. To our delight, over 140 additional abstracts were received during the month of December, most of them received just before the December 31 deadline.

The winter and spring months of 1989 were filled with much activity as we attempted to put the final program together. We structured the original four-day conference program much the same way we structure the conference today. That is, we have at least one general session (or plenary session) daily for all to attend to hear a major address on a key issue in AIDS care. The remainder of each conference day was filled with various ninety-minute concurrent workshop sessions on an array of topics. These sessions were given by social workers whose presentation abstracts were selected for inclusion by the program committee. Topics of these sessions typically included areas such as AIDS case management, advocacy, strategies for serving vulnerable populations, AIDS and mental health concerns, social policy issues, medical updates, strategies for funding services, global issues, and cultural competency issues. There were also informal networking sessions scheduled, as well as receptions and social events. At our first conference there were just over 100 presentations given. We still offer just over 100 sessions each year. In recent years we have added the less competitive category of "poster session" for those who wish to more informally discuss their work with colleagues. At these poster sessions, the presenter uses a mounted poster, which highlights key points of his or her topic and engages in informal discussion of the topic to those who visit the poster "station." In recent years we also have included an advanced content track for those with three or more years of experience. Recent conferences have also offered off-site visits to local AIDS service organizations.

As spring 1989 dawned, we began to see registrations for the conference slowly (and then more steadily) arrive in our office. The day before the conference was to open I received a phone call from officials from the Immigration and Naturalization Service who informed me that a Danish social worker had arrived at Boston's Logan Airport and was detained because customs officials found AZT in his suitcase. At that time there was a strongly enforced U.S. policy that prohibited entry into the country of those who were living with AIDS. The exception to this policy was for individuals who wished entry into the country in order to attend an AIDS conference. I confirmed to government officials that our Danish colleague, Knud Josephsen, was indeed registered for the conference. He was eventually allowed to proceed. He attended the conference and offered to tell his story to us all.

By the time we opened the conference on June 12, we had received 431 registrations from AIDS care social workers. These attendees were from thirty-one states throughout the United States, and we also had a remarkable number of international delegates, most of whom made the journey from Montreal to Boston. Our international group included AIDS social workers from Canada, Australia, Ireland, Wales, England, Uganda, Denmark, Japan, Norway, Sweden, Zimbabwe, Finland, Poland, India, and Switzerland. A spirit of solidarity quickly emerged among all of us, and Gary Lloyd commented at one point that the conference seemed like a big, wonderful family reunion. I think all of us were deeply moved and realized that this conference was unique, long overdue, and indeed we all felt privileged to be part of this historic event. What added immensely to these feelings was Knud Josephsen's powerful testimony in our closing session in which he recounted the emotional pain and humiliation he felt while being detained at the airport. He went on to tell us more about his life—the hopes, the fears, the challenges of what it meant for him, and indeed, all who were living with AIDS in 1989. Knud Josephsen died in 1993.

As we said our good-byes on June 15 and 16, a grassroots movement seemed to be springing forth. Conference attendees were quite zealous in their belief that this conference should not be a one-time event. Several approached me and asked if I would consider exploring ways in which this conference could occur regularly. They indicated that what happened during this conference must be sustained and must continue. Dozens of people expressed this sentiment to me. Many offered to do what they could to help in future conference planning tasks and activities. Although I was deeply touched by this enthusiasm, I must confess that a large part of me was ready to let go of the conference. I was not completely ready to undertake such a complicated and difficult activity again on such short notice. After some lengthy discussions on this issue with Gary and Manuel, we decided that the three of us would work as a planning team for two more years. We agreed that with such a geographically diverse audience perhaps we should think about moving the conference to different cities. We agreed to plan a 1990 conference on the campus of Manuel's university, San Jose State University. If successful, Gary would then consider bringing the meeting to New Orleans in 1991. Dean Hopps authorized me to continue to serve as the principal organizer for the conference and to permit me to use my budget resources, as well as the infrastructure of my office, to accomplish the varied planning tasks and activities.

Within a few days after completing the final tasks associated with the Boston conference, Gary, Manuel, and I set out to begin the planning for the San Jose conference. Similar to Boston, we held that meeting on a university campus and made university housing available. The dean, faculty, and staff of Manuel's school, San Jose State University College of Social Work, went to great lengths to make our conference in their city a success. Similar to our first conference, we received approximately 150 abstracts from individuals wishing to present their work. As registrations came in during the winter and spring of 1990, we once again found to our surprise that we had approximately the same number of registrations: 418 in 1990 compared to 431 in 1989. We had fewer attendees from other nations, but nonetheless had eight nations in addition to the United States represented, including a six-person delegation from Australia, a four-person delegation from Egypt, and an eleven-person delegation from Canada. Social workers from thirty-eight states in the United States were represented at the San Jose conference.

In 1991, we held the conference in New Orleans but decided that it might be more efficient to use a hotel that year so that all sessions could be under one roof rather than spread out in several buildings, as was the case on the two university campuses we used in 1989 and 1990. This was a successful strategy, and we were fortunate to have this hotel-based meeting held at the charming Hotel Monteleone located in the middle of New Orleans' French Quarter. This third conference also proved to be a successful venture, with over 100 presentations offered and 452 individuals in attendance. We have returned to New Orleans with great regularity since it has proven to be such a popular destination for our attendees. Four of our fourteen conferences have been held in this wonderful city, and we find that our registration numbers usually rise during the years we use New Orleans as the conference venue. The dean, faculty, and staff at Gary's school, Tulane University School of Social Work, have consistently helped us each time and have shown us true "Southern hospitality" during all of our stays in New Orleans. Gary also has been especially generous during these stays. He has hosted wonderful "crawfish boil" parties at his lovely home in the French Quarter for those who have contributed to the planning of each of these New Orleans conferences. Gary also has helped us to gain access to some of New Orleans' wonderful musical artists who have provided entertainment at various functions during the conferences.

After successfully completing the conference in 1991, Gary, Manuel, and I evaluated where we were at that time. We had agreed to plan these first three conferences, yet the need seemed to remain for this conference to continue beyond that third year. After some debate and hesitation, the three of us agreed to continue to work together and to plan the conference as an annual event for as long as the need seemed to exist.

CAN THIS CONFERENCE CONTINUE?

When Gary, Manuel, and I decided to continue this venture beyond year three, it became clear that some additional sources of external funding needed to be obtained if we were to move forward. The cost of postage, printing, advertising, and other "up-front" expenses continued to rise tremendously each year. In addition, if we were to continue the plan to have the conference at hotels and not on university campuses, significant new expenses such as audiovisual rentals, meeting room charges, and costly food and beverage expenses needed to be budgeted. Although my Boston College budget continued to be a vital resource, there were real limitations that needed to be recognized. We also did not want to increase registration fees as a way to offset new expenses, since most of our conference attendees were already on very tight budgets. What to do?

While we were in the midst of these issues regarding the future viability of the conference, I received an unsolicited phone call from an executive at the pharmaceutical company Burroughs Wellcome. His name was Fred Gregg. Fred had learned of our conference from colleagues and was interested in learning more about the role of social work in AIDS care, since his company was gaining an appreciation for the fact that psychosocial professionals, as well as medical professionals, worked closely with AIDS patients around questions and decisions pertaining to medications. Gary, Manuel, and I provided some information to Fred Gregg during several consultations, which helped him understand better the role of social work in AIDS care. In appreciation, the company made a very generous unrestricted educational grant to Boston College in 1991, which enabled us to continue the conference. This generous support from the company continued until 1999, despite the fact that Burroughs Wellcome underwent a merger in 1995 (its name then changing to Glaxo Wellcome). A further change in corporate structure occurred in 1999, which necessitated a moratorium on certain funding commitments, including the continued funding of our grant. I am pleased to report, however, that in 2001 we have obtained conference support from the new corporate entity, GlaxoSmithKline. I am hopeful this is the beginning of another longstanding "win-win" relationship for both of us.

The generous grants just mentioned helped us greatly in keeping the conference alive through the 1990s and into the present. Nonetheless, additional funding sources needed to be explored as well so that the conference would not run a deficit. Although registration fees and the funding previously mentioned did significantly offset those Boston College budget resources allocated to the conference, still more funding would be needed if we were to reach our annual goal of breaking even. Over $300,000 in grants, contracts, and in-kind services have been awarded to Boston College during the past decade, which has enabled the conference to meet its goal of breaking even financially each year. Additional supporters in the past ten years have included:

> Health Resources and Services Administration—HIV/AIDS Bureau
> Centers for Disease Control and Prevention
> National Institute of Mental Health
> New England AIDS Education and Training Center

Midwest AIDS Training and Education Center
Delta Region AIDS Education and Training Center
Southeast AIDS Training and Education Center
Tulane University
San Jose State University
University of Illinois at Chicago
AIDS Project Los Angeles
Massachusetts Chapter, National Association of Social Workers
Agouron Pharmaceuticals, Inc.
Bristol-Myers Squibb
Chicago Department of Public Health
Stadtlanders Pharmacy
CVS ProCare

A LOOK AT 1992 TO THE PRESENT

The conference has indeed continued beyond those first three years. The fourth annual conference was held in 1992 in Washington, DC. Additional conferences have been held in:

San Francisco, 1993
New Orleans, 1994
Chicago, 1995
Atlanta, 1996
Los Angeles, 1997
New Orleans, 1998
Chicago, 1999
San Diego, 2000
Philadelphia, 2001
New Orleans, 2002

We are now planning our 2003 meeting, to be held in Albuquerque, New Mexico. The 2004 conference will be held in Washington, DC.

We estimate that over 6,000 AIDS practitioners have attended the conferences over the years. Each year the conference continues to draw 400 to 500 attendees. Each year approximately 10 percent of our attendees are people living with HIV/AIDS, and we are able to waive the registration fee for those individuals. This initiative for people living with HIV/AIDS is known as the Manuel Fimbres Project, named in honor of our friend and colleague.

I am very pleased that we consistently receive positive evaluations regarding the presentations given at the conference each year. Many presenters have taken material from these excellent conference sessions and developed their ideas into articles that have been published in distinguished social work and other professional journals. I have had the honor of serving as editor and co-editor of four books that address AIDS and social work (published in 1993, 1996, 1998, and 2000). All four of these books contain chapters by colleagues who have written about topics that they have presented at previous conferences.

CONCLUDING THOUGHTS

The "take home" message in this chapter is that what began as a product of chance and serendipity has become a conference that is alive and well. It has been a distinct honor for me to work closely for so many years with AIDS social workers and with countless other people and organizations that have supported the need for, and the work of, this conference. I truly did expect when I began this venture that the conference would be a one-time event. As I write this chapter, however, we are about to mail the "Call for Presentation Proposals" announcement for the 2003 conference; this will be our fifteenth annual conference. I also have recently completed contract negotiations with the hotel that will serve as the venue for our 2004 conference in Washington, DC.

The work of organizing this conference brings bittersweet feelings for me. On one hand, I have made so many new and wonderful friends over the years and have experienced great personal and professional satisfaction. On the other hand, the fact that there is a continued need for this conference only underscores that this epidemic is far from over. In this country as well as abroad, HIV/AIDS continues to disproportionately impact those least able to seek and receive adequate care and treatment. In many ways it would make me happy if there was no longer a need for this conference, because then, no longer would HIV/AIDS be a reality in our world. This obviously will not be the case for decades to come.

So the fight goes on. Social work continues to play a vital role in fighting this disease. We plan to continue the conference as long as it is needed. I look forward to the years ahead and hope that newer and younger colleagues help us keep this necessary resource alive and well so that AIDS social workers will continue to have a place to go to learn from one another, to be refreshed, and to be renewed, a place where, in Gary Lloyd's words, the big, wonderful family reunion can continue. Recently, our new dean at Boston College Graduate School of Social Work, Dr. Alberto Godenzi (himself an AIDS researcher), has reaffirmed the importance of the conference and stated that he supports us in continuing our work as the need exists.

I wish to thank the dozens of friends and colleagues who have helped me over the years with the many tasks and activities that needed to be carried out in order for each conference to succeed. I would also like to remember my dear friend and colleague, the late Willis Green Jr., who helped us to make the conference a truly inclusive experience for all. I leave you with the challenge that the late Dr. Jonathan Mann, founding director of the World Health Organization's Global Programme on AIDS, gave to us when he was the closing speaker at our conference in Chicago on June 3, 1995: "AIDS is about society more than it is about a virus. We must move forward, but to do so requires that we confront ourselves—our own status quo, our fears, our uncertainties."

I hope our conference continues to be vital and alive for as long as it is needed, a resource that helps AIDS care social workers move forward in the ways that Jonathan Mann encouraged us to back in 1995. I hope it continues to be a place where we can learn from one another and, perhaps most important, a place to nourish one another.

Chapter 10

Motivating the System from Within

Barbara Willinger

I was an experienced, seasoned hospital social work supervisor when I began working with AIDS patients in 1989. I knew hospital systems and, in fact, had designed a few that facilitated and improved patient care; however, I had never tried to impact a citywide system. Little did I know then that in the next twelve years I, personally and through the efforts of a social work committee, would impact a city and state system.

In 1985 New York City responded to the AIDS crisis through the development of a specialized unit then called the Crisis Intervention Service AIDS Case Management Unit, known by 1988 as the Division of AIDS Services (DAS). The agency was initially staffed by dedicated, committed line staff and administrators who chose to be involved with AIDS clients; they were for all intents and purposes the cream of the crop in the Human Resource Administration (HRA). Issues of stigma and fear were practically nonexistent in that agency.

For the first year in my new position as a social work manager, I struggled to make sense of DAS. The system seemed a labyrinth in which referrals moved at a snail's pace, much too slow compared to the devastation of AIDS that we, in the hospitals, experienced. In retrospect, I wonder if my sense of confusion was a displacement of my attempts to make sense of such a confounding illness.

How can anyone forget the 1980s—when GRID burst upon the American landscape, when fear gripped people's emotions, when the epidemic was finally given the name AIDS, and when people, primarily gay men, were admitted to hospitals with crippling and often terminal opportunistic infections, such as *Pneumocystis carinii* pneumonia, toxoplasmosis, or cryptococcol meningitis, to name only a few? Any of these might result in decreased ability to care for oneself or the need for intravenous therapy resulting in home care services and/or nursing services. Some of our patients had lost their homes; some never had homes to lose. Many could no longer continue to work and either had health insurance that was insufficient to cover their outpatient needs or had lost their benefits. DAS was the touchstone for all and any of these services, including financial assistance. Homeless clients were placed in SROs (single room occupancy) hotels in which one kitchen and bathroom were shared by many. Despite the clarity of a patient's need, arranging for these services usually took days to weeks after the patient was medically cleared for discharge. The delays seemed related to the lack of available resources and/or the conundrum of the DAS system.

Joseph was a sixty-two-year-old African-American homosexual male who had recently retired. The meningitis that precipitated his admission to the hospital led to the suspicion of AIDS, which was confirmed through testing. Joseph had been living with a friend, waiting for a senior citizen apartment to become available, but circumstances unrelated to his AIDS diagnosis precluded his return there. Technically, Joseph was homeless. In addition, Joseph received Social Security benefits, but his need for and the cost of home care services necessitated an application for Medicaid. The conundrum in this case was that a referral to DAS for home care services could not be made until Joseph had an address—which finally occurred a week after he was medically cleared for discharge. It took another ten days in the DAS system for home care to be put in place.

Juan, a married thirty-year-old Latino male, required TPN infusion (total parenteral nutrition over a twelve-hour period) in order to return home to die. This plan necessitated home care and nursing services. His wife was caring for their children, ages two and four. The medical documentation was completed and sent to DAS two weeks prior to his readiness for discharge. Daily phone calls were made to DAS to track the progress of the application since this was a race against death. Family anxiety over Juan's deterioration manifested itself through anger at me "for not moving quickly enough." A parallel process ensued with my own anger and frustration being voiced to DAS. Nothing seemed to work. Juan died in the hospital, his illness more powerful in the end than the good intentions of many people.

Why couldn't the system move faster? Why couldn't DAS administrators get it to move? What didn't I know? Why couldn't I make it move faster? After a year of supervising and doing the work, I felt no closer to understanding or knowing how to negotiate the system. Out of my confusion arose an idea to personally speak with the director of DAS and have her explain the system to me; she had been accessible and responsive in previous telephone conversations. What I expected to be a one-on-one meeting became a roundtable discussion with her and some of her administrative staff. The timing was right; it was the period when people described themselves as "warriors, fighting the enemy, a shared enemy" and people bonded together easily and in creative ways. We shared the hardships on both sides, hospital and city bureaucracies, in accessing care for people with AIDS.

Our meeting ended with an agreement that if I could rally other hospitals, the director would commit herself and her site administrators to monthly discussions of obstacles that mitigated against timely access to services. Thus was born the Hospital/DAS Task Force which met monthly for over five years. Although we had our differences, we more importantly had the shared goal of making life and death easier for those infected with and affected by HIV.

Collaborative efforts ensued between us. For example, because of the paucity of available SROs, patients remained in hospitals until a vacancy occurred; this period could vary from days to weeks. However, if a patient appeared at the DAS central intake site, as happened on numerous occasions, the DAS worker was obligated to house that individual, thereby bumping a patient who was already waiting in a hospital. Hospitals engaged in that practice ultimately discontinued sending patients to DAS as a result of our efforts. This change resulted in mutual respect between hospital social work and DAS staffs and decreased the number of crisis responses by DAS. Hospital social work supervisory staff now had access to DAS administration when problems occurred. DAS had a "face," as did we in the hospitals, and for some time the level of frustration on all parts diminished.

When multidrug resistant TB became an issue, the contagion of fear again spread as it had in the early days of AIDS work. This time, however, the DAS staff was frightened that they would die from the spread of and contact with someone who had this form of TB. Patients were being hospitalized in isolation for long periods of time. For many patients, particularly those engaged in substance-using behaviors, this became intolerable; at some point the drug cravings kicked in. Many patients would "elope," leave against medical advice. Those already known to DAS returned there for new housing, yet DAS had no idea of their diagnosis. Once the task force noted this pattern, members agreed to call DAS immediately to alert the staff so that the patient could be returned to the hospital. This action solidified the working relationship between the two groups.

Two sentinel events occurred, however, that initiated major systemic change within the DAS system. The first occurred in 1994 when the mayor attempted to revamp, if not obliterate, the entire DAS system. By this time the nature of the epidemic and needed services had resulted in a proliferation of community agencies, many of whom may have felt that DAS was nonresponsive to clients but recognized its importance all the same. The mayor created a citywide task force comprised of representatives from various community agencies who were selected from an already existing coalition; DAS administration was also represented. Clearly missing from the table were the hospitals; we were not seen as a politically active force to be reckoned with. However, we were finally recognized, because of our close alliance with DAS, and I, in my capacity as chair, was asked to represent our task force. Who better than the hospitals could describe the process of obtaining home care for patients? Who better than the hospitals could describe the interminable wait that existed because of the current system and how it negatively impacted the length of a patient's hospitalization? Who better than the hospitals could describe the impact this wait had on dying patients and their families or those struggling to hold onto their fragile health? The DAS system was ultimately saved because of the shared cooperative efforts of agencies, hospitals, and consumers, with many changes emanating from that politically convened group, including the streamlining of the home care referral process.

The task force was also instrumental in changing the referral form that gained entry into the DAS system. Since its inception, DAS had utilized a four-page form, the M11q, as medical verification of a patient's HIV/AIDS diagnosis. The form had originally been created and continues to be used for the evaluation of home care services for all applicants. Since the M11q included medical information, DAS, from its inception, used it rather than creating a new form. The form requires a physician's signature and a psychosocial evaluation of the patient's needs. Over the years the form took on a life of its own and also became the access to community agencies, confirmation of diagnosis, and referral to most social service agencies. Supply and demand for the M11q quickly overtook social work's capacity to facilitate timely completion of the form. We therefore advocated for a shorter, more standardized referral form.

Our discussions with DAS administrators, who agreed, were taken to their superiors. In the interim, task force members created a simple letter of diagnosis that we used in referring our patients to other agencies. These discussions about a more user-friendly form persisted for five years and with changing DAS administrators. Finally, in July 1999, a new referral form was generated. The persistence of a small group of social workers had again impacted a citywide system.

The task force was disbanded in 1998 due to the downsizing and dismantling of many social workers within AIDS hospital programs. However, the co-editors of this book continued an informal relationship with DAS administration and in 2000 were asked to reconvene the committee. Although we continue to meet, the interrelationship with DAS is to disseminate information rather than to problem solve systems. The system is now too vast a bureaucracy. However, having access to DAS administrators and site directors still facilitates patient problem solving on a macro level.

Using our impact on the citywide system as a model, in 2000 the task force decided to try this on a state level with the AIDS Institute Case Management section. The AIDS Institute is a state organization that has promulgated standards of care to HIV/AIDS providers in hospitals and community-based organizations. The latter, community-based organizations (CBOs), require medical updates on their patients after ninety days and then every six months. Their forms vary from agency to agency and are quite lengthy. Hospital social workers and case managers are responsible for coordinating the completion of this information. Every member of the task force complained of pushing papers and diminished patient contact as a result of the multitudinous requests. In addition, while we were sharing information with the CBOs we often were unaware of what the nature of their contact was with our mutual patients. We questioned why medical updates were needed every ninety days—CD4s and viral loads rarely changed that rapidly since many patients/clients during that period are responding to the medications. Again, our timing was right; the AIDS Institute had been considering this. Therefore, our approach to them was well received and after a series of meetings an agreed-upon form was designed by the task force and the AIDS Institute. In addition, the hospitals were able to introduce a new form that requested information from the CBOs. Now a collaborative relationship could exist between hospitals and CBOs—one in which information could be shared and discussed rather than the focus being only on the collection of information. Our work has not ended. The hospital staffs still find themselves educating the CBO case managers as to the existence of this form. The task force has made several requests to the AIDS Institute that a confirmatory letter be sent. Change always is and continues to be a slow process.

In the more than twelve years in which I have worked with patients with HIV/AIDS, medical care has expanded its frontiers of knowledge and more and more medications are and will be available. Similarly, systems have expanded, changed, and grown. Who would have thought that a relatively small group of dedicated social workers could and would impact both city and state systems? Not I, but we did.

SECTION III:
THE HEYDAY

Chapter 11

From Medical Social Work to the Constant Object: The Long and Winding Road

Diane Pincus Strom

I am a child of the 1960s. Growing up in postwar blue-collar prosperity, I am a "Bronx girl," raised in the midst of what is now called cultural diversity, but was then known as a "mixed neighborhood." I had the opportunity to observe differences in family dynamics, nuances of religious practices, and variations in role expectations and values. I began to understand how our cultural origins influence the way we define ourselves, and how, regardless of viewpoint, we all struggle for the same things: a decent lifestyle, a healthy environment, and the warmth, love, and acceptance of those close to us. Living in a mildly observant Jewish household, formal religion was a small part of my day-to-day existence. Nevertheless, we were taught about the importance of doing the right thing, the parameters of which were spelled out for us in those temple services we did attend:

> We will raise up those who fall, heal those who are sick, free those who are in need. . . . we will support the poor, feed the hungry, house the homeless, befriend the lonely, and give hope to all people. (Service Prayer)

Thus, my social work education began early.

Like so many of my peers, I attended City College of New York (CCNY), at the time a tuition-free institution, and in the mid-1960s comprised of a student body more than a little left of center. It was here that I learned about activism and advocacy. We were antiwar and pro-choice; we sat in, loved in, and burned our bras and draft cards. As a sociology major, I studied disenfranchised populations, poverty (and the war against it), inequality, and the importance of empowerment and self-esteem. In one of those life-altering experiences that takes less than a minute, my fate as a social worker was sealed following a conversation with a nine-year-old Puerto Rican girl. The child attended the Saturday morning CCNY community center run for the neighborhood kids, where I volunteered. "I love coming to this place," she told me. "I'd really like to go to college here when I'm older. Do you think I could?" "Of course," was my eager, supportive reply. "Good," she said. "Where do I have to go to become Jewish?" I was stunned by her statement and learned suddenly what she, in her young life, had already known for a while: access isn't equal; whole groups of people are excluded based on who they are or what they believe; and many need help leveling this inequitable playing field. I knew then, too, that the insight I gained from this child would form the basis of much of my life's work.

I learned something else at CCNY. I learned about rituals of mourning. Having gone through the assassination of President Kennedy when I was still in high school, my college years saw the losses of Malcolm X, Martin Luther King Jr., Robert Kennedy, and Medgar Evers. It was a time for memorial services and candlelight vigils, for anger and sadness. Who could have predicted these were feelings that would later become all too familiar?

By the early 1980s, I had completed my MSW and was working on a hemodialysis unit in an inner-city hospital. The patients, mostly African American and Latino, all carried a diagnosis of end-stage renal disease (ESRD), essentially kidney failure, the cause of which ranged from primary kidney disease to diabetes, hypertension, trauma, and substance abuse. The treatment sessions on an artificial kidney machine three times a week, four hours per session, were intrusive at best, traumatic at worst. As the social worker, I targeted my interventions carefully and, whenever possible, in order of importance. Assuring that the patient could receive all necessary treatments and medications was of uppermost concern (e.g., home care, access to pharmacy, equipment, wound care), followed by concrete and social needs (e.g., insurance coverage, income benefits, immigration status, housing, transportation, meals on wheels), and psychosocial support (e.g., counseling, treatment of depression, family therapy). Hemodialysis was the first and only (to this day) disease entity to confer automatic Medicare coverage to eligible patients (in response to a dramatic, emotion-packed demonstration of dialysis on the floor of the House Ways and Means Committee in the late 1960s). By 1972, a handful of resources was available to Medicare patients with ESRD, but available only in limited amounts to the Medicaid population (O'Brien, 1983). It was the social worker's job to manage each situation to ensure that the patient's needs were met by utilizing existing resources. Creative thinking and system negotiation were often the keys to successful intervention, and we were pretty good at it. We believed we were practicing social work at its best. We didn't know it then, but we were also doing case management. As hard as the work was, it started to get harder.

Herbert G., thirty-eight, was an African-American man who worked as an administrative assistant. He had been a dialysis patient for about a year when he developed *Pneumocystis carinii* pneumonia (PCP). Despite the intensive efforts of his caretakers, he deteriorated rapidly, developing infection after infection. Mr. G. wasted away before our eyes. As the social worker, I arranged home care at each discharge, made sure he had all of his benefits, arranged for his transportation and medical equipment, spoke with him about his anxiety and fear, and offered support to his family and friends. But no one could stop the course of the illness; no one even understood what the illness was. His death was ultimately not a surprise to us, but we couldn't figure out how we'd gotten there.

Chevon M., a twenty-eight-year-old African-American woman with a long history of intravenous drug use, prostitution, and incarceration, was struggling to establish a "normal life" after she was released from prison. Shortly thereafter, she was diagnosed with ESRD and began dialysis. Shortly after that, she began to waste away, at a rate unattributable to her kidney disease. Her hopelessness, anger, and considerable need for care required intensive intervention, including emotional support, monetary benefits, home care, and, later, assistance to her teenage daughter for grief and bereavement. Similar to the case of Herbert G., we didn't know what had happened to cause her death.

We look back at these and many other cases and understand only in retrospect that we were dealing with AIDS. At the time we didn't have a clue. By the mid-1980s, as we understood more about HIV, we realized this was a whole different ball game.

Early social work with patients who were HIV infected had two distinct though related components. On one hand, there was enormous work to be done in the realm of emotional support related to anxiety and depression around diagnosis and fear of pain, death, and dying. Many of us, myself included, felt competent in that arena since our prior work with patients with ESRD, cancer, and heart disease had dealt with similar issues. On the other hand, there was considerable need for concrete services, such as housing, food stamps, and transportation. This, too, was familiar territory. It is the difference between these components that has led to controversy over what falls under the heading of case management and what falls under the rubric of social work and whether they are, in fact, one and the same. This has been (and continues to be) a most difficult question to resolve. What was clear, even in the1980s, however, was that caring for HIV-infected patients moved us to another place, introducing subtleties and complexities that made both social work and case management intervention more difficult.

First, HIV infection is often a result of high-risk behaviors. Despite the early designation of the "four H risk groups" (i.e., heroin users, homosexuals, hemophiliacs, and Haitians), we knew even then that HIV infection was not a result of which group one is in, but rather what risky behaviors one practices. What that meant (and still means) was that as soon as a patient's HIV diagnosis was revealed, so was the fact that the patient had somehow engaged in a risky activity. The first question on everyone's lips was always "What did they do to get this?" The question implied that the patient should somehow assume blame for having chosen to become ill and set up a "them versus us" relationship with the infected individual. Patients felt doubly exposed, first for the revelation of their illness and second for the exposure of their lifestyles. Shame and secrecy, then, became key components of our work. I'm reminded of Marshall, a client whose mother could care for him only by telling the neighbors he was dying of cancer, for fear of losing her home if her neighbors found out about the AIDS diagnosis and for fear of losing support should the rest of the family or friends find out her son was gay.

Second, HIV can be transmitted to others, and in the mid-1980s it was not widely known how that transmission took place. There was considerable reluctance on the part of families, health care workers, and community agencies to involve themselves with AIDS patients, in large measure due to fear of contagion. One patient, Matt, kept cleanser in his hospital room so that when staff and family visited he could scrub the chairs and allow everyone (including himself) to feel more comfortable using anything he might have touched. Often Matt would sob and tell me he deserved what he got for being a drug user, but he would never allow anyone else to suffer again because of him. This fear of contagion was a major influence on how care was rendered. Dietary workers, as yet uneducated about HIV transmission, refused to bring trays into patients' rooms. Elevator operators wouldn't allow patients into their elevators. One city employee, who had come to interview a client on the inpatient service, opened his briefcase to reveal a fully functioning gas mask that he intended to wear to protect himself during the session. When we wouldn't allow it, he left, and we did the intake ourselves in his place.

Third, in a related vein, was the issue of stigma and confidentiality. Patients feared, with good reason, that if their conditions were known in the community they would suffer ostracism or worse. For example, Clayton D. went home postdischarge and didn't return for his follow-up appointment. His brother went to his house, knocked on the door, and said, "Clay, you missed your appointment at the AIDS clinic." By the next day, Clayton and his family had been evicted. In other parts of the country, children with AIDS were being excluded from attending school, and some legislators were advocating tattooing and quarantining as a public health response. We began to speak in codes and whispers—not the best way to help a client feel empowered and accepted.

Fourth, this is overwhelmingly a disease of young people. None of us was used to a caseload of fifty patients all under the age of forty and all expected to die within the next year or so. The nature of transmission being what it is, it was not unusual to see entire families wiped out because they had shared needles (in one instance, five brothers infected one another, leaving their mother and three sisters to care for them), or a husband who had infected his wife and their children (in one case the parents and four of five children were infected and died, leaving an eleven-year-old boy on his own).

Fifth, anyone was vulnerable. As we all frantically checked our own histories, we lost four social workers, the mother of one social work assistant, two doctors, and countless others whose cause of death or disappearance was never revealed.

AIDS was relentless; there were no resources for dealing with it; and the cases were mounting up. It was a time for hoping that people knew how to reach out and do the right thing. Not everyone rose to the occasion. (One young physician once asked me why I was so concerned about "these people." "AIDS is not the problem," he said. "It's the solution." In that one comment our relationship was forever ruptured. He left about a year later, and I welcomed his departure.) Fortunately, many did rise to the task and still do.

In 1985 I was asked to participate in the submission of an application for the hospital to become a New York State Designated AIDS Center (DAC). New York State, which has been a model in responding to HIV since the early days of the epidemic, had created the AIDS Institute as the Department of Health agency to address AIDS-related issues.

The AIDS Institute recognized that caring for patients with AIDS called for interventions that were labor intensive and time consuming. Hospitals, for their part, were already stretching their resources as far as they could and were not eager to place additional burdens on themselves by providing special programming for patients with AIDS. The AIDS Institute realized that if hospitals were going to adequately provide AIDS care, they would need additional resources, specifically an enhanced payment rate to cover the increased expenses. This recommendation was very attractive to some hospitals, since it offered the opportunity to cover the costs they were already incurring anyway. The more AIDS patients they were treating, the more appealing was the proposal, and we were seeing more than any other facility in the borough.

The standards for becoming a DAC were complicated. Physical plant requirements were described in detail, staffing ratios recommended, and minimum team membership standards prescribed. A payment rate was negotiated on a per diem basis. This became a critical concept. It meant that for each day the patient was hospitalized, the hospital was paid the negotiated rate. This was different from all other diagnoses, which were paid on the DRG system (diagnosis-related groups—a flat fee for a particular diagnostic cluster of conditions, regardless of how long the patient stays in the hospital). The best news for us was that the case manager drove the whole system.

The AIDS Institute understood that medical care was only a piece of what the AIDS patient needed. To assure that all areas of care were addressed, the institute mandated that each patient receive case management and tied these services to the receipt of payment. The subtlety here was that hospitals which agreed to become a DAC had to direct a portion of revenue to the hiring of case managers or they would not be eligible for the enhanced rate. Since most hospitals assigned the role of case manager to the social worker, provision of social work services, for the first time, had a direct fiscal implication. Overall, this was an enormously empowering experience for hospital social workers. On another level, however, there were ripple effects within the departments and the unintended creation of a two-tier system of social work care. Those social workers working with populations other than HIV still struggled with the large ratios they had always had, and they resented the "favored child" status of those doing AIDS work. Those in the AIDS program were buoyed by the recognition they received and were not always appreciative of the work of their colleagues. It was a tense time. More recently, however, decreased length of stay and reimbursement rates led most institutions to opt out of the per diem system in favor of DRGs. Not surprisingly, AIDS case management no longer enjoyed the status it previously held and, little by little, the ratios grew. In fact, in many institutions, patients with HIV are now seen as a regular part of all social workers' caseloads. Arguments can be made for which is better—specialty care by social workers with particular HIV expertise or general care by social workers with a range of skills, of which HIV is one of many. Either way, it is important to note that this decision is fiscally driven rather than the result of professional analysis and recommendation.

Although the AIDS Institute's recognition of the importance of case management was exciting, it also raised many questions. The term *case management* was confusing and meant different things to different people. We were providing medical social work services as we always had, including discharge planning, linkage for benefits and services, counseling to patients, family, and significant others, and following through with ongoing services postdischarge in the ambulatory setting, all while taking into account the added dimensions of HIV. In many ways it was business as usual in terms of day-to-day activities: we met with patients, collaborated with team members, contacted agencies, and documented our work. How was this different? Were we doing it correctly? Was this the coordination we were supposed to do?

An understanding of case management and its history may be useful here. The concept of coordinating services was first evident in the United States in 1863, when Massachusetts established the first board of charities. The term *case management* itself was first used in the 1960s in relation to coordination of health and human services. The definition of case management has generally been "the coordination of complex, fragmented services to meet the needs of the client while controlling the costs of services" (Kersbergen, 1996, p. 169) or a similar construct that attempts to balance the needs of the patient with the cost of care (Katz, 1991; Rodriguez and Montvale, 1986; Brennan and Kaplan, 1993; Fleishman, Mor, and Piette, 1991; Sowell, 1995; Moore-Greene, 2000; Chernesky and Grube, 2000; Twyman and Libbus, 1994; Piette et al., 1990, 1992; Cobere et al., 1992; Buie, 1991). During the 1970s case management was most often associated with chronically mentally ill patients as an effort to reduce readmission to psychiatric facilities and to enhance quality of life (Rohde, 1997; Cruise and Kuo-Tsai, 1993). Though the success of these programs was inconsistent, the overall impression was that the model was useful and potentially of value to patients with HIV (Cruise and Kuo-Tsai, 1993).

In 1992 the AIDS Institute defined case management for us and set the standards for the provision of case management. The definition was further refined years later as follows:

> Case management is a multi-step process focusing on coordination and expedient access to a range of appropriate medical, psychological and social services for the client and family. The goal is to promote the independent functioning of the individual to the fullest degree possible. The case management process consists of assessing specific medical, psychological and social needs and strengths; developing an individualized service plan; obtaining the services specified in the plan, monitoring the patient's status; and making necessary adjustments in the plan as the patient's service needs and resources change over time. (New York State Department of Health AIDS Institute, 2001, p. 1)

It is noteworthy that, although it may be implied, the AIDS Institute does not spell out the relationship of case management to containment of cost, preferring to take the role of patient advocate, much to the appreciation of social workers and clients.

The introduction of the case management standards was doubled edged. On one hand, we now had guidelines regarding how to implement case management, and these were enormously helpful. On the other hand, we were now going to be reviewed and measured on these standards, so our efforts had to become both more formal and more rigorous, especially in terms of documentation. The guidelines defined the elements of case management (including minimal activities and time frames for implementation) and left it to us, the DACs, to develop the mechanisms to put these elements into practice. The elements were logical and sprang from sound social work theory, calling for intake/assessment, development of an initial service plan, implementation and monitoring of that plan, reassessment and update of the plan, crisis intervention, and, finally, case disposition or closure (New York State Department of Health AIDS Institute, 2001). We developed forms for intake and criteria for determining eligibility, implemented checklists to assist in the initial assessment process (and later in reassessment), and mandated weekly "sit-down" interdisciplinary team rounds where all cases were discussed and treatment plans completed. We formulated an initial service plan and updated it regularly as the patient's situation shifted or several months had passed since our last look. Finally, from time to time we closed cases that no longer required case management, either because all service needs were being met, services were no longer required, the patient had died, or the patient was lost to follow-up.

Meanwhile, another controversy began to brew. We were all aware that although case management and its implementation were mandated, it was not clear who the case manager was supposed to be. There were no standards that required the task be performed by a social worker. Discussions on who should be the providers of AIDS case management were passionate. Models of care differed from location to location and demonstrated great variability in terms of who was identified as the case manager, including physicians, nurses, social workers, and nonprofessional staff (Buie, 1991; Piette et al., 1990, 1992; Brennan and Kaplan, 1993; Coleman, Brown, and Gestoso, 1996; Moore-Greene, 2000; Flynn et al., 2000). There is no doubt, nor was there ever, that social work training uniquely equips social workers to negotiate the arenas required by case management. What is less clear, and what we as social workers struggle with still, is that case management is a coordinating function and as such has to assure that all necessary services are received. The case manager *does not,* and, in fact, *should not,* personally supply those services. This means, for example, that if a patient requires ongoing psychodynamic counseling, the case manager refers that patient to an agency that provides counseling services and follows up to confirm that services were received. The case manager does not become the provider of that counseling. It is easy to see how this can be conflictual, because who better to do counseling than a social worker? In fact, although social workers do long-term, psycho-dynamic counseling, case managers, even though they may be social workers, should not. This is no small issue, and it continues to go unresolved.

Despite these ambiguities, case management was clearly the intervention of choice. Cases were complex and numerous, with referrals coming in at a rate that was virtually unmanageable. Plus, the work was emotional. Supervision of staff sometimes focused as much on dealing with our own emotions as with the dynamics of any given case. Staff support groups were a necessity, as were opportunities for crying, grieving, or simply stomping about in anger and helplessness. As the cases kept coming, the variation of need remained remarkable.

Walter P., a twenty-one-year-old Puerto Rican man, was hospitalized for complications related to *Pneumocystis carinii* pneumonia. Recently diagnosed with AIDS, Walter had been released from a short prison stay just two weeks before. Sullen and at times hostile, Walter finally revealed that he believed his source of infection was his brother, Ricky, with whom he had shared needles and who had died due to AIDS-related complications a year earlier. Walter had watched Ricky deteriorate while being cared for by their mother. He was terrified of the same thing happening to him and, worse, he couldn't bear to tell his mother about his own diagnosis because he felt she would fall apart. To make matters worse, he couldn't even stay with his mother, as he had burglarized the apartments of several of her neighbors and he was afraid they would assault him if they saw him. He was too sick to work, had no place to live, was without insurance, was markedly depressed, and, as we later learned, had a warrant out for his arrest for a robbery he had committed prior to his recent incarceration. He also was in severe discomfort due to drug withdrawal, and he urgently required drug treatment.

Melinda V., twenty-seven, a former IV drug user, appeared at the clinic with her four daughters, ages three through seven. Pale and wasted, she asked for help in finding a family to adopt the girls and keep them together. Although her own mother was willing to help, Melinda felt her mother's dysfunction had played a significant part in her own drug use, and she didn't want her children raised in that household.

Joey R., twenty-two, was hospitalized for PCP and CMV (cytomegalovirus). He was wasted and barely able to hold a conversation. He had left Puerto Rico five years earlier and lost touch with his mother, who had tried to stop him from going. He missed her and wanted only to see her before he died. He had no one else to care for him, was unsure where she was living now, and was overwhelmed with sadness over how disappointed she would be.

These situations were not only complex, they were painful. Housing problems were almost impossible to resolve; there were no residences or apartments for people with AIDS. Other clients, such as Clayton, were actually being thrown out of their homes. Even when families or friends responded, it was frequently inadequate.

José F., thirty-nine, had been an intravenous drug user for more than fifteen years. His family had long since given up on him, refusing to permit him into their homes. His situation had deteriorated to the point that he was homeless and without any benefits. When he became ill, his aunt agreed to give him dinner every night and to do his laundry. He ate with her and her family and then was given a clean blanket and pillowcase, which he used in the alley where he slept. He felt grateful that his aunt was willing to help him at all.

Even as concrete requirements became overwhelming, they were easier to deal with than the intense emotional and psychological needs. Some cases were especially intense.

Betty, forty-eight and living in Newark, had previously been married for twenty-three years. At the age of forty-four she was widowed. She dated briefly and, at forty-seven, remarried. In the interim she had been involved with two men. A successful office manager, Betty participated in her company's blood drive. She was shocked to learn, as a result of their blood screening, that she was HIV positive. Within ten days she was fired and her new husband (who was uninfected) asked for a separation. Having lost her job and home, she came to the Bronx to live with her mother, who lost no opportunity to blame Betty for her situation. In addition to her many concrete needs, Betty also wished to find a home where her daughter, Dara, twenty-two, could live with her. Dara had been using drugs and was getting mixed up with the "wrong crowd" in Newark. Dara learned she herself was HIV positive and became increasingly depressed. Betty took on the care of Dara's three-year-old daughter. We applied for housing for this family (a virtually impossible task at the time). After months of phone calls and follow-up letters in an effort to get some response, we learned that Dara had been attacked and killed by a group of drug dealers.

As we tried to negotiate these many needs and systems, we began to notice a pattern in the types of problems in which we had to intervene and the range of solutions we had at hand. First were those situations arising from the patient himself or herself and calling for a direct educational, counseling, or treatment response. Examples include depression, lack of understanding about transmission, and shifts in medical condition. Second were those circumstances involving the provision of ongoing medical care, negotiating the medical system, and requiring interdisciplinary collaboration to assure optimum access to treatment. Examples include setting appointments, obtaining test results, and helping staff to feel comfortable caring for the patient. Third were problems concerning the patient's immediate and extended world and necessitating a response from a community-based organization, a family member, a benefit provider, or others. Examples are obtaining entitlements (such as SSI), locating housing, receiving transportation assistance, or permanency planning for children coping with their parents' HIV. Last were issues involving the overall community that might not directly impact an individual patient but had implications for our patients as a group. Examples include providing education to community centers and churches, arranging delivery services from local pharmacies, and working with community-based agencies to gain their commitment to making home visits to those patients too sick to leave the house.

We got better at case management, developing an understanding of the mandated elements and refining our practices so that coordination of care was achieved to whatever level was possible at the time (Epstein, 1988; Strom, 1989). Our expertise in assessment, developing and implementing a care plan, collaborating with team members, and long-term follow-up grew. We learned that not only did we have to work with our patients to identify their needs and provide the necessary care and services (of which few were available), but we also had to work to develop services where they did not exist, advocate in those arenas that were reluctant to develop or provide care, and educate those who were openly hostile to the idea of serving patients with AIDS.

A brief phone call subsequently taught me the wisdom of never saying no to an opportunity for collaboration. The Bronx, particularly hard hit by the epidemic in the late 1980s and early 1990s, provided the perfect medium for interagency partnerships. A newly formed community-based organization (CBO) had been recently funded to provide nonmedical services to patients with AIDS. The director of case management chanced to call me, looking for an affiliation with a DAC, so that clients at his agency who were not yet in care could be referred. I said yes. From that phone call and the subsequent meetings developed the Bronx AIDS Services and Education Society (BASES). This group, comprised of representatives of four hospitals, several CBOs, clinic programs, Visiting Nurse Services, New York City Department of Health, and, later, New York State Department of Health AIDS Institute, became leaders in advocacy for services for patients infected with HIV. From BASES sprung many of the currently existing HIV networks and work groups. Equally important, this group was key in identifying client needs and developing programs that provide housing, home care, legal services, social support, and nutritional services. Alliances and friendships that formed there, more than fifteen years ago, exist to this day. Most of us are still working in AIDS programs.

One important innovation was the introduction of the concept of the case management technician. The creation of this role opened the door for the inclusion of peers and other community members in many aspects of case management. Not only was this enormously helpful to clients, who frequently could relate culturally and linguistically to these peer workers better than to their social worker/case manager, but also benefited the peers themselves who were able to enter the workforce and begin a continuum of training that could potentially take them from peer to professional (Strom, Wayne, and Chambers, 2001). These workers continue to be a critical component of case management, outreach, and educational and support activities, in large measure because of their willingness to perform those functions (i.e., escort, home visits) that master's-prepared social workers are sometimes reluctant to do. In fact, case management models that utilize the MSW as a team leader and supervisor, while the bulk of the patient-related work is performed by bachelor's-prepared and peer workers, are exceptionally successful, appropriately tapping into each worker's level of expertise and experience.

Over the years, controversies have continued around issues of who should do case management, where case management should originate (i.e., hospital-based versus community-based organizations), the optimal utilization of time in the provision of case management, staffing ratios, and more (Piette et al., 1990; Abramowitz, Obten, and Cohen, 1998). Simultaneously, case management in HIV has evolved as the illness itself has changed from an acute, terminal disease to a chronic condition. The wider accessibility of programs, benefits, and services, together with availability of new, clinically promising therapies (e.g., protease inhibitors), has shifted the focus of many interventions from the inpatient service to the ambulatory clinic or community-based organization (Merithew and Davis-Satterla, 2000).

In 2001, the New York State Department of Health AIDS Institute reformulated their case management definition and standards for the provision of case management in response, at least in part, to some of these controversies and changes:

> Case management is a multi-step process which ensures coordination of medical and specialty care and access to a range of appropriate medical, psychosocial and social services for the client and family and which promotes and supports the independent functioning of the client and family. Case management can be accomplished through a designated case manager or a team approach within the Comprehensive Ambulatory HIV Program (CAHP) agency, or, with the client's concurrence, by a case manager in another community based setting. (New York State Department of Health AIDS Institute, 2001, Appendix 3, p. 1)

In 2001 the AIDS Institute also promulgated a new paradigm for HIV care that examines critical issues in caring for people infected with HIV (Noring et al., 2001). Still a leader in patient advocacy, the AIDS Institute identifies eight principles of HIV care:

- Knowledge of HIV status
- Access to health care services
- Access to HIV treatment information
- Patient-provider collaboration
- Special populations
- HIV treatment support services
- Access to HIV treatment
- Responsibility to individual and public health (p. 691)

This refocus, which incorporates both ethical and clinical considerations, reflects the many changes we have seen in HIV care since the early days of the epidemic. No longer is there a total absence of benefits and services, at least not in most urban areas. The general public knows more about HIV and although there is still enormous stigma attached to an AIDS diagnosis, there is greater awareness of information about transmission and treatment. An entire generation has grown up with AIDS as a part of its world. It is not the "unknown" it once was. Nevertheless, the case manager remains a key component in the treatment of people infected with HIV. The refocus on treatment adherence, maintenance of the patient in care, access to state-of-the-art treatments and family-centered programming, and the recognition of the mental health and substance abuse needs in HIV care may differ from those times when we were unsure of what we were dealing with, when for some the proposed solution was a tattoo and imprisonment. On the macro level, things have improved greatly. On the micro level, however, for each individual patient, there is the same configuration of medical, emotional, and social need, the same fear and anxiety, the same requirement for support and care. Thanks to twenty years of experience, we are better equipped to do the job.

REFERENCES

Abramowitz, S., Obten, N., and Cohen, H. (1998). Measuring HIV/AIDS case management. *Social Work in Health Care* 27: 1-28.

Brennan, J.P. and Kaplan, C. (1993). Setting new standards for social work case management. *Hospital and Community Psychiatry* 44: 219-222.

Buie, L. (1991). Making sense of medical case management: Perspective from a case manager. *Journal of Insurance Medicine* 23: 256-257.

Chernesky, R.H. and Grube, B. (2000). Examining the HIV/AIDS case management process. *Health and Social Work* 25: 243-253.

Cobere, P.C., McGovern, P., Kochevar, L., and Widtfeldt, A. (1992). Measuring satisfaction with medical case management—A quality improvement tool. *Journal of the American Association of Occupational Health Nurses* 40: 333-341.

Coleman, K., Brown, L., and Gestoso, L.P. (1996). Hospital-based social work HIV case management: Reducing continuity of care barriers. *Continuum* 16: 16-22.

Cruise, P.L. and Kuo-Tsai, L. (1993). AIDS case management: A study of an innovative health services program in Palm Beach County, Florida. *Journal of Health and Human Resources Administration* 16: 96-110.

Epstein, D. (1988). Managing counter-transference: A guide for health care professionals. Poster presentation: Fourth International AIDS Conference. Stockholm, Sweden.

Fleishman, J., Mor, V., and Piette, J. (1991). AIDS case management: The client's perspective. *Health Services Research* 26: 447-470.

Flynn, M.B., McKeever, J.L., Spada, T., and Gordon-Garofalo, V. (2000). Active client participation: An examination of self-empowerment in HIV/AIDS case management with women. *Journal of the Association of Nurses in AIDS Care* 11: 59-68.

Katz, F.G. (1991). Making a case for case management. *Business and Health* 9: 75-77.

Kersbergen, A.L. (1996). Case management: A rich history of coordinating care to control costs. *Nursing Outlook* 44: 169-172.

Merithew, M. and Davis-Satterla, L. (2000). Protease inhibitors: Changing the way AIDS case management does business. *Qualitative Health Research* 10: 632-645.

Moore-Greene, G. (2000). Standardizing social indicators to enhance medical case management. *Social Work in Health Care* 30(3): 39-53.

New York State Department of Health AIDS Institute (2001). *HIV Guidelines.* Appendix 3: Case management guidelines. New York: New York State Department of Health.

Noring, S., Dubler, N.N., Birkhead, G., and Agins, B. (2001). A new paradigm for HIV care: Ethical and clinical considerations. *American Journal of Public Health* 91: 690-694.

O'Brien, M.E. (1983). *The courage to survive: The life career of the chronic dialysis patient.* New York: Grune and Stratton.

Piette, J., Fleishman, J., Mor, V., and Dill, A. (1990). A comparison of hospital and community case management programs for persons with AIDS. *Medical Care* 28: 746-755.

Piette, J., Fleishman, J., Mor, V., and Thompson, B. (1992). The structure and process of AIDS case management. *Health and Social Work* 17: 47-56.

Rodriguez, A.R. and Montvale, N.J. (1986). Psychiatric case management offers cost, quality control. *Business and Health* 3: 14-17.

Rohde, D. (1997). Evolution of community mental health case management: Considerations for clinical practice. *Archives of Psychiatric Nursing* 11: 332-339.

Sowell, R.L. (1995). Community-based HIV case management: Challenges and opportunities. *Journal of the Association of Nurses in AIDS Care* 6: 33-40.

Strom, D. (1989). Developing comprehensive services for HIV infected intravenous drug users: A guide for case managers. Poster presentation: Fifth International AIDS Conference. Montreal, Canada.

Strom, D., Wayne, S., and Chambers, D. (2001). Professionalizing a peer-based workforce: The intersection of social casework, patient care and community development. Presentation: HIV and Diversity. V: Changes in the HIV/AIDS Epidemic: Social Work Responses, Wurzweiler School of Social Work, Yeshiva University. New York, NY.

Twyman, D.M. and Libbus, M.K. (1994). Case-management of AIDS clients as a predictor of total inpatient hospital days. *Public Health Nursing* 11: 406-411.

Chapter 12

You Cannot Make This Stuff Up

Alan Rice
Barbara Willinger

The editors thought this would be a good place for an interlude. What you have already read and what follows revolves around the seriousness of the work with patients, family, and significant others. Every agency has its own culture, as does every hospital, and the exigencies, which many of us have encountered and relate here, are often what "got us through the day." It's what has often been referred to as hospital "black humor."

When you work in a hospital setting, situations and events happen that require you to sometimes take a deep breath and appreciate them for their worth. At times the events can be very humorous, at times, they can be very humbling, but, at all times, you have the feeling that these events can take place only in a hospital. They also help us realize that in spite of the misery, unhappiness, and sorrow that working with AIDS can cause, there is always a lighter side to the work that should be remembered.

In the early days there was less concern about being politically correct, and the definition of harassment was still being developed. Today's workplace is indeed a different environment. Hospitals are no longer excluded from the laws that govern work etiquette. Workers can be immediately terminated for saying some of the things that were said in the early days of AIDS. We are not certain whether this is good or bad; however, we know it is a different work environment, and there seems to be more stress now than there was in the past. Today hospitals are organized more like big business, with the "bottom line"—profits—always in the forefront. However, as long as hospitals treat human beings and are staffed by human beings, they can never be mistaken for a factory making computer chips.

The following social workers provided the vignettes for this chapter: Jay Boda, Holly Dando, Charles Finlon, Alan Rice, Mary Tucker, and Barbara Willinger.

The following are stories shared by various social workers who have worked in hospitals. Some are short. Some are long. All should be appreciated for what they are: an interlude to help us through the day.

Discharge Planning Can Be Very Complicated

I was covering the ER when I was paged to see a patient that was recently discharged from the hospital back to his single room occupancy hotel (SRO). Lowell had returned, however, since he felt unable to care for himself. Although his self-assessment was accurate, he was asymptomatic, and the ER doctors did not want to readmit him. He was not the most cooperative patient during his hospitalization, and if there was a way to keep him out of the hospital, the doctors preferred that. I was asked to then arrange home care for him, so he could be sent back to his SRO.

I had recently established contact with a private home care agency and thought they might be able to assist me. Lowell had private insurance paid for by his father, despite their estrangement for years due to Lowell's drug addiction. I took a chance and called this home care agency. They listened to my story and, like good business people, viewed this as an opportunity to show me what they could do. This was in 1984, when many patients needed home care and had the insurance or the money for these services.

Marge and Barbara came to the ER. Marge was the nurse, Barbara the sales representative. Marge made the assessment and decided they could provide the service the patient needed, even in the SRO. In order to discharge the patient safely from the ER, Lowell initially needed twenty-four-hour care. Again, this was 1984, when safety came first, and length of stay and keeping patients out of the hospital was secondary. It was Barbara's job to negotiate with the insurance company and with Lowell's father. The insurance company would pay for only eight hours per day of home health aide coverage, so Barbara had to call the father to see if he would cover the balance. The patient had told us that his father was wealthy, so money did not seem to be the issue. Somehow, Barbara was able to get the father to agree, although Lowell and the father never spoke then and did not speak at all until the patient was near death. The father continued to pay for Lowell's insurance and home care services. Lowell was not admitted to the hospital that day and, because of the home care provided, he had very few hospitalizations until he died.

As a result of this incident, the staff gave me the nickname "miracle worker." My credibility as a social worker was established, but the ER staff expected that I would *always* be able to prevent readmission to the hospital for nonmedical reasons/social admissions (obviously not always possible). The other important thing that happened was the beginning of a relationship with Barbara that has existed to this day. In the early days, I was able to use her agency a great deal. As the population changed and more of the patients became Medicaid eligible, I had to use another New York City nursing agency for home care for AIDS patients. One thing that has never changed is how quickly Barbara responds when I call her, and we always talk about Lowell and the home care services arranged from the ER.

In 1986, a social worker could manipulate the system for the good of the patient, especially when it came to discharge planning. The following illustrates what I call a win-win situation. A patient known to me from previous admissions was admitted to the AIDS unit. He was very sick. John was a gay man whose family lived out of state. His support system consisted of other gay men who divided their time to take care of him at home. In addition, John had home care services from the New York City Medicaid Home Care Program. One of the reasons his doctor admitted him was to give a respite to his support system. He stabilized quickly, although he was clearly terminal. However, being "medically ready" to return home meant that I had to create a safe discharge plan. It was my job to refer John back to the New York City Home Care Program for continuation of his services, which was eight hours a day of home health care. The remainder of the services was to be provided by his support system. Although John was lucid some of the time, he could no longer make real decisions for himself. One of the friends came to talk to me days before John was supposed to be discharged. He told me that he was the spokesperson for the patient's support system and wanted me to know that they could no longer provide the type of home care service that they had provided for him in the past. It had become too difficult for most of them, some being sick themselves, others just burning out. I suggested increasing the home care. He said it seemed to all of them that John was dying—why couldn't he just remain in the hospital until then? I explained that although the patient might be dying, according to the doctor he was "medically ready for discharge." "Medically ready" is a misnomer. It means only that a patient no longer requires acute care. Without the support system continuing to provide some of the home care services, I would have to ask for an increase to round-the-clock home care service. I explained this to the spokesperson, who said he thought having the patient at home at all would be too difficult for the rest of them. I had no choice but to make the referral for the increase of home care services; however, I thought of a way to keep John in the hospital until he died. If the New York City Home Care Agency would reject the patient for home care services, my only option then was a referral to the only nursing home in New York City accepting AIDS patients. Needless to say, there was a very long waiting list for patients to be admitted to this facility. I had an established relationship with the director of the Home Care Agency, and I called him to come to the hospital to evaluate John for an increase in services. When he arrived, I met him on the unit. I guess I must have had "a look" on my face; poker was never my game. I explained the situation and asked him to reject the case as not being a safe discharge. He understood and said he would. He walked into the patient's room and said immediately, "Case rejected." I documented the situation and changed the plan to nursing home. I completed all the paperwork required and informed the friend. He asked me what would happen if a bed at this nursing facility became available. I told him that according to his doctor John didn't have much time left, and we should just wait and see what happens.

John died in the hospital several weeks after this, with all his friends around him. They were able to be there for him at the end because they could choose when to see him, not having to provide the intense level of home care services that they had previously done. The one friend whom I was dealing with told me it was a great thing I did for the patient and for them. I didn't think so; I thought it was my job to find the best discharge for each patient. This was a win-win situation. How did the hospital win? I worked for them, and the hospital's reputation as a humane place for AIDS patients increased tenfold.

Bravery at Its Best

A gay man was hospitalized with end-stage AIDS, a diagnosis not used much anymore. Among the many systems breakdowns that he incurred was blindness due to CMV retinitis. He was bedridden, having multiple seizures during the day. His lover of many years was by his side for most of the day and early evening. The lover was from Italy and had his own business that allowed him to be away from his job at length, although he was still able to make money. His care and dedication was something to behold, but this person had a secret that he insisted all of the medical unit staff promise to keep until his lover died. He was going to return to Italy after his lover died so that he could die himself. He also had AIDS and KS, but the patient was unaware of this because of his blindness. The patient's only concern was that the lover take a break after he died. The staff kept their promise.

Pay Attention

I walked into Mr. S's room needing to complete an assessment that I had started several days earlier. I knocked on the door and thought I heard "come in." When I entered the room the patient was somewhat in a sitting position, so I sat down and began to ask some questions from where I had left off. I must have been thinking of other things, because it took me several seconds before I realized that this patient was not answering. I then took a better look, and it appeared that he was not breathing. I went a little closer and then thought I had better get the nurse. I went to the nursing station and said, "I think you better check out Mr. S. I think he is dead." He was.

Does It Really Matter?

I received a call from Jewel (in the terminal stage of AIDS) who was clearly in a state of panic, crying hysterically. It took some time to calm her down enough to discover what was wrong. This was a woman who contracted HIV through sharing needles and was a longtime drug addict. Her son, now eight, lived with her parents, as she could not take care of him due to her drug addiction. When she discovered that she had AIDS, she went into detox treatment, cleaned up, and was able to remain drug free. She reconnected with her son, and they were both living with her parents. When she became calm enough she told me that she needed to go back into detox. I asked her what drugs she was using. All of them had been prescribed by her doctor, including Percoset. I asked her how many Percosets and how often. She told me she was taking exactly what the prescription advised. I was confused. I asked her what the problem was. She told me she had worked too hard to become and remain clean and now she "was using again." A lot of people, drug addicts included, are not aware of the difference between abuse and addiction. I explained to her that being addicted to the Percoset did not mean she was abusing it. In fact, it sounded like she was doing what she needed to allieviate her physical pain, which is why the doctor prescribed this drug to begin with. She remained adamant about needing a detox and not wanting to die a "drug addict." Her son was not going to remember her that way. I arranged for admission to the detox unit, where she was able to detox from the Percoset; however, in the hospital she became more ill and never left. She said to me that helping her detox was the best thing I ever did for her; she would now be able to die "drug free." She did.

Strange Connection

Judy had multiple admissions to the hospital but refused to give any information to me; all that was known about her was that she "looked" abused and was homeless. One day, as I was crossing the street, Judy stopped me and asked for money. In that split second I noticed a truck bearing down on us, and I pulled us out of harm's way. When Judy was next admitted she gave me her family's names and numbers. I was able after some time to locate them. The family was grateful to be reunited with her before she died;

they had been looking for her for years, even though they never understood her destructive behavior.

Staff Bloopers

One week after beginning as an inpatient worker I met Chip, a very isolated man with HIV who had various complaints, including unremitting stomachache. He was well known to the team from several previous admissions, usually for similar complaints. Since no medical explanation had been found previously, most staff referred to him as a "malingerer." Chip showed me his advanced directive/living will that clearly stated he wanted no heroic measures; no one had been named as a proxy. Within a brief time Chip developed lactic acidosis and needed transfer to the ICU. The problem was that the doctor intubated Chip, a life support measure against his expressed wishes in the advanced directive which had been clearly spelled out in the medical record. Despite my advocacy for his "rights," hospital staff ignored his wishes and involved the police to find his family—all to no avail; no one claimed his body when he died. It took me a long time to reconcile my feelings of anger at the staff for not "respecting" his wishes, as well as to understand and accept my own feelings of helplessness.

Tom, married with two children, was admitted to the ICU with altered mental status changes. The medical staff suspected HIV. The medical resident asked the patient's wife to "sign the consent form for HIV testing"; he was unaware that this is illegal in New York State—only the patient can give consent. When the result was positive I was called in since the staff did not know how to proceed. The staff were in a quandary, given their actions, but at the same time were concerned about the wife and her two children. Tom was still not mentally clear. This time I was able to resolve the dilemma for all, since according to the state law physicians can inform spouses that they may have been exposed (without identifying the source of exposure) to a transmissible disease, such as STDs or HIV. In fact, the staff became less circuitous and indicated that her husband had PML, a brain infection sometimes associated with HIV. This story had a happy ending in that the wife and children tested negative.

Advocacy Responsiveness

Randy was a gay male who had few friends. He lived in a hotel and kept medical appointments regularly. I had completed his advanced directive/

living will, in which he indicated he did not want to be resuscitated. A copy of this document was on his chart, and I had also verbally informed the team. During an admission for PCP Randy went into cardiac arrest during the night. I came in the next day, only to find him in the ICU on a ventilator. In this instance the ICU staff listened to Randy's wishes as I strongly advocated for the removal of life supports. Prior to the removal I contacted his friends and I and other team members who knew him came in and bade him farewell. The supports were removed Friday afternoon. When I returned to work Monday, Randy was sitting up in bed and able to talk to me. He had come back from the dead. Needless to say we were all shocked but happy for him. We also thought that this would make it almost impossible for Randy to do another directive. I was right. The next time he needed transfer to the ICU he lingered for a week—on the ventilator.

Jean was a single Haitian male journalist on his way home from Japan; he had stopped off in New York City and was hospitalized, only to be diagnosed with AIDS. I met him during this hospitalization. His shame and fear of being found out remained palpable throughout the next two years. I continued to see Jean every two weeks—I was his only contact in the city. He refused to speak with former friends. Concrete service provision occurred, but his isolation and loneliness were heartbreaking to me. He finally allowed me to refer him to a Haitian agency on the condition he be visited in his "hotel" room. During the time I saw him he shared his dreams and sadness, as well as information about his family history, past and present (and that he was sending $100 monthly to his siblings in Haiti; he received $500 each month for his needs). I assisted him with a will and arrangements for cremation. When Jean did not come to see me for a month and did not respond to telephone messages, I decided to pay a visit to his hotel (one of the seedier ones in the city). The manager told me Jean had been found dead in his room one month ago; his body had been taken to the medical examiner's office (MEO) for autopsy and to be claimed. I immediately went to the MEO, only to learn that several hours before, Jean had been buried in Potter's Field (the site for unclaimed bodies). I contacted a funeral home, showing them Jean's will and asked that they dig him up and cremate him as he wished. I eventually sent his ashes to Haiti—bringing closure to my relationship with a very gentle gentleman.

A Funny

Our computer system is known by an acronym—CLIMACS, which stands for clinical information management something or other. I was sitting with a patient who needed some information from another computer program in the network. I turned from him, toward the computer, muttering to myself, "Just let me get out of CLIMACS." He raised an eyebrow and responded dryly, "I hadn't been aware you were in climax." I must admit we both laughed as I clarified the difference.

What Year Is It?

I was at a dinner party and found myself seated next to a bright, sophisticated thirty-eight-year-old married New York woman. When she asked me what kind of work I do, I decided to be truthful. (Usually I couch my HIV involvement.) I was shocked and amazed when she asked me, "Can't you catch it?" At least she allowed me to educate her about HIV transmission. Did this occur in the 1980s? No, it was 2002.

GROUP INTERVENTIONS WITH HOSPITALIZED PATIENTS

Chapter 13

Rethinking Group Process—Or Do We?

Alan Rice

It was October 1985, and I had been working as the sole AIDS social worker at Beth Israel Medical Center (BIMC) in New York City since July 1983. I had realized early on that working with AIDS patients included not only assisting the patients but also providing for the needs of their support systems consisting of parents, spouses, lovers, friends, colleagues, and hospital employees. These support systems were beginning to tire.

Up to this point, my day-to-day work consisted of discharge planning (although not often, as many patients came to the hospital and died there), individual counseling, and some family counseling, if the patient allowed. There were so many secrets at that time and disclosure raised many issues including being diagnosed with AIDS, being gay, and being a drug user, to name a few. Many patients would not allow me or any other staff member to speak in depth with their particular support system, for fear of disclosing their secrets. The more contact I had with patients, the more interaction I had with the patient's family and significant others. As the only AIDS social worker, the hospitalized patients were always assigned and reassigned to me. This allowed me to establish ongoing relationships with the patients and their families and significant others. (Did the term *significant other* exist before AIDS?) The patient *and* his or her support system was my caseload, and I did not have enough time in my day to address everyone's needs. People kept asking me if I knew of any family support groups. I was unaware of any such groups, so I decided to start one for the families and significant others of the patients in the BIMC AIDS program.

"How difficult could this be?" I asked myself. Just arrange for a room, a time, send some flyers around to the different units in the hospital, and I will have a room full of families and significant others. Life should be so simple. In a hospital, the chance of finding an empty room for one hour, every week is almost an impossible task. It took me weeks to locate such a room. Time was another problem. I thought I would have the group at lunchtime, which was good for me. This would not be the case. This lesson of what is good for me is usually not good for others would return often during my work with AIDS. What was best for the potential group members was later in the day, preferably after 5 p.m., as many people worked. I compromised with a group time from four to five in the afternoon. It was not the best time for me as it took away my availability for any crisis that happens at the "witching hour" of the hospital day. These are the times in a hospital when events might happen such as a suicide attempt or another type of crisis, and they usually seem to happen during nursing shift changes or when other staff is ready to go home. For me, it was at five.

There were many other questions to be answered before that first group took place. Was there going to be a charge for this group? How did my supervisor feel about an inpatient social worker leading a group for family and significant others of patients not necessarily hospitalized? Was this group for BIMC patients' family members and significant others or was it for anyone who is affected by AIDS, regardless of whether that person was connected to a patient at BIMC? Would there be documentation, either in the patient's medical record or in a separate chart for group members? Would this group be opened or closed? Is a commitment needed by group members? Would it be time limited or ongoing? Would there be a cap on the number of group members? Is one family considered one group member? Should there be separate groups for parents, wives, lovers, etc.? So many questions, so few answers—this was becoming a theme of AIDS hospital social work in the early 1980s. I decided the best thing to do was to begin and to evaluate the process after a number of groups and weeks. The support group I organized was set up as an open-ended, ongoing, free support group for anyone close to an AIDS patient, regardless of where or if the patient was hospitalized. The group met for one hour every week and no commitment was required.

My thought before the first group was, "What are you getting yourself into?" This was similar to the thought I had when the AIDS social work job was offered to me. Although I had led groups before, I had the feeling that this group was going to be unfamiliar territory. I had already been involved in a controversial situation when I began to lead a group for gay men with AIDS at the hospital. Some in the AIDS community questioned if I should be leading such a group, as I was not gay. How they even knew of my sexual orientation is still a mystery to me. Others, specifically the gay men in the group, rushed to my defense, saying that all that mattered was that I was a skilled professional. All of this was captured in bold print in the second and third issues of the new New York City PWA Coalition Newsletter. I wondered if I would get a similar reaction from the AIDS community again, since I did not have a family member with AIDS. It seemed as if standard social work practice was being challenged at every turn.

The first group met on a Tuesday at the designated hour. This began a long-term relationship between me, as the designated group leader, and the core members of this group. The core group members consisted of the elderly parents of a gay man who lived in Key West; a mother whose IV drug using son was being treated at another hospital in New York City; a gay man, a BIMC employee, whose lover was treated at another hospital; the wife of a BIMC patient, whose husband was a hospital employee with a past history of substance abuse; and a friend/ex-lover of a gay man that was treated at another hospital in the city. Support groups aim at commonality. What common ground was there between these group members except that a loved one had AIDS? Would that be enough to sustain this support group, or would this seeming diversity cause this group to be counterproductive? Only time would tell.

After the initial meeting, at which group rules were established, I realized that this was going to be unlike any group I had ever led. There was very little need to follow traditional group process, as the group engaged from the very first meeting. The core group was in crisis and immediately connected to one another and to me as the leader since they finally had an arena to verbalize and vent their feelings. The problem of establishing group trust between the group leader and the group members themselves was a nonissue. This took care of my concern regarding the group's diversity being counterproductive to their interaction.

Being the only AIDS social worker at a large inner-city hospital that was now averaging between thirty-five and fifty AIDS patients a day plus covering the outpatient AIDS clinic, one would think I could have used that hour for other things. Perhaps this was true, except I found myself looking forward to Tuesday afternoons. As I look back on this experience, I think I felt this way because this group was a source of support for me as well, although in my mind and actions, I clearly was the professional leader. I know only that when the group ended and I left to go home, I felt a renewed energy and spirit that helped me through the rest of my week. Talk about countertransference, or rather let's not talk about countertransference.

Over the life of this group, there were numerous different group formations as members came and left. Some came for one session, sometimes calling me that morning. The group was advertised in the New York City PWA Coalition Newsletter and through the Gay Men's Health Crisis hotline, the major AIDS community service provider in New York City. Most of these short-term members used the group for their own perceived crises. Many times, their family member or significant other was in another hospital dying, and they needed somewhere to talk about this. This group member dominated that session and rarely returned. The assumption by the group was that the patient had probably died. Talk about changing the flow of group process. Flexibility was needed, by the group and especially by me, which was difficult since I was still in the process of learning this skill. I had to take a crash course, or I would not have survived the group or AIDS work. At one point I even asked the core group if they objected to this transitional type of group member. (Here is that countertransference again.) The group was very strong and unified in its response, allowing me insight into the power of the group. They said that if they, the group members, could help someone, it was their honor and privilege to be able to do this, even if they never saw this person again. This actually left me speechless, an unfamiliar state for me.

As the group leader, I took on many different roles. I was a group facilitator, a resource as a hospital social worker, and an AIDS educator. This was, after all, 1985, when transmission routes of HIV were not as clear as they are today. Many of the group members were trying to decide whether the patient could live with them, and there was a lot of fear surrounding this issue. There were times that I took on all three roles in one group session.

The common issues that the group struggled with were as follows:

> *Control and empowerment:* How much does the support system do for AIDS patients versus how much do you allow the patients to do for themselves in order to empower the patient? Mothers were afraid of babying their adult children; lovers and spouses were afraid of turning into the patient's parent.
>
> *What do you talk about?:* Even an innocent question such as, "How do you feel?" can become a major issue. Asking the question might result in finding out how the group member is really feeling, something you might not want to hear. Not asking might be interpreted as not caring.
>
> *Hope versus reality:* This was a major theme for the group as it constantly attempted to walk that fine line. Each group member wanted

to help the patient retain as much hope as possible, yet the group always had a sense of reality that this disease was fatal.

Parallel process: Group members experience the same set of feelings as the patient does.

Anticipatory grief: This was another major theme and was the most difficult issue for the group. This concept deals with preparing for the patient's death by beginning to examine and cope with some of the feelings surrounding the event. For the most part, the group avoided this issue as it was just too painful. When it was brought up, typically by a drop-in group member, the group was able to be supportive toward one another. They never backed away from an issue; this one was just not often brought up.

Be careful what you say: Members were always concerned about saying the wrong thing and upsetting their loved ones. They feared this would lead to a quicker death. A secondary issue arose regarding how much negative behavior the support system should tolerate, such as a patient's drug use, verbal abuse, or other negative behaviors pertaining to their relationship. Sessions were spent helping members find ways to express their feelings to the patients and ultimately their "death fears" diminished.

Anger: Much time was spent on anger as it related to the political aspect of the disease. Although clearly this was displacement, at least the group members were expressing their anger.

AIDS respite: People who make up the support systems have a difficult time recognizing that they need a break from AIDS and their role as primary caregiver and have an even more difficult time taking that break. The concept that they have their own lives was too much to think about without feeling guilty. The group members were able to give permission to one another to take that break, and some actually did.

AIDS was a terminal illness in 1985. This presented an additional problem, as there would eventually be group members whose family member or significant other died. The group was defined and existed as a support group for family members/significant others who had someone living with AIDS. Instead of addressing this issue before it happened, I decided to allow the group to dictate what it wanted to do when that time came. Not surprisingly, when the son of one of the core group members died and she continued to attend the meetings, the group rallied around this woman and supported her through this grief period. The group was again serving its purpose and eventually this woman decided on her own to stop attending.

By the middle of 1990, the original core of the group no longer existed. There were many weeks when there was no group at all. By this time, I was the social work supervisor of the AIDS Program at BIMC. My responsibilities increased and my time for this group decreased, especially since there were no regular group meetings. In addition, by now there were many more resources available to the support systems of persons with AIDS, which influenced the number of people attending my group. Hospitals, outside of psychiatric clinics, are known to treat sick people, not to provide outpatient support groups, especially groups led by a medical social worker. I made the decision to discontinue the group and finalized this by removing it from the PWA Coalition Newsletter and GMHC hotline.

As I reflect on the title of this chapter, for me there was a rethinking of the group process. I will never forget the experience of leading this group, sixteen years after its beginning. I have yet to encounter another like it. This speaks to the members of this group, their ability to use the group for their needs, and their willingness to allow a young social worker a life-changing opportunity.

Chapter 14

HIV Support Groups in a Hospital Setting

Charlene Turner

Mr. W walked into my office one Friday afternoon and explained in a some-what agitated manner that he had received an AIDS diagnosis. He explained that he was all alone and wanted me to guarantee that he would have a decent burial. After considerable discussion, Mr. W seemed calmer and did not appear to be a suicide risk. He refused any suggestions to speak with a psychiatrist. He was not open to revealing contacts of family or friends but did give me his telephone number and address. For some reason, I attempted to reach him over the weekend (perhaps just a social work instinct), but my calls went unanswered. On Monday, he was discovered in our hospital's intensive care unit with a self-inflicted gun-shot wound to the head.

What a dramatic statement about the need for support. This incident oc-curred at the beginning of the AIDS epidemic, when there was consuming fear and dread surrounding this disease. Indeed, in the beginning, patients (and many health care providers) viewed an AIDS diagnosis as a death sen-tence. In response to this context, our support group was formed in 1986 at Grady Hospital.

Grady Hospital is the public teaching hospital for the Atlanta area. It is one of the largest facilities in the Southeast, with a mission of serving the underserved. Although the establishment of the AIDS Clinic at Grady in 1986 had considerable support, there were many detractors, including some health care workers who wanted nothing to do with "those patients."

GROUP FORMATION

The early stages of the group's formation were focused on practical mat-ters such as recruitment of members, advertising the group, and obtaining the support of the medical treatment team. Once several patients were identified as prospective group members, the challenge was finding a suitable meeting room. (Space is a constant, valuable commodity in hospitals.) The only available suitable meeting room was owned by Chaplaincy, so we negotiated for the space for one hour per week at noon on Fridays. (The one-day clinic met at that time.) The room provided great privacy (in the form of poor ventilation, no windows, etc.) *but* we had a designated meeting place. In addition, we served a lunch of bologna and cheese sandwiches initially. This HIV support group at Grady lasted close to ten years. As the clinic population grew, the group began meeting in space owned by the HIV clinic. We kept the meeting at a consistent day and time, but the lunches were elevated to ham and cheese.

The potential group members were interviewed prior to the first meeting to determine their suitability, and they were given information on what group participants might expect. There was no particular restriction on who could become a group member; it just turned out that the group's composition over the years was gay males who were newly diagnosed when they joined the group. The group was potentially open to any patient attending our HIV clinic. Initially, this openness presented no problem; however, once the group developed and the core membership was established, my ideology led me to consider closing the group. The group members, on the other hand, always expressed strong feelings against closing the group to "anyone suffering with AIDS," so the group remained open. In fact, we took in an African-American patient from another hospital when that hospital's social worker called and asked permission to send him to our group because he was the only African American in her group. At that time 10 percent of our membership was African American. The group members were willing to risk their anonymity in order to keep the group open. The average attendance through the years ranged anywhere from six to ten members. However, there were a few sessions when we had as many as eighteen to twenty participants. Groups with eighteen to twenty people proved so large that discussion was hampered and still dominated by the core group of participants.

GROUP FACILITATION

The group had cofacilitators from the beginning, with changes over the years as social workers changed jobs. Different social workers hired to work in the HIV clinic were then asked to cofacilitate the groups. I was also Director of Social Services and took the groups on as an additional responsibility because of my special interest in them. Near the end of the group cycle, my cofacilitator was a white, gay male, which turned out to be the best combination with me, a straight, African-American female. Our styles were very different but complementary. He was more theoretical and generally nondirective, while I tended to be directive and active in the group's deliberations. However, we agreed on the broad purposes of the group:

- Increasing the patients' general awareness of themselves and knowledge of their illness
- Assisting them in adjusting to the illness and its impact on their lives overall
- Providing practical support and tools for living with HIV
- Offering a supportive climate for positive interaction

The group always started at noon and lasted for one hour. We had a general format for most meetings: introductions if there were new members; "checking in" with the group (members expressed how they were feeling emotionally, physically, etc.), and discussion following whatever concerns were raised in each meeting. Essentially, there were no established agenda items. The discussion flowed from whatever concerns were raised during the check-in time. The facilitator would "tune in" to the spoken and unspoken messages that were given during the check-in, listening for commonalities, major dilemmas, or interpersonal problems. Often a question was posed to all group members based on what the facilitator heard, and this generally got the group discussion moving.

From time to time, based on specific issues presented by members, we invited speakers or held educational sessions. For example, the medical director of the clinic came to talk about the various clinical trials and the treatment modalities being offered in the clinic at that time.

At the close of each group meeting, I normally summarized the group's discussion. The intent was to provide some statements that would offer insight and points for continued reflection to carry from each group.

GROUP THEMES AND ISSUES

In the beginning, the group consisted mainly of gay white males. The themes at that time related more to acceptance of the illness by significant others and the fear of suffering and dealing with loss, including loss of employment, loss of loved ones, and loss of good looks. As the group's composition shifted to primarily African-American men, many of the issues changed. Although acceptance by the religious community was a common theme for both, it became a more prevalent issue among black group members.

The change in the economic status of the members also closely paralleled the shift in the racial makeup of the group. In the early stages, the focus was on estate planning and how to live a more modest lifestyle with reduced income. In the later stages of the group, the emphasis was on educating members about housing and welfare resources.

Confidentiality

Confidentiality was discussed at the beginning of each group meeting and a verbal agreement by members was acknowledged. Some sensitive issues and tests of confidentiality arose from time to time, for example:

- Since we initially used the Chaplaincy space, several requests for student chaplains to "sit in" on group meetings had to be denied. Later, when the clinic grew larger and the group began meeting in the clinic conference room, staff members had to be told that they could not just openly visit the group unless invited.
- Confidentiality was a prevalent issue as long as group members insisted on keeping the group open. However, new members did not have to reveal any pertinent information about themselves in the group until they were comfortable. Thus, we had a married group member who came to three sessions and revealed only his first name. He was consumed with the fear that his wife and grown daughter would learn of his illness and desert him. He dropped out after those few visits and could not be contacted since he had given me no information.
- Group members often spoke of times when their confidentiality had been breached. One member from a rural Georgia town revealed that his doctor had written a letter to the patient's estranged wife informing her of his AIDS diagnosis. He felt betrayed and was encouraged by the group to pursue his legal options.

Family Issues

The issues surrounding family relationships were paramount throughout the years. Acceptance or nonacceptance of a gay lifestyle by close family members was foremost in the minds of most patients. At the beginning of the epidemic several group members were totally estranged from their families and sought to establish their own "family" support system. Thus, the group took on special meaning for those members. Members were encouraged to exchange phone numbers and offer support and encouragement outside of meetings. This connection proved especially useful when members missed several consecutive meetings.

Despite the fact that members had developed "new" families, most spoke, with much pain, of longing to be accepted by their natural families and held on to the hope that someday the estranged relatives would reconsider and reconcile with them.

Intimacy versus Isolation

Given the age range of most members (early twenties to late fifties), it was only natural that much discussion centered on the need for companionship versus remaining isolated. Isolation for many members translated into complete sexual abstinence. Most members expressed considerable concern about passing on the virus to someone else even when practicing "safer sex." This arena was amenable to role-play that addressed scenarios:

- Monogamous gay couple (one HIV positive; the other HIV negative)—Do they continue to be intimate, or do they now abstain from sex altogether?
- Intermittent gay or bisexual sexual partners—How soon do you reveal your HIV status and how do you do it?

The intent here was for members to think through various situations and come up with the right answer for themselves. The facilitator and most group members supported the idea of "safer sex." The group expected that members would not take advantage of unsuspecting sexual partners, and the group dealt in rather harsh terms with any member who hinted at deviating from the group's norm. The facilitators, however, allowed the group to press the deviant member only to a point, since we didn't want these members to leave.

This issue was highlighted by a tragedy when a group member was murdered. He had attended the group for several months and was an integral member. New to the vicinity, he had attempted to quickly establish relationships. Unfortunately, according to newspaper accounts, he took the wrong person home, where the violence occurred. This was a chilling time for the group (the facilitators included). We decided to acknowledge the deceased member and his contribution but then led the discussion to personal safety guidelines. This discussion also raised the issue of dying from something other than AIDS.

Fear of Suffering and Dependency

Before beginning the group, I anticipated that the focus would be on the fear of dying. Most patients, particularly in the early years of the epidemic, had generally come to accept that they might be "dying," but an even bigger concern was related to suffering, which was also closely tied to being totally dependent on someone else for care. Members were encouraged to complete advanced directives and to have discussions with their physicians and their agents about the contents of these directives to ensure that their wishes were fulfilled.

Initially, the group's expectations were that members would visit one another when hospitalized. Getting those visitations to occur, however, became increasingly difficult. In confronting the group with this fact, it became clear that it was too hard on those visiting, as they envisioned themselves in the same position. So, the protocol changed. The leaders visited the hospitalized member and reported to the group, and, depending on how the person was faring, others would or would not be encouraged to visit.

Spirituality and Religion

Issues relating to religion and spirituality were prevalent throughout the group's history. However, it became more of a focus as the group became predominantly African American. The general perception among white members was that they had a large degree of acceptance from their religious institutions—even though there were pockets of resistance and hostility. On the other hand, black members spoke of condemnation and hostility by the black church, with great anguish and pain. Most members were raised in a traditional religious community and had a great need to continue that association but spoke of alienation due to their churches' strong opposition to a gay lifestyle. Many spoke of the "hypocritical" nature of some of the local religious leadership, as they knew "closet" gay or bisexual individuals within those ranks. There was continuing debate about the Scriptures and whether homosexuals were condemned to hell versus God being a loving creator who judged all individuals on the basis of who lived a good life and treated others well. The group members were encouraged by the leaders to adopt the view that religion and spirituality were very personal beliefs. Whenever there was a hint of AIDS being God's punishment for a certain lifestyle, the group was encouraged by the leaders to think about Rabbi Harold Kushner who wrote the book *When Bad Things Happen to Good People* (1997).

Group Profiles

Over the many years of facilitating the group, numerous individuals made a measurable impact on the group and vice versa. The three individuals profiled here were consistent and active group members until their deaths.

Dennis was a gay white male in his early forties. He was a former executive at one of the leading banks in the country, married to the "storybook southern belle," and the father of two teenage sons. By his own account, that life was miserable because he was "living a lie." He felt free of so much "baggage" now that he had acknowledged his homosexuality and, even with his AIDS diagnosis, felt relieved of pressure. In moving away from all of the traditional middle-class trappings, his ex-wife allowed no contact with his children, the most painful aspect of all, and his family of origin had also disowned him. So, the group was particularly meaningful to him.

He poured his heart and soul into the group's development—organizing lists of members and contact information, tracking absent members, organizing special events. Perhaps most important was the extent of "sharing" he was willing to do in the group, generally done in an inspiring manner. He took it upon himself to bring a closing item to each meeting—an inspirational poem or special reading of some kind. He never missed a single meeting in two years until he left town and even then continued to visit the group periodically.

Dennis and I developed a special bond: he taught me so much about being gay—"If I could be any other way, I would not have chosen this lifestyle"—and he would relate the painful price he had paid for being gay. He once spoke to the social work staff at an in-service program relating to AIDS and homosexuality, and as he told his story, the audience wept openly. He then made some humorous remark and told them to stop the weeping, as he had "done enough already." Others in the group admired Dennis for his intellect, his ability to relate to all group members, his sense of humor, and his true compassion for them. His courage, honesty, and sense of integrity were most remarkable. If he were still alive, he would have approved of this chapter because it might help others to develop similar support groups.

Phil was referred to the group by a social worker in another state who knew about the group. The preinterview with Phil centered on the need for confidentiality and whether he wanted to become a Grady patient. He was the oldest member of the group and came with the idea that the group was something to do while he awaited death, having read somewhere that AIDS progressed more quickly in people who were at middle age.

Major issues for Phil were his reputation as a professional social worker and whether he wanted to openly acknowledge his homosexuality. Interestingly enough, Phil was not prone to put on his social work hat and attempt to cofacilitate the group. However, he was very supportive of the group process and instrumental in helping to explain the value and purpose of the group. The group provided him unconditional support and gave him the courage to be true to himself. For example, he progressed from being an uptight, three-piece-suit individual to comfortably wearing turtlenecks with necklaces.

Dennis was especially helpful to Phil because they could identify in so many areas—the professional careers, the position of wealth, and strained family relationships. A major hurdle for Phil was informing his adult children of his HIV status. His disclosure finally came after much work in the group and role-playing as to how it might be handled. The group was quite focused on this event in his life and celebrated when he reported telling them without encountering the hostile response he had expected. Another major event in Phil's life was the birth of a grandson. This event seemed to provide him a new lease on life. Initially his goal was to live to see the baby born and then it was to see him reach his first birthday. Phil lived to see his grandson enter elementary school. He later credited the group with having "saved" his life—and he did outlive all of the group members who started at the time he came to the group.

Jay, a streetwise hustler, was indeed an interesting group member. He preferred to be called "Pam" and was well accepted by the group, despite his educational level and flamboyant style being quite different from those other members. He was in and out of jail for various reasons, including petty thefts and public drunkenness. The group seemed bent on changing some of his behavior. In particular, Pam would brag about his sexual exploits. Some group condemnation was allowed when Pam described these reckless behaviors. As Pam continued coming to the group over a period of years, the bragging lessened. When he no longer boasted of his many exploits, he became rather silent but remained a faithful member. His attachment to the group was evident by his attendance at all funerals and hospital visitations and calling whenever he needed to miss a meeting.

Lessons Learned

My termination from the group was brought on by a change in my job responsibility. It was extremely difficult, but the group did continue. In retrospect, I learned some lessons that should be considered by other facilitators.

It is important to establish basic rules and guidelines from the onset. We tended to establish rules as situations occurred, which made it more difficult. Some summary recommendations for rules:

- Permit no guests unless the group approved them ahead of time.
- Do not allow verbal abuse or disrespectful comments. The facilitator is the judge of whether a comment is disrespectful.
- Written confidentiality agreements should be used instead of verbal ones.
- No sexual harassment of any member is allowed during the group.
- Members who encounter one another outside of the group are not required to acknowledge one another.
- Members who arrive at group intoxicated are not allowed to attend the meeting that day.

Most of these rules were considered or established after a situation occurred that made it necessary. The group was purposely conducted without many rules as it was so varied and diverse, and we made a great effort to be inclusive of any patient attending our clinic.

The group helped me grow as a person and as a professional. I learned a great deal about the medical aspects of the disease process, but I learned more about the social, emotional, and physical losses involved in the process. I learned to be even more accepting of people whose lifestyles might be different from mine but who possess the same desires and hopes as anyone else in society.

The group provided me the most treasured experience of my professional career, and for that I'm truly grateful to all "my guys."

Chapter 15

Group Intervention in the Early Days of the GRID Epidemic: A Reflection of One Social Worker's Personal Experience

Lori Wiener

INTRODUCTION

On June 5, 1981, the Centers for Disease Control (CDC) published a report in the *Morbidity and Mortality Weekly Report (MMWR)* of a new disease that was striking gay men. This report was one of the first publications describing what we now know as the AIDS pandemic. Since the first cases of AIDS were reported, AIDS has claimed the lives of more than 21 million people worldwide, and tens of millions more are believed to be HIV infected. In the United States alone, 400,000 people have died, and more than one million individuals have been infected.

At the time of the CDC report, social workers in large city medical centers were experiencing firsthand the devastating impact of this new disease. They were there supporting physicians, nurses, and hospital administrators as they expressed anxiety about an increasing number of gay men being admitted to hospitals with some sort of enigmatic illness ranging from swollen lymph nodes (lymphadenopathy), a rare form of a life-threatening pneumonia only previously seen in cancer and other severely immunocompromised patients *(Pneumocystis carinii),* disfiguring skin lesions often initially presenting on the nose and feet (Kaposi's sarcoma), unrelenting diarrhea that did not respond to any standard treatment (cryptosporidium), chronic fevers and weight loss *(Mycobacterium avium intracellulare),* and changes in the patients' mental status (dementia). Social workers were also there supporting the men who were previously vibrant, productive, and healthy as they were developing these opportunistic infections and dying. Media accounts of the contagious nature of this new "gay" disease were rampant, and many of the men did not feel they could call upon their families of origin, as they had not disclosed the fact that they were gay. Social workers—trained in crisis management, community advocacy, the alleviation of emotional anguish, understanding the role of family dynamics, and the negative impact of prejudice and social discrimination on coping and adaptation—assumed a leadership role from the first days that this disease emerged.

Within the first eighteen months of the epidemic, key medical breakthroughs occurred. Most major routes of HIV transmission had been identified: sexual contact with an infected person, needle sharing among intravenous drug abusers, and transfusion of blood and blood products. In 1983, prevention recommendations were issued, and the virus was labeled HTLV-III (now known as HIV). By 1985, a blood test had been developed, the CDC had issued recommendations for screening the blood supply, and medical professionals became aware of the transmission of AIDS during pregnancy. Nevertheless, the disease, especially the issue of transmission, continued to be perceived as a "medical mystery."

Many of the authors in this book have been on the front line in the fight against HIV/AIDS since the first CDC report was published. The twentieth anniversary of this disease recently passed, and it provided us with a time to step back and reflect on the tremendous scientific and treatment advances made. It was a time to remember the family members, friends, and colleagues we have lost to this disease. It was also an opportunity to honor all of those who dedicated their lives to eradicating this horrific disease and had the courage to march on when there appeared to be no hope in sight.

Perhaps the best way to honor those lost, as well as those who held steadfast during the darkest hours, is to make certain that we vow to never forget the past. This chapter describes one social worker's experience attempting to provide comprehensive psychosocial services to persons living with what was known as GRID (gay-related immune deficiency) in the early to mid-1980s at a large New York City hospital, Memorial Sloan-Kettering Cancer Center (MSKCC). Being a part of that history means having to recall very distressing events, such as sitting with patients as they were interviewed by scientists from the CDC about the explicit details of their sex life and drug use. During these interviews, the scientists wore masks, gowns, and gloves. Other patients suffered a great loss of dignity, as the explosive nature of their diarrhea required them to be hooked up to a rectal tube. Most of the patients feared losing their vision due to KS lesions, cytomegalovirus (CMV), or toxoplasmosis. Unfortunately, many did. It also is a time to remember the heroic moments and the enormous strength of the gay community to reach out, support their own, and fight back on personal, community, state, and federal levels. It was a war, and those involved were on the front line of the battlefield. Our weekly meetings, patient sessions, and groups were often scheduled around funerals. Every patient died.

COMMON EMOTIONAL REACTIONS

Early in the epidemic, GRID was characterized by a profound and irreversible suppression of the immune system. Persons diagnosed with this disease confronted multiple and severe medical crises and psychosocial stresses. Some of these stresses waxed and waned as a result of the disease's often fluctuating course of intermittent opportunistic infections. However, most of the major stresses associated with the disease remained quite constant throughout the illness and are still the main issues persons diagnosed with HIV must address today.

Disclosure

Despite the many symptoms a person might have been experiencing early in the epidemic, each individual endured a long period of uncertainty until the diagnosis was made. This time period, from early symptoms to diagnosis, was characterized by heightened anxiety and significant psychological distress (Morin, Charles, and Malyan, 1988). Individuals were confronted by the threat the disease posed to their long-term survival, the question of when and how they became infected, whether they had transmitted the disease to others, and with whom they could confidently share the diagnosis. The majority of people diagnosed with this disease in the early 1980s were homosexual and bisexual men. These men were young (twenty-five to forty-nine years of age), were working on career goals, had limited insurance, and were not at a point in life that they would expect to develop a potentially fatal illness. For most of these men, the thought of sharing their new diagnosis with family members raised enormous fears of rejection, as only a minority of them had previously shared their sexual orientation with their families. Despite attempts to help these men reach out to their families, most never did share the true diagnosis. Some courageously contacted their families and informed them of the nature of their illness, only to be rejected.

Many others, though, who did reach out to their families, received a positive response, but the bulk of the support came from their network of friends, gay community organizations, and the medical staff. In fact, 62 percent of the patients seen at a major medical center in New York City during the first four years of the epidemic reported minimal or no contact with their families (Christ and Wiener, 1985). Disclosing the diagnosis to employers carried a cruel social stigma and raised many of the same concerns, such as "implied" homosexuality or substance use. By disclosing their diagnosis, these men risked rejection from their families and loss of employment when they were most in need of emotional support, a sense of security, and reliable income.

Mental health providers found themselves trying to help patients change their sexual practices by abstaining, using precautions, and/or disclosing their diagnosis to their sexual partners. It was often very difficult for providers to be empathic when hearing of someone who engaged in risky sexual practices. The therapeutic task was to persevere while understanding what the patients' sexuality meant to them, whether an intimate expression; a form of social contact; a feeling of closeness, warmth, or caring; or a means of expressing a number of emotions, including anxiety.

Disfigurement, Debilitation

The debilitating and disfiguring aspects of GRID caused a great deal of anxiety and fear. Typically, individuals experienced fever, significant weight loss, and malaise. In some cases, these symptoms were not associated with a concomitant opportunistic infection but rather were the result of the underlying disease itself. Kaposi's sarcoma, one of the original GRID diagnoses, most often presents with multiple reddish-purple lesions. The head and neck are common sites for these lesions, which are visible and can be readily observed and identified by others. Because physical appearance can be highly valued and also plays an important role in some professions in which many gay men are frequently employed (e.g., the arts, theater, broadcasting, fashion, and law) these physical changes were extremely upsetting and could present major obstacles in continuing employment.

Debilitation was additionally threatened by central nervous system manifestations. It was estimated at the time that between 10 and 20 percent of all persons living with this disease developed slowly progressing dementia, manifested by confusion, disorientation, and memory deficits. It was often hard to sort out whether a person's paranoid ideation, depression, and/or social withdrawal were associated with central nervous involvement or the psychological response to the stresses of an incurable, disfiguring, and disabling illness.

Death

By 1984, GRID was known as AIDS, and the virus that causes the destruction of the immune system was no longer referred to as HTLV-III but instead as HIV. Despite the fast pace that medical research was taking to understand this disease, a cure was still not found and the full range of responses to terminal illness was seen in persons living with the disease. Because of their young age, most persons living with AIDS had never experienced the death of a loved one, much less preparing for or even considering their own deaths. Although some patients responded to the diagnosis of AIDS with such statements as "I've been given a death sentence, so why don't I just live whatever time I have to the fullest?" others contemplated suicide or asserted a strong belief in euthanasia if treatments failed to help them. However, many other persons living with AIDS during this time remained hopeful: "I've beaten everything so far, and I am going to beat this too. No matter what it takes," or "It is only a matter of time until research renders answers, treatments, and cures" (Ferrara, 1984, p. 1287). Most, however, experienced an unpredictable vacillation between feelings of hopefulness and periods of despair. For patients with AIDS, the optimism of an experimental treatment protocol was often quickly replaced by images of physical deterioration, dependency, and isolation from loved ones. The role of the social worker during this time was to provide supportive counseling and education about the disease, treatment options, and coping skills. Counseling also continually addressed loss of self-esteem, and finding "best ways" to inform family members or employers about the illness. The therapeutic alliance established during counseling provided the patient with an opportunity to share frustration and fears associated with limited treatment options, side effects, treatment compliance, and ways to plan for the future. Relaxation techniques, visual imagery, and other behavioral techniques were offered to individuals in conjunction with individual counseling. Along with comprehensive need assessments, individual support, and linkages to community resources, the social worker was in a key position to draw on the collective strength of the patients through the use of support groups.

GROUP INTERVENTION

After the patient's basic needs had been met and individual issues were addressed, each patient was invited to participate in a group. Many patients had a continued need for reassurance and valued the opportunity to observe and speak with others who were experiencing the same illness. Isolation and stigma were common themes throughout most groups, and the experienced, mutual support provided many of these individuals with a new sense of purpose and meaning. Dinner invitations, telephone contact with members who were acutely ill or depressed, and the sharing of coping methods such as visual imagery or body massage were common. The groups were effective in reducing feelings of isolation and provided an atmosphere where patients were comfortably able to share experiences in a safe environment. The group members not only served as role models for others, they were also often able to reinforce their own self-perceptions of successfully coping with AIDS and maintaining control over their lives.

Although members were encouraged to attend each of the groups regularly, each group was open, with flexible membership and attendance. Similar to today, not all individuals are comfortable joining a group. In the early to mid-1980s, joining a group meant that the patient accepted the diagnosis and was willing to confront the words, faces, and physical conditions of the other group members, as well as potential disfigurement, wasting, and death.

Lymphadenopathy Group

The lymphadenopathy group first met in October 1983 and grew out of a workshop offered to persons living with lymphadenopathy. This particular group met monthly and was led by a social worker assigned to the infectious disease clinic and a nurse. It was primarily a support group for gay men with symptoms associated with AIDS who were being medically followed at New York City hospitals. The symptoms that these men reported included chronically swollen lymph glands, thrush, unexplained weight loss, fatigue, and recurrent infections. A spectrum of patients participated in these groups, from individuals with relatively minor symptoms to those who very probably had AIDS but who had not yet had a classifiable opportunistic infection. Approximately one group meeting in four featured a speaker, often from within the hospital but sometimes from the gay community or other appropriate community resources.

The topic most frequently discussed at these group meetings was the patients' attempts to live with the uncertainty of their medical conditions. These individuals had not received a diagnosis of AIDS; although it was known that they were at increased risk, their precise chance of eventually developing AIDS was unknown. This uncertainty added an additional burden of ambiguity in group discussion of sexuality, sexual responsibility, contagion, and whether to discuss such an uncertain medical status with lovers, friends, family, and employers.

AIDS/KS and AIDS (Non-KS) Education-Support Groups

The AIDS/KS and AIDS (Non-KS) groups, which began in October 1982, were the most well attended. Enrollment was open to all patients being treated at MSKCC. There were no requirements pertaining to gender, sexual preference, or inpatient versus outpatient status. The groups met weekly for one hour and were led by two social workers. They were primarily designed to be supportive in nature and encouraged a high degree of cohesion and relatively little confrontational and "here-and-now" interpersonal exploration. Nevertheless, group sessions included a considerable amount of self-disclosure, sharing of mutual concerns and fears, and discussion of various coping strategies. For example, group members shared skills such as specific meditation exercises aimed at reducing anxiety, pain, and sleeplessness.

Group meetings focused on information about community resources, discussions of death and dying, family relationships, employment concerns, relationships with friends and acquaintances, treatment options, and how to live as richly as possible in the face of a potentially life-threatening disease. As Yalom and Greaves (1977) so eloquently describe, members' perspective on life had been radically altered by their experience; trivial and inconsequential concerns were seen for what they were, and liberation and autonomy rather than resignation and powerlessness occurred for many of the group members.

Two social workers skilled in group dynamics served as facilitators in this group. Due to the many questions about the disease and the high degree of anxiety, they developed an approach that combined education with support. Every third week an educational session was planned that was followed by a traditional support group. The group members decided what topics were of interest to them, and the appropriate speakers were then invited to the group. Topics included safer sex practices in and out of bathhouses, how to apply for disability, making a will, holistic approaches to healing, relaxation techniques, nutrition, a "101 class" on HTLV-III, specific opportunistic infections, makeup tips to cover KS lesions, counseling techniques for disclosing the diagnosis to family and friends, how to become involved in community activism, treatment choices, and how to begin to address end-of-life issues. There was a tremendous tendency at this time in the epidemic for individuals to receive inadequate or incorrect information from the media. The educational portion of this group helped increased trust between the group members and the medical team. Some of the founders and active members of Gay Men's Health Crisis (GMHC) frequently attended the education sessions and provided invaluable information and support to the group members. Nevertheless, an integral part of this group was mourning members who grew sicker or died. The atmosphere of support and cohesion in the group fostered visits and cards to members when they were hospitalized. Frequent phone contact among members between meetings also took place, and the leaders kept an up-to-date listing of the phone numbers of the group members who wished to be called. When a group member died, the group leaders took the initiative to inform the members of the patient's death during the subsequent group meeting rather than allowing them to hear about it informally, if they had not already heard. The leaders' openness increased group members' trust and confidence, even though the information was disturbing. The leaders tried to reduce over-identification by discussing different manifestations of the disease. Group members were encouraged to express their reactions and questions were answered, but then the group refocused on the present and how the members could continue to cope with the disease and improve their own lives.

This particular group had to work through a number of unfortunate events since its inception. The patient who assisted in the formation of this group died suddenly prior to the second group meeting. Eight months into the group, a person living with AIDS who had been known to many of the group members committed suicide and a group member found him. Another patient with no history of central nervous system disease had a grand mal seizure during the group time and remained unconscious in the group room despite medical assistance. As can be expected with a disease with such a high mortality rate, many members died. However, the identification with the collective group appeared to be a factor that continued to strengthen the group's cohesive forces. As leaders, we fostered a climate of permissiveness and acceptance, with a related sense of solidarity that also appeared to play a major role in enhancing attendance and group involvement in general (Scheidlinger, 1980). One quote that will stay with me forever came at the end of a difficult group session. A particular group member described his sense of disfigurement and rejection by his partner with tremendous emotion. As he was speaking, another group member held his hand and stated, "I know the statistics. We've seen enough people die, lose jobs, lose families. I feel as if I'm surrounded by glass protection. It's fragile. But the one thing that holds us together is each other."

Couples Group

Most of the AIDS patients seen at MSKCC at this time were geographically distanced from their families of origin. The majority were also gay, a fact that most of their family members did not know. As a result, their "family" or closest support network usually consisted of close friends or a significant other/lover. These individuals were also in need of support. There was no test available at this time to determine HIV infection, and the issues for couples predominately focused on fear of transmission, loss, and separation. A number of partner/caretaker groups were being formed in the community, but no format seemed to allow couples to share their concerns together. A couples group was formed that was open to persons living with AIDS and their partners. This open group met every other week for approximately one year and was led by the author. The purpose of the couples group was to allow for discussions associated with illness, intimacy, treatment decisions and side effects, changes in lifestyle, communicating with the patients' biological family, and legal issues. An educational format was used in this group as well, but on a much more informal basis. For example, a speaker was invited when the group members felt the need for specific information. In this group as well, it was necessary to continually balance issues relating to dying with those related to living. Respecting the hope for life and living while making realistic plans for a life filled with illness and loss and maintaining intimacy and open communication were the key elements addressed in this group.

Bereavement Groups

When a person living with AIDS died, the significant other was often left with a limited support network. Many of these surviving individuals had withdrawn from past social ties in order to spend more time with the patient. Most had not shared information with their families, employers, or co-workers about the patient's illness or homosexuality and relationships. As a result, these survivors were often left feeling alone and frightened following a partner's death. Unresolved legal issues were not uncommon, and such lack of resolution often caused tremendous emotional and financial distress. A bereavement group was formed for the partners of the AIDS patients in an attempt to provide an atmosphere in which they could share their concerns and learn to cope with the process of bereavement. Other issues focused on mourning and grief around coping with loss, monitoring their own health, the process of developing new social supports, and sharing with others about their own "at-risk" status. Many later joined an AIDS support group when they too presented with the disease. For these individuals, having to live through their own illness without a partner there for support, as they had supported their partners, was exceptionally difficult. The group, which met bimonthly and continued for over a one-year period, became their family.

Staff Support Groups

Physicians, nurses, and others involved in patient care are prone to occupational stress, fear and anxiety, prejudices, and guilt as a result of working with AIDS patients (Christ and Wiener, 1985). Nurses would report their social life being negatively affected when people they were dating were not comfortable with them caring for people living with AIDS. Crisis intervention, educational forums, multidisciplinary rounds, and weekly "stress" groups were developed and proved to be effective with health care providers. These groups addressed facts and fears associated with transmission; reactions from families and friends; the impact that multiple losses of patients, who were often the same age as the staff members, was having on the staff members' emotional well-being; the difference between being sad and being depressed; and the need to grieve. Today, twenty years later, staff support groups address many similar issues, though the hope for long-term survival mitigates the stress associated with caring for these individuals. Although the chance of becoming HIV infected through a needle stick injury is less than 1 percent, transmissions have occurred. Balancing risks, maintaining appropriate emotional boundaries, and understanding the complexities of adhering to difficult drug regimens are the main issues addressed in staff support groups then and today.

In summary, during the early years of the AIDS epidemic, support groups demonstrated the complex experiences and needs of persons diagnosed with a new, socially stigmatizing, often progressively disfiguring, and always fatal disease. Despite tremendous fear, these men illustrated remarkable reserves of strength and resilience. Nevertheless, their coping skills were clearly strained by the demands of the illness and media coverage of a "gay plague." For the partners of the individuals we were working with, groups were aimed at helping them cope with their own uncertain medical status, confront the potential losses in their lives, and work toward building a future for themselves with or without their loved ones. Today, support groups continue to be a part of almost all medical and community support programs. The emergence of highly active antiretroviral therapies has improved the length and quality of life for many of those infected, but with advances in treatment have come new challenges. For most, within groups the focus has changed from learning to live with a limited life span to learning to live with a chronic disease. This includes preparing emotionally and financially for periods of well-being and for periods of incapacitation. Support groups continue to be well attended, and it is encouraging to see new research in the literature that at least preliminarily supports our own observations from twenty years ago—that HIV-related support groups significantly influence survival (Summers et al., 2000).

YESTERDAY, TODAY, AND TOMORROW

Personal Reflections

Looking back on the early days of this epidemic resurrects powerful memories. My emotions vacillated among frustration over watching some individuals continue to engage in high-risk behaviors, awe over how so many individuals mobilized politically and socially against AIDS, sadness when family and friends withdrew, and grief when each of these people I came to know so well passed away. I remember feeling angry when people questioned whether I, as a woman, would be the "right" person to provide services to these men. I remember feeling alone when medical professionals raised the fact that I was a heterosexual woman, questioning whether my empathy and commitment were genuine. I remember feeling spiritually isolated when my own family questioned whether I really "needed" this pain in my life, as I experienced loss after loss. Throughout all of these emotions, I knew that the work that I had begun was important, effective, and essential. I knew that I was making a difference. It was exceptionally difficult, personally challenging, and life affirming at the same time.

To be in a therapeutic relationship with a dying person makes us aware of our finiteness and our limited life span (Kübler-Ross, 1969). Past losses are reactivated with each death, and constant reminders of one's own mortality surface as we prepare the individual we are working with to leave this world. Within group sessions in particular I was often aware of my own grief, anxiety, and anger, but I am sure that any defense against any of these countertransference responses, whether denial, repression, reassurance, overprotectiveness, false optimism, or intellectualization, would have markedly interfered with my usefulness to the group. My conscious awareness of the sources of these responses was what made it possible for me to respond appropriately in terms of the groups' needs. In essence, the issues of death and loss inevitably provoke countertransference responses in the therapist, but I have learned that acceptance and utilization of these can be most therapeutic for the therapeutic process and for the group as a whole.

Today, it has become increasingly apparent that the medical aspects of AIDS are only one component, albeit a crucial one, of the life of a person living with HIV/AIDS. This disease will be with us for a long time. As social work pioneers, we have continued to be leaders during this epidemic both here and abroad. Through the hard work of many dedicated individuals, we have made great strides in devising and providing prevention strategies, have challenged stereotypes, hopelessness, and barriers to good medical care, have administered outstanding mental health services, have been instrumental in educating our own, and have conducted ongoing psychosocial research. Being on the cutting edge has also provided us with a gift, a true appreciation of the preciousness of life—a gift often not afforded to most people until they are presented with the loss of their own good health or that of those close to them.

In twenty years, AIDS has changed the face of the United States and the world. We can use this milestone to once again bring attention to the devastation and impact HIV/AIDS has had locally and globally. There are more people living with HIV than ever before, and nearly one-third of these individuals are unaware of their infection status. In 1990, Michael Shernoff wrote an article titled, "Why Every Social Worker Should Be Challenged by AIDS." He concluded with the statement, "When the history of AIDS is finally written, let the social work response be recorded as one of the finest during this immense public health crisis" (p. 7). The social work response so far has been exemplary. In many ways, our work has just begun.

REFERENCES

Christ, G. and Wiener, L. (1985). Psychosocial issues in AIDS. In DeVita, V., Hellman, S., and Rosenberg, S. (Eds.), *AIDS: Etiology, diagnosis, treatment and prevention* (pp. 275-298). Philadelphia: J.B. Lippincott Company.

Ferrara, A.J. (1984). My personal experience with AIDS. *American Psychologist* 39(11): 1285-1287.

Kübler-Ross, E. (1969). *On death and dying.* New York: Macmillan Publishing Company.

Morin, S.F., Charles, K.A., and Malyan, A.K. (1988). The psychological impact of AIDS on gay men. *American Psychologist* 39: 1288-1293.

Scheidlinger, S. (1980). *Psychoanalytic group dynamics.* New York: International Universities Press, Inc.

Shernoff, M. (1990). Why every social worker should be challenged by AIDS. *Social Work* 35(1): 5-8.

Summers, J., Robinson, R., Capps, L., Zisook, S., Atkinson, J.H., McCutchan, E., McCutchan, J.A., Deutsch, R., Patterson, T., and Grant, I. (2000). The influence of HIV-related support groups on survival in women who lived with HIV. *Psychosomatics* 41(3): 262-268.

Yalom, I.D. and Greaves, C. (1977). Group therapy with the terminally ill. *American Journal of Psychiatry* 134(4): 396-400.

Chapter 16

The Missing Support:
Group Interventions with AIDS Patients

Barbara Willinger

In 1979, St. Luke's-Roosevelt Hospital Center, an inner-city voluntary institution, admitted its first patient with AIDS, although at that time AIDS had not yet been defined. As we and other hospitals began to see patients with this baffling illness, initially known as gay-related immune deficiency, the New York State Department of Health responded to the crisis. The AIDS Institute was created in 1983 and subsequently promulgated standards of care for providers and hospitals requesting designation as an AIDS center. In agreeing to provide specialized patient care, institutions were reimbursed by Medicaid at higher levels. At St. Luke's-Roosevelt Hospital, coordinated care was delivered by a multidisciplinary, hospital-based team consisting of doctors, nurses, social workers, a nutritionist, a psychiatrist, a pastoral care worker, and an occupational therapist. In 1987, St. Luke's-Roosevelt became one of the earliest hospitals designated as an AIDS center. At that time, most AIDS patients survived no more than three years.

The initial infected population, whose risk behavior was homosexual activity, gradually shifted to a group whose infection was the result of substance abuse behavior, by both men and women. From 1987 through 1989, the delivery of service to patients was by the usual means of multidisciplinary team collaboration and social work case management services focusing on counseling and discharge planning. Those were the days that patient hospital stays were lengthy, from two weeks to several months, depending on the severity of the opportunistic infections and/or the discharge needs of the patient. This time period allowed patients to become well known to staff and for staff to encourage and support the development of "community." This was particularly meaningful to our patients who, because of their margin-

The author wishes to acknowledge the contributions from Abe Moskowitz, CSW, and Jim Giacone, OTR.

alized lifestyles, were often estranged from their families. These patients lived in single room occupancy hotels where drugs were rampant and friendships sometimes based on who supplied the next "fix" or exchange of services.

This chapter focuses on the creation and expansion of inpatient groups during a time in AIDS history when hospitalization stays were lengthy and social work staffing was prolific.

THE EXISTING GROUPS

Between 1987 and 1990 two groups existed for patients: a weekly creative arts project group and a community meeting group. The creative arts project group was originally led by the occupational therapist and later co-facilitated by a social worker once staffing increased. The activities provided ranged from simple ones for those with difficulty concentrating, such as selecting colors for a predrawn poster, to complex tasks such as creating a lasting memory for a friend, relative, or significant other. Projects carried over from one week to another to ensure the sense of time and future planning. The community meeting was led by the occupational therapist and a nun. This group encouraged patients to problem solve difficulties they experienced in the hospital, such as miscommunications with staff or other patients. Patients who had left the hospital could return to these groups and did, since our outpatient program was small and completely medically focused.

Carmen, a friendly forty-one-year-old Hispanic woman, had been drinking since the age of thirteen. When diagnosed with AIDS, she gradually decreased her alcohol intake with the support and encouragement of staff until she was able to reach and maintain abstinence. She formed close relationships with the nursing and social work staff and over time with other patients. Although she had to return to her hotel at discharge, she continued to come to groups, to participate and listen to others, and to assist patients who needed errands done. Many patients looked up to her as a role model; her self-image had changed as a result of the sense of caring from the community.

Issues that arose in the groups were brought to the attention of the team, and, over time, social workers saw an inroad in which their expertise with groups could be utilized. "Turf issues" did not exist. Mutual respect and support did, which facilitated social work integration into the community group in 1990. The role of social work was to enhance exploration of affective states and further mediate interpersonal and group dynamics. Leadership by three distinct disciplines had the positive effect of broadening and deepening the group interactions and of developing an experimental frame of reference in which diverse group activities were attempted. The latter included implementation of a relaxation exercise to end the group, a humor hour in which patients and leaders had to relate a funny story or joke, and the development of rules of behavior for the unit solarium. The tripartite leadership worked because of the close professional relationship and mutual respect that existed.

PROGRAM EXPANSION

In mid-1990 the combination of increased staffing in social work and psychiatry afforded the program the opportunity to reexamine its population, the changing nature of the disease, and the deficits in external systems. We were then seeing many cases of HIV dementia, as well as an explosion of pulmonary and extrapulmonary tuberculosis (TB). Juxtaposed were the continuing cases of the newly diagnosed, many of them severely ill because of multiple opportunistic infections. Because of the early success of the original two groups and the community feeling that the staff and many patients shared, it seemed a natural extension to expand group services. Lonergan (1982) refers to group interactions as humanizing the hospital experience, which can lend to the elevation of self-esteem and possibly lead to the renewed stability of the psyche-soma balance. In addition, we understood that participation affords patients the opportunity to be active participants as well as helpers; this position counteracts the often-assumed position of regressive passivity and dependency experienced by many hospitalized patients (Lonergan, 1982; Beckham, 1988; Child and Getzel, 1989).

GROUP EXPANSION

The first newly developed group was a patient information psycho-educational group that had a ten-week module. Social workers facilitated the group. Each week there was a different topic and speaker, some from within the program, others from within the hospital at large. The topics ranged from "AIDS 101" to disclosure issues to the effects of substances on the immune system to permanency planning. These issues are as germane today as they were then and could easily be incorporated into an outpatient group. Again, the concept of community and support were endemic to the group. Although Lonergan (1982) notes that "the content of the group is not as important as the critical process of interaction that results" (p. 12), in this instance the psychoeducation and information were crucial.

Bobby, a forty-one-year-old single intravenous drug user (IVDU), diagnosed in 1989, suffered from HIV dementia. He had developed a support network with several patients and returned to the group after discharge. When the weekly topic was disclosure, Bobby, unlike others, resolutely indicated he would never tell his mother—"I've hurt her enough with my drug use." He also felt she was too old to bear the sadness of the news. Instead, he made it clear that he had created a substitute family through his relationships with staff and patients.

In contrast was Sam, a thirty-three-year-old IVDU, who told his family his diagnosis only after he had secured permanent housing, in case he was "rejected." On the contrary, he was supported and accepted by them.

At the other end of the spectrum was Alan, a forty-eight-year-old teacher, who informed his family a year after diagnosis. This came about through intensive individual counseling, since it also meant revealing his homosexuality. He shared with the group his relief at no longer carrying a secret.

Each of these men struggled with the fear of rejection linked to the shame of their lifestyles. It is the author's experience that these very same fears exist today as exemplified by a newly diagnosed fifty-year-year old male who refused to disclose his diagnosis to his siblings who visited him daily in the hospital. He died within two months of the initial diagnosis of HIV/MAI (*Mycobacterium avium intracellulare*) having refused medications and treatments seemingly because of his intense shame and pride. This man did not have the benefit of group support; perhaps if he did, his hospitalization stay might have been different.

In today's treatment of HIV/AIDS, providers focus on when to initiate antiretroviral therapy (ART), and much is being discussed and written about adherence. In the late 1980s and early 1990s the arsenal of medications was smaller: AZT, ddI, d4T, Bactrim, pentamidine, and gancyclovir, to name only a few. Even then adherence was important and controversy about the medications, particularly AZT, existed. The "word on the street" at that time, according to many of our patients, was that "AZT killed—a conspiracy to kill off the black people." Our inpatients needed a place to vent their concerns and to be educated. With that in mind, a medication information group was established, led by a nurse and social worker, both Caucasians. It was imperative then that the leaders understand and deal with the sense of mistrust that periodically erupted and was spoken about by some of our African-American patients. In addition, and just as important, the power of the group influence was evidenced when our African-American patients assumed the role of leader and supported the benefits of AZT based on their own personal experience. For social work in the current climate, the health or adherence educators have replaced medication groups.

The continuing goal of the groups then was to educate, to empower, and to build community—a community of hope, understanding, mutual concern, and shared efforts. This seemed, and still seems, important for those patients whose lives have been twisted by their use of chemicals, crack, cocaine, heroin, and alcohol. Although one could view the chemically dependent population as having few internal resources available to cope with the devastation of HIV/AIDS other than to self-medicate, group leaders observed behaviors that flew directly in the face of total defeat. Several patients used the lengthy admissions as a "breathing space," a chance to confront self-destructive behaviors or dysfunctional situations. For others, the knowledge that they would die, and die ignominiously, viewed by themselves and others as "junkies" or "alkies" moved them to examine and experience their needs and desires long anesthetized by chemicals and the deadening life of the streets. The groups provided a venue in which these issues could be addressed within the powerful healing currents of the group process. Patients variously described these meetings as "information sharing," "getting in touch," "reinforcement for life," and "relaxation."

Many of the patients returned to the groups, indicating not only their attachment to the unit but an unspoken acknowledgment of wanting help to live. These patients visibly confronted the wasting away of others, the incoherent talk of the demented, and the empty bed of a patient who was there the previous week. Death and dying were frequently given voice. In this specter of living and dying, patients came to see that they were related to as people—for what they said and did, for what they were able to give to one another, and not because they could provide a "fix" for someone else.

THE ABSENCE OF NEED

By the mid-1990s the number of admissions decreased; hospital stays were briefer; and the arsenal of effective medications increased. Our unit was moved and integrated within a general medical floor. No longer could the program support the existence of groups as they had been operating. We tried to continue the psychoeducational information group but soon realized that staff constraints and fewer patients militated against continuation. In an effort, however, to maintain some sense of "community," as well as to carry on the conceptual benefits of group participation, social work developed a new group module that focused on the shared characteristics of HIV/AIDS and substance use. The goal of this three-session module (to be held on consecutive days) was to promote awareness of "triggers" to substance use and their illness. For example, through the use of a "game" format, patients could identify their anxieties about their illnesses and the possible use of illicit substances to self-medicate. Coping strategies would be made available, and at the end of the third session patients would be presented with options for self-interventions, such as referrals to hospital providers or outside agencies.

Although the patient response was favorable, the group did not last. The number of available patients was too small, and we could no longer count on the nursing staff to bring patients to the group room. The groups, which were once a necessary "missing support" in the care of HIV/AIDS patients, were no longer viable due to the changing contingencies of the illness and the hospital structure. This was a difficult reality for me, as the supervisor, and for my staff to accept. Its impact was far ranging, from changing the focus of the work from inpatient to outpatient to the dissolution of close-knit relationships that had been emotionally sustaining.

The group function now appears to reside in community-based agencies and day treatment programs that currently exist for HIV/AIDS patients. Although the sense of "community" still exists within our clinic, the term has taken on a broader meaning. As of now, no groups exist for adult patients within our clinic other than one led by a peer counselor, with good attendance, I may add. However, to whatever extent hospital outpatient clinics are able to develop groups, be they support, education, or adherence focused, the power and influence of the group process is a tool for ongoing healing and self-actualization.

REFERENCES

Beckham, D. (1988). Group work with people who have AIDS. *Journal of Psychological Oncology* 6(1-2): 217-221.

Child, R. and Getzel, G. (1989). Group work with inner city persons with AIDS. *Social Work with Groups* 12(4): 65-80.

Lonergan, E.C. (1982). *Group Intervention.* New York: Jason Aronson, Inc.

Chapter 17

Twenty Years of the Epidemic: A Social Work Administrator's Personal Perspective

Susan W. Haikalis

1981 TO 1985—THE CRISIS TO BE, STILL UNKNOWN (3,500 CASES WORLDWIDE BY 1983)

The day in late August 1981 that a thirty-six-year-old gay man was admitted to the intensive care unit at Mount Zion Medical Center (San Francisco) will never be forgotten. It was our first encounter with an AIDS patient. As he struggled to breathe and then was placed on a ventilator, the medical personnel were totally stymied. How could this healthy, athletic young man, who two days before had been sailing in Puget Sound, be so sick and then die? The intensive care staff assumed the autopsy would provide an answer, but the findings made no sense. He died of complications from PCP (*Pneumocystis carinii* pneumonia), a disease seen in patients who had severely compromised immune systems—usually secondary to long-term chemotherapy for a cancer diagnosis. With this patient, the epidemic began for me.

Over the next five years, other gay men, their friends, and their partners, and a few women, were admitted to Mount Zion and other Bay Area hospitals with opportunistic infections or cancers. The single commonality was that almost every person was gay and had engaged in sex either with another man who was sick or with a man who had also had sex with a person who had become ill. Very few medical treatments were effective, and frequently the psychosocial issues became the primary ones for hospital health care professionals.

Social workers came to play a major role in interactions with these individuals because they saw the person holistically. They were often the staff who helped the patient deal with this frightening, unknown illness that more often than not meant death in the very near future. What did this "death sentence" mean to relationships with families of origin as well as families of choice? Crisis intervention became a part of everyday work. Social workers helped mothers and fathers cope with learning not only that their son was gay but also that he was dying. Social workers were also there to support the partners. It was the social workers who took the lead in challenging the intensive care rule that permitted only immediate family to visit patients in the unit. Many hours were spent providing counseling and mediation in the early years between parents and partners, trying to stay focused on the needs and issues of the person who was sick.

In the early 1980s, biomedical ethics committees in health care settings became more commonplace. In San Francisco, the AIDS crisis played a major role in the development of these committees. Patients were young (in their thirties and forties), were often in excellent health until very recently, were professionally and financially successful, and were used to making their own decisions. With social workers supporting their right to self-determination, the medical community slowly became more willing to see the patient as an equal partner in making medical decisions, particularly those that impacted their quality of life. Social workers spent much of their time on the issues surrounding death and dying.

Without a reliable test for the HIV virus, clients waited for the "time bomb" to explode, i.e., for symptoms to manifest themselves. They read in the San Francisco gay press each week literally hundreds of obituaries, including those of friends and acquaintances who had died of the disease. All of this had a profound psychosocial impact. As a result, social workers had to learn to balance grief and stress counseling with direct services and advocacy. They also learned to become effective advocates for their clients—fighting for their right to health care and benefits, for their partners to be treated with respect, for the right not to be evicted or fired because of their medical status, to be able to see their children, and, if a child, to be able to attend school.

Social workers also lobbied the community at large to provide services to meet the needs of this population. Hospices were developed both for direct services in the person's own home, and as specially designed freestanding facilities. Agencies were founded to provide emotional counseling, financial benefits counseling, housing, emergency financial help, political advocacy, and information and referral/hotlines. Because of the waiting period of five months for Social Security disability to begin, benefits counseling became a critical factor in working with clients. Social workers and other legal advocates argued for granting presumptive eligibility for SSI to AIDS patients, which allowed people to have a source of income and Medicaid coverage during their last few weeks or months of life.

Clinical supervision challenges were multilayered. Transference and countertransference issues were frequently addressed by supervisors and have continued to be basic issues throughout the twenty-year history of the epidemic. Staff members frequently saw themselves in their clients—the same age, the same ethnicity, and the same socioeconomic levels. Boundary issues also became an important consideration in supervision. San Francisco is really a small town—only seven by seven square miles. It was not uncommon to know acquaintances of clients and to meet people in social interactions who had connections with clients. How to feel comfortable setting boundaries was a frequent focus of supervisor-social worker discussions.

The social worker had to provide a far more holistic approach in working with the HIV/AIDS client than with other "special" client populations. The worker had to help the client deal not only with such a frightening diagnosis but also with how to deal with many of life's other issues:

- How would a partner be affected?
- Would the relationship continue, and if not, would there ever be another relationship?
- How should clients deal with family-of-origin issues—not only parents but also siblings?
- How should clients deal with employers if returning to work was reasonable?
- How could clients learn to live on a substantially reduced income?
- How would a landlord deal with the client?
- What were the best methods to manage mental health issues that were frequently exacerbated by being diagnosed as HIV positive?

Through the years, the psychosocial aspects of being HIV positive have increasingly become the focus of our work with clients. In 1981, the laws to protect personal privacy were woefully inadequate. However, over the past twenty years additional legal protections have evolved. One significant change is that people cannot be discriminated against because of their sexual orientation or HIV status. In California, specific legislation was passed after the HIV test became available that made it illegal to write in a medical record that the patient was HIV positive. Such legislation was the result of individuals losing health insurance and life insurance because insurance companies learned of their status through medical records.

When HIV testing became available, it was quickly understood that the procedure itself could have a significant impact on an individual. In San Francisco, the UCSF-AIDS Health Project, a counseling agency, developed a thoughtful process to help prepare clients for the test and possible outcomes. A specific consent form was developed that helped the client understand what the test was and what the results would mean. Clients are required to read the consent form and sign it prior to having their blood samples taken. A formal counseling strategy was also developed that included the pretest content to be covered and a requirement that the client return a week later for the results, again with posttest counseling. Clinically, whether the result was positive or negative, it gave the counselor an opportunity to help clients learn about choices available to them—i.e., if negative, understanding the need for safer sex and how situations may affect their decision making, and if positive, understanding their choices in treatment. As the epidemic has progressed and people with HIV have gained greater control of the virus through treatment, leading normal lives, including continuing a sexual life, has meant that clients have needed information and support in making healthy choices.

In addition to one-on-one supervision in which these issues were addressed, it became common for social workers to lead support groups to discuss these frequently encountered situations. As the epidemic expanded, the psychosocial complexities only increased, combining AIDS-specific issues with the problems of poverty, homelessness, mental illness, and substance use. One group that formed in the early days of the epidemic, the Social Work AIDS Network (SWAN), became a significant source in the support, education, and training of colleagues working in this challenging field.

1985 TO 1995—A DECADE OF HOPE (10,000 AIDS CASES IN THE UNITED STATES IN 1985)

The decade from 1985 to 1995 was a period of increasing treatment opportunities combined with a hope that a viable vaccine would be on the market within ten years. When the HIV test became available in 1986, there was some ambivalence among practitioners: Was it better to know one's status or to wait until there was an effective treatment? One argument for taking the test was that knowing one's status permitted an individual to make more informed decisions about safer sex and to access medical treatment if desired. Another was that individuals had the right to know their HIV status so that they could plan their lives accordingly.

One proactive program utilizing the new HIV test offered by Mount Zion Medical Center was the Look-Back program for people who had received blood transfusions from the late 1970s to 1986. As awareness increased that HIV could be transmitted by blood transfusion, the blood banks began following up on their donors' health status to determine the numbers of people who were ill or had died of AIDS. They also offered to work with Mount Zion to follow up with the patients who had received transfusions from these infected donors.

The hospital administrators turned to the social work department to collaborate with the laboratory to follow up with former patients. Patients were seen for pretest and posttest counseling, and laboratory results were coded so that there was no report kept in their medical records. Any additional follow-up was to be referred to the patient's primary medical provider under rules of strict confidentiality. However, no positive results were found. It was assumed that among patients from the neonatal intensive care unit HIV-positive babies would be identified, given the high number of transfusions, but this was not the case. For some time blood used for infant and/or mother transfusions had been tested for the presence of cytomegalovirus (CMV), and CMV-positive blood was discarded. Later studies showed that many individuals who had CMV in their blood were also HIV positive. Thus, the CMV test had reduced HIV transfusion transmission risk to many individuals who were patients in this specialized unit.

In the early 1990s, while working at another large medical center in San Francisco, the need to evaluate a large number of patients for possible exposure to HIV occurred, and again the social work staff was asked to quickly develop a program to address the crisis. A lab technician had told a friend that he had intentionally infected pregnant women over a four-year period, and he intended to blackmail the hospital. The friend called the hospital; after an assessment, it was determined that the lab technician may have actually done this. In response, the hospital decided to offer HIV testing to anyone who had had lab work at the hospital and was concerned about his or her HIV status. A twelve-hour hotline with multiple lines was set up within two days, with staff from the social work department and mental health unit. Again, everyone was offered pretest and posttest counseling utilizing the standard protocol. Four thousand people were seen in a four-week period with follow-ups offered for up to six months. No positive results occurred, but follow-ups indicated that people were very satisfied with the thoughtful, supportive counseling provided by the social work staff.

Fortunately, no incidence of HIV was discovered as a result of either of these two testing programs. Both examples illustrate the need for social work staff to be aware of possible emergency situations and to be prepared to develop emergency procedures and protocols that impact the lives of thousands of individuals—both HIV positive and negative.

In 1987, the first drug treatment for AIDS patients, AZT, was introduced. Initially there was great enthusiasm that AZT was a kind of panacea allowing HIV-positive patients to survive longer, to be healthier, and to stay alive until a cure was developed. However, it soon became evident that for some clients the side effects of AZT were so severe that they could not tolerate the drug. Experimental drug trials became the norm in San Francisco. Many clients wanted quicker access to these "new" drugs and were willing to deal with the as yet unknown side effects. They were already dying. Many of these patients were willing to take the risk that they might die sooner in exchange for the chance to live longer, healthier lives. These new drug therapies and their side effects offered yet another challenge to social workers. We had to be aware of our own morals, values, and rescue fantasies again and ensure that we were not displacing them onto our patients—again, supervision became important.

As more drugs came down the pipeline, complicated treatments for opportunistic infections (OIs) required creative post-hospital care planning. Clients did not want to stay in the hospital and turned to their social workers to together devise a plan for coping once released. Such planning often entailed coordinating care with partners, friends, relatives, and neighbors—having nurses both in the hospital and through home care teach them techniques that had previously been done only by nurses in a hospital setting.

By 1989, communities across the United States began experiencing a new HIV-related phenomenon. The epidemic began expanding to other population groups, specifically injection drug users and their sexual partners. Again, enlightened communities with the help of concerned social workers advocated for programs to help prevent transmission of the HIV virus, and needle exchange programs began to emerge. One successful program was San Francisco's HIV Prevention Project (HPP), a program that had the support of the local health department, the city/county board of supervisors, the police department, and most of the community. The University of California-San Francisco Center for AIDS Prevention studies have consistently shown that needle exchange programs significantly reduce HIV transmission in this population and do not increase drug use. San Francisco was fortunate to be in the forefront of instituting such programs and to offer counseling and support to program participants. Unfortunately, 1989 was also the year that the epidemic reached 100,000 AIDS cases in the United States (Center for Mental Health Services, 2000).

In 1990, Congress was successful in passing landmark legislation addressing the HIV/AIDS emergency in the United States. Millions of dollars were allocated, especially to those areas in the United States with specific threshold levels of people living with the HIV virus. This emergency legislation became known as the Ryan White Care Act, named after a teenager in Indiana who had become infected with HIV from a blood transfusion during treatment for hemophilia. Primary advocacy for this legislation came from public policy advocates at the San Francisco AIDS Foundation, who had experienced firsthand the enormous cost to its community of thousands of people becoming ill and dying without services and programs that could help them. Working with such congressional leaders as Senator Edward Kennedy, this landmark legislation was passed. The effect of the legislation has been profound and has provided millions of dollars to communities, such as San Francisco, which have been especially impacted by HIV/AIDS.

As the epidemic continued into the 1990s and more treatment options became available, the cost of primary medical care (including drugs), housing support, home care services (including hospices), and specialized mental health and substance use programs escalated. Clients were living up to eighteen months to two years after diagnosis and, as a result, were confronted with major costs. Social service departments were especially hard pressed to find ways to help clients cover these costs.

However, identifying financial resources was only one aspect of the challenges facing social workers and their supervisors. Counseling and intervention skills were required to address a number of issues, noted in the following list, as the life span of clients increased and the effects of the disease continued:

- Balancing medical treatment needs with quality of life issues
- Dealing with anticipatory grief in self and others
- Making decisions about guardianship for children; taking care of unfinished business
- Coping more effectively with conflicts between biological and chosen families
- Changing body image (In San Francisco, people who had AIDS could be readily identified on the street just because of wasting syndrome.)
- Loss of friends and family due to AIDS
- "Shattered dreams"
- Confronting increasing impairment, disability, and even the possibility of retirement of the patient and his or her partner

1995 TO THE PRESENT—LIVING WITH REALITY AND COPING WITH NEW CHALLENGES (500,000 AIDS CASES IN THE UNITED STATES IN 1995)

By 1995, new classes of HIV drugs became available, and an effective test for detecting the level of the HIV virus in the body had been developed. Within a few months people were learning to manage complex medication regimens, often taking thirty to forty pills a day. It soon became clear, however, that adherence to the treatment protocols had to be better than 95 percent each and every day. How were the homeless and mentally unstable to cope? Again, new programs had to be instituted to help these people learn how to maintain a consistent medication program.

Unfortunately, significant side effects also began to appear for clients who had been on long-term therapy. These included nausea and diarrhea—the latter so severe it was almost impossible to leave the house. Unusual body disfigurement, increasing cholesterol levels, adult-onset diabetes, osteonecrosis (particularly requiring hip replacements), and increasing cardiac symptoms were not uncommon. In one recent study, men in their forties who were on HAART (highly active antiretroviral therapy) when compared with those not on HAART had a five times greater incidence of heart attacks (Center for Mental Health Services, 2000).

What does all of this mean for HIV/AIDS social workers? They are constantly challenged to help some clients manage a chronic disease and to help clients with grief and loss when they experience a virus breakthrough that does not respond to a change in their drug regimen. On any given day, a social worker may be helping a client who has been living on disability for the past five years decide to return to work because his or her viral load (VL) has remained undetectable for a year, their CD4 levels are in the normal range, and they feel fine. On the same day, a social worker will be working with another client who returned to work six months before but is experiencing problems with the effectiveness of his or her treatment, evidenced by increasing VL and dropping CD4s.

There continue to be so many unknowns in the disease progression and treatment that HIV social workers continue to need, and benefit from, supervision that helps them look at the impact of these challenges on their work with clients as well as on themselves.

For some programs in large urban areas, it is not uncommon for the majority of clients to have both significant substance use problems and long histories of mental health problems. Across the United States, the HIV/AIDS epidemic is disproportionately affecting people of color, particularly African Americans and Latinos, as well as women and young people. These populations will continue to present complex challenges to social workers.

In one small HIV treatment adherence program in San Francisco—Action Point Adherence Project—over 90 percent of the clients have substance use histories, and over 70 percent have a mental health diagnosis. Few clients have had a significant work history, so any disability income is limited to SSI (Supplemental Security Income), which pays $750 a month plus medical coverage through Medicaid. Social workers in this program work closely with nurses to help clients learn treatment adherence to a HAART regimen, to reduce their substance use, and to deal more effectively with their mental health needs. This small storefront program has had some success in its almost three years with clients whose primary drug of choice was alcohol or heroin, including those on methadone treatment. Clients who use speed and cocaine and continue frequent use have not done as well. Clients who are seen regularly by staff and work on an identified plan also appear to be doing better with their adherence, evidenced by follow-up lab work. Stable housing for both Action Point clients and similar clients in a nearby ASO (AIDS service organization) that provides primarily social work (with treatment support available) also correlates with adherence success.

As the third decade of the HIV/AIDS epidemic begins in the United States, it is estimated that one million individuals are HIV positive, many of whom do not know their HIV-positive status (San Francisco AIDS Foundation, 2002). The impact of the HIV/AIDS epidemic affects everyone. Social workers in all fields of practice must accept its impact on their work with individuals, families, groups, and communities.

After twenty years, working with HIV-positive clients and with the staff dedicated to providing support and guidance to them, the work continues to be challenging and incredibly rewarding. The original goals remain: vaccines will be developed and will be effective; treatment will become easier and allow people with HIV to have hope and live satisfying lives; and the nations of the world will make a joint effort to end this pandemic. Social workers continue to be challenged by an epidemic which is constantly changing and which pushes them to become effective leaders in helping clients, communities, and nations have choices that meet their needs.

BIBLIOGRAPHY

Center for Mental Health Services, Substance Abuse and Mental Health Services Administration (2000). Coping with Hope: HIV/AIDS Treatment Decisions/Aderence (Curriculum).

National Association of Social Workers (2002). HIV/AIDS Spectrum: Mental Health Training and Education of Social Workers Project. HIV/AIDS and Substance Abuse: The Social Work Response (Workshop).

San Francisco AIDS Foundation (2002). *BETA—Bulletin of Experimental Treatments for AIDS,* 15(1).

Chapter 18

Supervising Pediatric HIV/AIDS Case Managers: Lessons Learned

David Strug

INTRODUCTION

This chapter describes my experience as the social work supervisor of eleven pediatric HIV/AIDS case managers (including social workers) from 1992 to 1997 at a Ryan White Title IV Care Act program called Horizons in an East Coast city. Title IV Care Act programs offer family-centered primary and specialty medical care, psychosocial services, logistical support, outreach, and prevention to underserved children, adolescents, women, and families most at risk for HIV/AIDS (U.S. Department of Health and Human Services Administration, 2000). Horizons' case managers assisted both HIV/AIDS-infected children and affected family members.

This chapter also describes both the successes and the limitations of my supervisory work with the case managers. At first, supervision helped to create an empathic and supportive milieu for a team of enthusiastic and effective pediatric HIV/AIDS case managers who felt very happy and energized by performing challenging work. The case managers' jobs were very meaningful to them, personally and professionally, because they valued helping and giving comfort to HIV/AIDS clients and affected family members. The case managers interacted with me and with one another in mutually supportive ways, forged strong bonds of identification with one another, and experienced a healthy grandiosity in relation to their work. Supervision helped to stave off burnout and worker attrition.

Several different factors ultimately came together causing the case managers to feel increasing unhappiness at work and increased conflict with the organization about three years after I started working at Horizons. Years of frontline work with terminally ill children and troubled families contributed

I wish to thank Craig Podell, LCSW, for his critical reading and helpful discussion of this chapter.

to growing feelings of frustration, anger, and burnout. A sizeable growth in their caseloads, a lack of opportunity for advancement, and limited salary increases added to their feelings of alienation. The combined effect of all of these work-related issues had a negative impact on the emotional well-being of the case managers and stifled the efforts made by me, by Horizons' directors, and by the workers themselves to avoid increased case manager burnout.

BACKGROUND

I was hired in 1992 by Horizons, an organization that was affiliated with the department of pediatrics of a major medical center. My job title was case management coordinator. I reported directly to Horizons' medical director who headed the organization and to another administrator who reported to the medical director. I had administrative responsibility of and clinical responsibility for the case management staff.

The eleven case managers I supervised worked at ten different Horizons-affiliated programs: eight hospital-based programs, one HIV/AIDS advocacy organization, and one foster care agency for the placement of infected and affected children. Horizons subcontracted with each of these affiliated programs. It gave them money from its Ryan White Care Act grant to pay the salaries of the case managers who were paid employees of their programs. Case managers came to Horizons' headquarters for weekly group supervision and for other meetings with me. I visited each case manager weekly at his or her program site.

Seven of the case managers were women; four were men. Seven of the case managers were African American or Hispanic; four were Caucasian. Three had master's degrees (two in social work and one in education); eight had bachelor's degrees. All eleven held the job title of case manager. Their age range was twenty-five to forty-three. They all described themselves as being very spiritual people.

HIV/AIDS was continuing its rapid spread into inner-city neighborhoods in the early 1990s. The disease was being diagnosed increasingly among IV drug users, their sexual partners, and heterosexual women and their children. By 1992, diagnosed cases attributed to heterosexual contact exceeded those attributed to injection drug use for the first time (O'Leary and Jemmott, 1995). The number of HIV-positive women in the United States grew by 600 percent from 1986 to 1990 (Gallegos, 1998). The most significant increases in AIDS incidence during this period occurred among African Americans (Centers for Disease Control and Prevention, 1998). Horizons' affiliated programs were located at institutions that not only served inner-city populations with very high HIV/AIDS rates, but also were geographically located in an area with the greatest number of cumulative pediatric HIV/AIDS cases.

Individual caseloads were high. Cumulative numbers for all case managers totaled close to 500. Their work was demanding. HIV/AIDS was only one of the issues that the families on their caseloads were dealing with, and sometimes it was not even the most pressing. Case managers' work extended beyond trying to find housing and arranging for transportation, respite care, home attendants, and medical equipment for families. Even more challenging for the case managers was the role they played in offering emotional support and counseling to children and especially to family members who often lacked basic knowledge about HIV/AIDS transmission, treatment, and prevention. In addition, my staff was responsible for maintaining detailed statistics on the clients with whom they worked and submitting them to me monthly. Despite these challenges, case managers undertook their work with enthusiasm, working tirelessly with the children and families on their caseloads.

THE SUPERVISORY MODEL

Horizons' case managers were emotionally starved for supervisory support at the time that I was hired. These workers had been without a supervisor for the previous six months.

There were three major components to case management supervision: individual, group, and a monthly grief and bereavement group session. Horizons' directors made case manager attendance at all three mandatory because they believed staff members would not voluntarily attend supervision that dealt with sickness and the death of children. Horizons' directors believed case managers needed an intensive level of individual and group supervision to be able to avoid burnout on the job.

Individual Supervision

Case managers were expected to discuss a particularly challenging case at our one-hour weekly individual supervision sessions at their affiliated programs. We analyzed family dynamics, talked about how to help families disclose an HIV/AIDS diagnosis, and considered community-based resources available to help families in need of services. In addition, a case manager was free to raise any other topic of interest for discussion in supervision. Several of the case managers talked about conflicts they experienced with departmental administrators at their affiliated programs or about feelings of professional isolation within the hospital-based departments in which they worked.

It was not always easy for my staff members to negotiate their multiple roles or to understand the different job responsibilities they had to perform for both their affiliated programs and for Horizons. They sometimes expressed confusion in our individual meetings about whether I, Horizons' directors, or the chief administrator at their affiliated program had the ultimate decision-making authority with respect to their employment. I explained that it was the head administrators at their affiliated programs who held ultimate authority; I clarified my role as a consultant who provided supervision to them. In addition, neither Horizons' directors nor I could directly hire or fire workers. Individual case managers accepted this but were not necessarily happy with such a complex work arrangement. Confusion about who was actually the "boss" arose from time to time and had to be addressed by me in supervision.

Group Supervision

Case managers also attended a weekly group supervisory meeting at Horizons' headquarters. One goal was to provide an empathic and supportive peer support group setting in which they could talk about their emotional reactions to working with sick and dying children and with needy family members. Horizons hoped group supervision would help the case managers cope with the emotional challenges of pediatric HIV/AIDS work. When an infected child became seriously ill or died, the case managers experienced the event as a psychological loss or blow that threatened their ability to cope on the job.

Bereavement Support Group

One group session every four weeks was designated as a "bereavement group meeting." This session was led by a social worker with expertise in grief and bereavement who was hired by Horizons specifically for this purpose. I also actively participated in this session, but in a much more secondary role than the facilitator. This was a very important session in which the case managers were free to express their deepest feelings about working with infected children and their caretakers. My presence did not appear to be an impediment to their openness.

The Group As an Empathic and Supportive Milieu

I believe the case managers had positive feelings about these meetings and felt emotionally supported for a long time. Both the bereavement group facilitator and I tried to create an empathic milieu through the projection of calm demeanors and through a demonstration of respect for and interest in the group members and their expressed concerns. The case managers also gave one another emotional strength to cope with death and dying by "mirroring" or validating one another's feelings in the group. In such interactions, they showed that they understood what each was enduring through their attitudes, words, and actions. The group members came to feel alike in essential ways that worked to sustain them in a manner that Kohut, the founder of the field of self-psychology, called "twinship" (Kohut, 1984; Strozier, 2001). One case manager explained:

> It [the group] is not like talking to a friend. Friends ask you questions like, "Oh, how do you do that work?" Everyone here is doing the same thing you are. It's like a form of identification 'cause outside you are talking to friends and other people about what we do and go through. They really can't identify with us, the way we do inside this group. This is our group, and we can come here and share.

Group members came, in time, to view one another as kin or family, not just fellow workers. For them, this identification as "family" was facilitated by the fact that they were similar to one another in age, ethnicity, gender, and socioeconomic status. A number of them became close friends and socialized outside the job.

Growing Frustrations in the Group

The group's process, however, began to change a few years after I began to work with the case managers. It went from being a supportive and harmonious forum in which case managers shared deep feelings about their work with their clients to a setting in which workers used the group to express anger and frustration at Horizons. They blamed me for what they saw as Horizons' shortcomings. Bolstered by strong twinship bonds, the case managers as a team lodged a series of criticisms of the organization. They complained about steadily increasing caseloads and stated that annual pay raises were not enough. They suggested that Horizons valued and rewarded their contributions less than those of other staff. They accused Horizons of not providing sufficient opportunity for job advancement. They criticized Horizons for not allowing them to move into supervisory positions. Several case managers were angry that they were required by their affiliated program administrators to perform some non-Horizons HIV/AIDS-related work. Their joy and enthusiasm for work now seemed clouded by these feelings. They identified with one another's unhappiness and discontent in the group more than with their positivity.

My role as supervisor made me a relatively easy target for their dissatisfaction with Horizons since they regularly interacted with me and met only rarely with Horizons' directors who made the major policy decisions at the organization. I came to be viewed as "siding with administration" and as insufficiently supportive of them. Differences in gender, ethnicity, and educational background between the case managers and me that never seemed salient before took on new meaning as our relationship became more strained. I had worked previously, as a behavioral scientist and clinical social worker, not as a case manager. I was a Caucasian male in my fifties and, as the supervisor, all of my Horizons job responsibilities were on administrative and supervisory levels. Unlike the case managers, I carried no individual cases. I felt the case managers distancing themselves from me. They engaged in more private interactions with one another before and after the group supervision and seemed to be talking less openly with me than they had previously. I postponed speaking with the case managers about this apparent disconnection for a while because I wanted to give myself more time to try to understand what was happening. In hindsight, I believe this was a mistake because I lost the opportunity to try to immediately resolve growing tensions. I discussed with Horizons' directors and with the bereavement group facilitator this perceived disconnection between the case managers and me. They encouraged me to talk directly with the case managers. I eventually did; however, it appeared to be too late. The situation between us did not improve appreciably.

I felt confused, angry, and hurt about being blamed by my staff for work conditions that were not under my control. I also wondered why it was at that moment that the case managers chose to complain about Horizons' supposed shortcomings. They focused almost entirely on what they perceived that they were *not* getting from me, and they ignored talking about what they had received. I tried not to show my dismay to avoid straining our relationship further, but a reactive frustration began to develop within me.

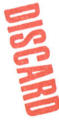

Understanding Changing Perceptions

I tried to be an empathic supervisor concerning the issues the case managers were raising, even though I was a target of their unhappiness. Some of the reasons for their discontent were clear to me and were acknowledged. I validated that their caseloads had grown significantly in tandem with the growth of the epidemic. A number of workers who originally had caseloads numbering twenty-five children and families in 1992 saw their caseloads almost double by 1995. Horizons' directors and I agreed it was unfair that a number of case managers were asked to perform additional non-Horizons

HIV/AIDS-related work in addition to their Horizons-related tasks. I made it clear that we were opposed to this practice and, in fact, I contacted a number of affiliated program administrators on numerous occasions in an effort to get them to stop giving case managers extra work. I explained to the case managers that I regularly met with Horizons' directors to discuss their concerns and to advocate for them, but I also had to tell them that it was not possible for Horizons to hire additional case managers, nor was it feasible to pay them more money because no funds were available. Even though they were previously informed of limited job mobility, the staff did not appreciate hearing of the impossibility of promotions; supervisory positions did not exist. My explanation—that limitations of grant funding made it impossible for Horizons to respond to a number of their expressed needs—did not satisfy them, and my efforts to be empathic seemed to have little impact on stemming their frustrations. Despite their complaints, however, none of the case managers chose to seek employment elsewhere.

There were, in fact, many positive aspects to the work at Horizons. Case managers were given a great deal of supervision, were sent annually to the National Pediatric HIV/AIDS Conference, and attended a weekly forum where they could meet with supportive peers away from their work sites. These were opportunities few case managers had at other HIV/AIDS social service agencies in the city. The case managers constantly had the attention of their supervisor and Horizons' directors who were extremely sympathetic and interested in satisfying their needs whenever possible. My staff knew this. I wondered why they were *so* dissatisfied. If they were so unhappy, why did they not choose to leave Horizons? They could easily have found work at other HIV/AIDS organizations, given their work experience. I concluded that underlying issues were fueling their discontent in addition to the ones they were actively voicing.

Primary and Secondary Traumatization

Increasingly, the case managers' discontent focused on the amount of work they had to do and on what they viewed to be the insufficiency of the material rewards given to them by Horizons. They spoke less in both individual and group supervision about the effect that their work with dying children was having on their psychological well-being. I concluded this was due to primary and secondary traumatization associated with their cumulative exposure to loss caused by the sickness and death of the children on their caseloads. The case managers expressed need for greater support from Horizons was a sign that they had reached, and perhaps had by then even *exceeded,* their capacity to perform such stressful work. I thought it was easier for them to state a need for greater material support than it was to openly discuss their painful reactions to losing infected children to HIV/AIDS.

By this time, the case managers had already seen too much physical deterioration of desperately sick children and too much death. They had witnessed an excessive amount of emotional pain in too many grief-ridden caretakers and had offered support to mothers of infected children on too many occasions. They were emotionally exhausted. They had helped countless families arrange for their children's funerals and had gone to far too many funerals themselves. One worker expressed how she felt:

> I guess everyone has a different level of tolerance about death, depending on how much you've seen. I have seen twenty-seven kids. I have seen more death ... I feel like a compact machine, almost like an accordion. It's a shock; you feel extremely drained by it, and then another child dies. It's a horrible feeling.

It was extremely hard psychologically for case managers to work repeatedly with anguished caretakers with whom they had forged strong emotional bonds. These caretakers had the need to share their despair with case managers in the terminal stages of their child's illness. Staff members had to bear both their own grief at seeing the child die and the caretakers' grief as well. Secondary traumatization of case managers was always a risk. One worker stated:

> It is [emotionally] tough on us workers having to come to grips—seeing someone you worked with who was healthy at one point and has gotten to the point where they are ready to pass on and have to deal with that. With the family members, discussing the funeral arrangements, and having to be there with that family member and seeing them cry, what they have to go through to make those arrangements; it is tough. It is not easy.

Other writers have described how HIV/AIDS workers frequently experienced anticipatory grief and mourning and had to confront their own mortality (Halin-Willinger et al., 1999; Winiarski, 1991). The horror and trauma of multiple deaths commonly produced "psychic numbing" (Lifton, 1979), anger, and irritability among workers (Schoen, 1998; Warren, 1998). "Secondary or vicarious traumatization," resulting in psychological avoidance, desensitization, and hyperarousal (McCann and Pearlman, 1990), came from assisting the emotionally suffering family, as well as the infected child, over time. Absenteeism, stress, sickness, and job turnover were common worker responses (Maslach and Ozer, 1995).

I increasingly saw the expression of case manager frustration to be a sign of emotional neediness and of internal turmoil resulting from having performed several years of traumatizing work in a death-infused environment. The collective expression of resentment at both the organization and me was cathartic for the case managers. The false perception that Horizons was able to offer the case managers more resources but was not doing so, I concluded, was a collective psychological construct of the case managers. They created an "organizational straw man" so to speak, which provided a target and an outlet for them to direct their feelings of anger, frustration, hopelessness, and despair. These profound emotions were expressions of my staff's inability to reverse the tragic course of HIV/AIDS in their clients' lives.

It was perhaps easier for the case managers to talk about what was not being given by me and by Horizons than to continue to explore and feel their inner pain. When I explored this possibility with them, it was, not surprisingly, rejected. Burnout and emotional exhaustion are not always recognizable by those who experience them. Even if one does recognize burnout, it is not necessarily easy to identify all the factors contributing to the condition. It was, I thought, perhaps too difficult for the case managers to realize that after several years of performing traumatizing work many of them had reached their limits in their abilities to continue doing such difficult work.

Horizons' directors and I tried to address all of the case managers' complaints in a variety of different ways, such as holding retreats and utilizing supervision to discuss their particular needs. Horizons publicly acknowledged the special contributions of all of the case managers at luncheons held in recognition of them and of other staff. Eventually, however, despite these and other efforts made by the organization, a number of the case managers who had worked for Horizons for up to four years started looking for and found work elsewhere. In 1999, I, too, left Horizons after being offered a teaching position. I made this decision in part because I felt somewhat burned out from this particular type of work, but also because I was offered a job that involved teaching at a school of social work. I had enjoyed teaching earlier in my professional career and wanted the opportunity to do so in this particular type of setting—a school of social work.

CONCLUSIONS

Horizons was, and remains, an excellent pediatric HIV/AIDS organization, but however well it succeeded in attaining its overall goals of helping children and families live with HIV/AIDS, it was, like similar programs, limited by the funding that supported its work. Staff at Horizons, including case managers, doctors, nurses, and directors, were always operating in a crisis mode. There was never enough money to hire a sufficient number of workers to significantly reduce work pressures. Increased workloads followed from the rise in the numbers of newly infected individuals, especially women and children living in the inner-city neighborhoods served by Horizons. Horizons' case managers, who worked tirelessly on the front lines of the epidemic, understandably grew emotionally exhausted as a result of their work with increasing numbers of infected children and their families. Case management supervision helped them to cope psychologically in a difficult work environment for a longer period of time than would have been possible without the intensive level of supervision they received.

In such a stressful work environment in which case managers are exposed over long periods of time to the death of children and the grief of affected family members, worker frustrations, emotional exhaustion, and burnout are likely to emerge among even the most enthusiastic and dedicated employees. In my opinion, this is even more likely to occur if caseloads are not capped, if salary increases are small, and if job advancement is not possible, as was the case with Horizons' case managers.

It is essential for HIV/AIDS supervisors to be alert to the beginning signs of burnout in their staff, including indications of fatigue, demoralization, and emotional exhaustion. It is important that supervisors talk with staff members about these conditions in a nondefensive, direct, and supportive manner at the moment they arise. The cumulative effects of stress on workers must be acknowledged and dealt with by program administrators and by supervisors before worker fatigue becomes irreversible. It is sometimes difficult but necessary and even ethically responsible for a supervisor to raise the possibility or probability of emotional burnout and to assist the worker to transition elsewhere.

My work at Horizons convinced me of how important it is for supervisors to find their own support systems, both professional and personal. I was not so much affected by the loss of infected children and by the despair of affected families as the case managers were. However, I was seriously impacted by the frustrated emotional reactions of the case managers and by their expressions of unhappiness that were directed at me. I found this experience at times to be psychologically dismaying and anger provoking. This complex set of emotions needs to be analyzed and worked through if the supervisor is to function effectively in his or her role over time.

Individual and group supervision should be available to all staff at HIV/AIDS organizations. It is essential that HIV/AIDS program administrators and policymakers find ways to mitigate the inevitable impact that primary and secondary traumatization and other work-related stressors have on the psychological well-being of staff and on worker attrition, even in a postprotease HIV/AIDS work environment. Protease inhibitors are currently either ineffective or cannot be tolerated for a variety of reasons for anywhere from 20 to 50 percent of all infected persons (Kelley et al., 2000). There is a high rate of failure to adhere to recommended treatment regimens by HIV/AIDS-infected individuals, especially children and adolescents (National Institute of Allergy and Infectious Diseases, 2001). HIV/AIDS staff will continue to work into the indefinite future with infected persons for whom protease inhibitors never worked, stopped working, or have worked only minimally. HIV/AIDS staff members are likely to experience the negative emotional consequences related to treatment failure with their clients into the indefinite future. Let not the lessons of yesterday be forgotten in the present.

REFERENCES

Centers for Disease Control and Prevention (1998). Trends in the HIV and AIDS epidemic, 1988: A turning point in the epidemic. *Morbidity and Mortality Weekly 43*(11): 1-20.

Gallegos, S. M. (1998). Providing services to HIV-positive women. In D. M. Aronstein and B. J. Thompson (Eds.), *HIV and social work: A practitioner's guide* (pp. 431-443). Binghamton, NY: The Haworth Press.

Halin-Willinger, B., Powers, M., Carlson, C., Lee, L., Beaudet, M., Bernson, M., and Kleinschmidt, J. (1999). Social work with hospitalized AIDS patients: Observations from the front lines of an inner city hospital. In M. Shernoff (Ed.), *AIDS and mental health practice: Clinical and policy issues* (pp. 221-234). Binghamton, NY: The Haworth Press.

Kelley, J., Otto-Salaj, L. L., Sikkema, K. J., Pinkerton, S. D., and Bloom, F. R. (2000). Implications of HIV treatment advances for behavioral research on AIDS: Protease inhibitors and new challenges in HIV secondary prevention. *Health Psychology 17*(4): 310-319.

Kohut, H. (1984). *How does analysis cure?* Chicago: The University of Chicago Press.

Lifton, R. J. (1979). *The broken connection: On death and the continuity of life.* New York: Basic Books.

Maslach, C. and Ozer, E. (1995). The measurement of experienced burnout. *Journal of Occupational Behavior 2:* 99-113.

McCann, I. and Pearlman, L. A. (1990). Vicarious traumatization: A contextual model for understanding the effects of trauma on helpers. *Journal of Traumatic Stress 3*(1): 131-149.

National Institute of Allergy and Infectious Diseases (2001). HIV treatment guidelines updated for adults and adolescents. *NIAID News,* February 14.

O'Leary, A. and Jemmott, L. (Eds.) (1995). *Women at risk: Issues in the primary prevention of AIDS.* New York: Plenum Press.

Schoen, K. (1998). Caring for ourselves: Understanding and minimizing the stresses of HIV caregiving. In D. M. Ironstone and B. J. Thompson (Eds.), *HIV and social work: A practitioner's guide* (pp. 527-536). Binghamton, NY: The Haworth Press.

Strozier, C. B. (2001). *Heinz Kohut: The making of a psychoanalyst.* New York: Farrar, Straus, and Giroux.

U.S. Department of Health and Human Services Administration, HIV/AIDS Bureau (2000). *Fact sheet: Title IV Ryan White Care Act* [Online].<ftp.hrsa.gov/hab/titleIVfact.pdf>.

Warren, J. R. (1998). Meeting the emotional health care needs of health care providers. In D. M. Ironstone and B. J. Thompson (Eds.), *HIV and social work: A practitioner's guide* (pp. 537-540). Binghamton, NY: The Haworth Press.

Winiarski, M. (1991). *AIDS-related psychotherapy.* Needham Heights, MA: Longwood Professional Books.

Chapter 19

Social Work with Hospitalized AIDS Patients: Observations from the Front Lines of an Inner-City Hospital

Barbara Willinger
Martha Powers
Chris Carlson
Lorna Andria Lee
Mary Beaudet
Miriam Bernson Adams
John Kleinschmidt

In the time since the AIDS pandemic burst upon the world, there have been many changes in the treatment of this illness that affect the length of a patient's hospitalization. However, what remains constant is the spectrum of issues facing our patients, including receiving the diagnosis, entitlement referrals, coping and living with HIV/AIDS, and eventually decline and death. In addition, our patients' lives are often further complicated by substance abuse, character pathology, poverty, racism, and tenuous family supports. Much of the work, therefore, on our inpatient unit can become crisis driven or focused on short-term, goal-oriented interventions. Although this type of work in and of itself is effective, the model used by this group of writers, as well as others, encompasses a broader perspective known as "continuity of care." This model allows staff the potential for involvement in the patient's life and the development of a therapeutic relationship over time, as well as for the exigencies of transference and countertransference reactions.

As patients struggle with the devastating effects of HIV/AIDS, so too, although differently, do staff. It is well documented that those who work with

This chapter was originally published in M. Shernoff (Ed.) (1999), *AIDS and Mental Health Practice,* Binghamton, NY: The Haworth Press (pp. 221-234).

persons with AIDS (PWAs) must be vigilant against emotional fatigue and demoralization (Rando, 1984; Robbins, 1983; Winiarski, 1991). This chapter is the culmination of discussions by a team of social workers and their supervisor about the common and disparate ways each needed and/or sought support. In addition, their personal accounts are placed in the context of an already-existing schematic progression of adaptation to working with the terminally ill from the perspective of the professional caregiver. Our experiences also support the work of Ross (1993), Anderson and Wilke (1991), McCann and Pearlman (1990), and Winiarski (1991), all of whom discuss the necessity of good clinical supervision to ensure professional longevity and avoid painful burnout and isolation. Clinical supervision is defined as a place and a person with whom the work can be processed.

HARPER MODEL: RESPONSES AND VIGNETTES

Kübler-Ross (1969) developed a series of stages defining patients' processes regarding their cancer diagnosis that helped clinicians to understand and frame their clinical work. Harper (1977) developed a schematic growth and development scale that described the normative sequence of emotional and psychological progress that health care professionals traversed to reach a comfort level which allowed them to work with patients facing death. Similar to the stages created by Kübler-Ross, in which patients can either fluidly shift from one stage to another or remain stalled in one place, so too the Harper model needs to be viewed as a process in which professional caregivers will proceed and regress. The model is presented by using illustrations of the authors' personal experiences juxtaposed with case vignettes.

The first stage described by Harper is the use of intellectualization. During this stage, the professional focuses on professional knowledge as a means to decrease latent anxieties of working with the dying patient and facing the resultant death. Within the parameters of the acute care hospital unit and one's adaptation to the setting, we have found that this process takes at least six months.

Chris, on the unit eight months at the time of this writing, is the father of two children and came to social work as a second career. His position on the AIDS unit was his first inpatient experience and, like most new workers, he found himself "treading into a new sea of systems, acronyms, and abbreviations." During the entry into AIDS work, paperwork can often symbolize realizable and tangible tasks on the patients' behalf that are more quantifiable than the counseling process often is.

Chris brought to social work his sense of community service and history of activism and of wanting to improve individual and community systems. Although intellectually aware that his "patients' set of circumstances are not mine to fix" he carefully worked on where to enter into each patient's struggle "against the undertow of helplessness" often associated with terminal illness. At the same time, Chris kept his own perspective about such helplessness. Processing these contrapuntal but always colliding forces became the initial goals of supervision and in staff support group.

Chris recalls experiencing much frustration in his first months, as he spent more time learning systems than working with patients. Along with the immersion in paperwork, Chris experienced the overwhelming emotional barrage of the cycle of illness and death: "I still couldn't, professionally speaking, keep track of my practice work, my use of self, and the patients' needs as I wanted to. But I knew I was progressing, both learning more and discovering my realistic limitations. I was establishing a foundation of understanding that we are hand in hand with the larger forces of disease, death and biology." The mastery of the initial stage facilitates the professional's concentration on the patient in a new way by allowing intense clinical relationships to be formed.

Harper's second stage entails the professional experiencing death on an emotional level while feeling traumatized as they confront the deaths of their patients and the reality of their own eventual mortality.

John was hired as an inpatient AIDS social worker after completion of his graduate training, which had included a field placement on an AIDS unit. He had come to social work only after becoming aware of his own HIV seropositivity. John's ultimate disclosure of his HIV-positive status to his colleagues and supervisor was to have ramifications in his professional relationships as well as for his own personal growth.

John began work with Robert when the patient was admitted to the hospital with severe shortness of breath. He was soon diagnosed with Kaposi's sarcoma of the lungs. Robert, a twenty-three-year-old African-American college student, had only recently learned of his HIV-positive status. Robert formed an almost instantaneous alliance with John. Most likely this grew out of Robert's intense anxiety and helplessness, as well as his need for mirroring and validation. The close relationship between worker and client was also aided by John's identification with, sensitivity toward, and empathy for Robert. Their work together focused on minimizing Robert's feelings of shame and guilt, his fear of losses, and his need to confront reality and to develop coping strategies. After two and a half weeks of hospitalization, Robert was discharged home. He returned to his family, who had not yet settled into an acceptance of Robert's health status or the fact that he was gay. Robert was given John's office telephone number for emergency contact. Within twenty-four hours he called, complaining of shortness of breath and friction with his family. He was instructed to call the EMS. John returned to the hospital after the weekend to find Robert intubated, with medical personnel frantically trying to help him before he was to be transferred to the intensive care unit (ICU). Within a few minutes, John was made aware that the prognosis was poor.

John's journey and struggle with the impact of his own HIV status was reopened by Robert's situation. In the ensuing hours, John sought support from his supervisor and co-workers at their weekly unit meeting and later at their staff support group. Because John had previously revealed his status to his supervisor, their individual supervisory time was utilized in helping John differentiate his own fears and anxieties from those of Robert. In this way, John could face his anticipated grief and mourning for Robert. This catharsis and processing allowed John to be with Robert and Robert's family in a professionally caring way that did not merge or confuse John's issues and boundaries with the patient's. Robert's situation provided John with his own watershed experience:

> catalyzing my accumulated losses—friends, patients, self—and it all poured out. Without the support of my peers and the disclosure of my health status to my supervisor, I couldn't have processed this case. Robert's illness allowed me to find a working distance in which to continue without overwhelming emotional vulnerability. The work has since normalized.

In the absence of being able to confront one's own vulnerability, Harper postulates the third stage as "grow or go," in which mastery of self is a challenge. Such mastery involves an increasing acceptance of the realities of death and dying as well as the notion that we cannot make our patients well. Professional caregivers experiencing this stage often vacillate between accepting death and denying its inevitability.

Martha had done a fieldwork placement in a counseling agency where she had worked with PWAs. She spent six months doing inpatient AIDS work with this team. She was then transferred to the program's outpatient clinic, where she met Cynthia after working there for a year.

Cynthia was well known at the clinic but had avoided medical appointments for several years and was noncompliant with any treatment plans. Martha's first contact with Cynthia occurred as a result of Cynthia's need for insurance clarification. After initial reluctance, Cynthia agreed to meet with Martha. In their ongoing sessions, Cynthia raged about the unfairness of having AIDS and her fears regarding disclosure to her family and friends. She maintained distance by wearing dark sunglasses and leaving sessions when she became too tearful. When hospitalized within a few months of their first contact, Cynthia was seen by another social worker. Upon Cynthia's return to the clinic as an outpatient, she vociferously expressed her anger and disappointment that Martha had not made arrangements to cover her while she was hospitalized. It became clear to Martha that a strong alliance and transference had developed that could, and needed to, include any social work coverage Cynthia required. From that time on, their meetings were sustained through painful affect, but Cynthia no longer wore her dark glasses.

During a subsequent admission, Cynthia lapsed into a coma. It was during this time that Martha learned about Cynthia from her family. Her source of infection had come from a man whom she no longer planned to marry, but with whom she still lived. She had been raised by her grandmother. Her biological mother, though involved in Cynthia's upbringing, was someone for whom Cynthia held contempt. Both women had recently been told by Cynthia of her illness. In the same meeting between Martha and Cynthia's family, it was agreed that Cynthia's twenty-one-year-old daughter must also be told about her mother's illness. Martha was cognizant of her own profound sadness, not for someone she had known for years, but for someone with whom she had only recently developed an intimate attachment. While experiencing this anticipatory grief, Martha began to realize that professional relationships often engender deeper feelings of connectedness that are not always obvious until the patients are near death.

Quite unexpectedly, however, Cynthia came out of her coma and talked of wanting to return home. As Martha proceeded with the arrangements, she also listened to Cynthia review her losses and the failures in her life. Cynthia asked Martha to help plan her funeral, eulogy, and cremation. Cynthia's health continued to decline during this time, and Martha waited for Cynthia's death.

Through supervision, Martha was able to unblock her feelings and identify her fear and pain as it related to the ebb and flow of Cynthia's deterioration toward death. When Cynthia died, Martha attended the funeral, feeling out of place since the only professional connection to Cynthia's family had been in their meetings at the hospital. Martha mourned and reviewed her work with Cynthia in supervision and support groups. In both settings, Martha began to let go of Cynthia and to find a place for her feelings, with the realization that she had assisted Cynthia in making peace with parts of her life.

Cynthia's case reflects the omnipresent struggle of professional versus personal self with which Martha had been grappling. Martha believed that "a professional stance always required distance." However, Cynthia's directness, despite her delirium and dementia, called for "complete involvement. I battled with myself, saying, 'Don't put lotion on her leg; don't wipe her brow; don't kiss her on the forehead.' But Cynthia brought me right in. There was no way around my full use of self. While Cynthia demanded the human, she needed the professional, and if I had been there halfway, she would have kicked me out of the room." Some staff are not able to traverse this stage and either remain within it, grappling with the issues of professional connectedness to patients, or decide to leave the setting.

The next stage that Harper describes is one of emotional arrival, involving moderation, mitigation, and accommodation. During this stage the worker leaves behind the debilitating effects of the previous stages. This is also the stage at which professionals more readily accept death and dying and are not incapacitated by the depression they may feel concerning their own good health.

Miriam had several years of social work experience prior to graduate training. Although not a novice to AIDS work, St. Luke's was her first full-time hospital AIDS employment. An energetic and physically active woman, Miriam likens her work with patients to running a marathon. She often describes the work as requiring her "to pay close attention to the job of putting one foot in front of the other." She seeks to assist each patient in gaining a sense of control over the disease process, as incorporated into the patient-worker contract. This can vary from mourning a loss of attractiveness and/or position within the social system to planning for the future of survivors or facing the arduous and crisis-filled disease process.

Miriam began her work with Elbia soon after the patient was diagnosed with AIDS. Elbia had grown up in an impoverished region of Honduras. She married early and immigrated to New York City, where she raised her four children while suffering periodic physical assaults by her husband. When her husband was hospitalized with, and later died of, AIDS, Elbia knew she too had been infected. Rather than finding her life made easier by the death of her abusive husband, she found herself a virtual hostage in the family apartment, which her children had transformed into a crack house. In her passivity and shame, Elbia had created a self-imposed prison. She confided to Miriam that being hospitalized allowed her to feel "safe" for the first time in her life.

Over the two months that Elbia remained on the unit, she opened up her life through laughter and tears. She shared a side of herself that she had always kept hidden. She experienced a strong sense of control and destiny regarding death, which had eluded her in her lifetime, from her belief in Santeria. Miriam knew that Elbia related to her and the staff as the transferential "good mother." This was confirmed in Elbia's poignant plea not to be transferred to a nursing home: "This is the only place where anyone has ever cared about me. . . . This is where I want to die." Although Elbia initially described her life as devoid of security, self-confidence, and environmental support—aspects of life highly valued by Miriam—by her life's end, Elbia had been able to attain these through the power of her relationship with Miriam and the other staff members. As it turned out, Elbia did not have to endure another perceived abuse/abandonment; she died in the hospital. Watching Elbia die was painful for Miriam, but this task is a frequent reality of working with AIDS patients.

Miriam was able to forge a deep relationship with Elbia that helped sustain her through the patient's long, erratic deterioration. According to Miriam, the lengthy hospitalization

> gave me the time to process things along the way, then to assist Elbia in working through her feelings of deprivation, and to die in peace. I was able to respect Elbia's strengths and remain her ally and partner in the process, rather than her caretaker.

In the fifth and final stage of development, Harper refers to deep compassion involving self-realization, self-awareness, and self-actualization.

> [A] concern for the dying patient is translated into constructive and appropriate activities based on a humane and professional assessment of the dying patient and the family. They understand and accept that in some instances, living can be more painful than dying. (1977, p. 435)

Barbara, the supervising social worker for this team, met Darren, a thirty-five-year-old African-American gay man, when he was initially diagnosed with Kaposi's sarcoma of the lungs. A call from the physician requested social work intervention due to Darren's "upset reaction" to the news. During the initial consultation,

Darren, a handsome young man, lay in bed with the covers pulled up to his chin. It was apparent that he was not going to engage in spontaneous conversation but rather needed and responded to gently asked questions, explanations about his medical condition, and statements regarding entitlements.

By the end of the first meeting, Darren had revealed that this was his characterological pattern to keep things to himself, "close to my chest." His friend later affirmed that Darren had shared a surprisingly significant amount of information with Barbara. Darren was discharged two days later and contact was sustained by telephone, as Darren struggled with the effects of chemotherapy and the ramifications of Kaposi's sarcoma. In the succeeding two months, Darren was hospitalized three times for about three days per admission. Although weaker, Darren refused home care. When questioned about this, he indicated that his family, with whom he lived, was unable to take care of him. One day Darren called Barbara, sounding breathless and as if he were choking. He asked nothing, seemed to be home alone, and consented to Barbara's calling 911. Barbara later discovered, when she called Darren back, that two family members were in fact at home but unaware of his current state. This was consistent with Darren's keeping his family "out of my business." Darren was admitted to the hospital. The family was grateful for Barbara's intervention, and Darren agreed to home care following this discharge from the hospital.

Time had run out for Darren, however, and within a week he was readmitted for the last time. The purpose of Barbara's intervention was to clarify with the physician the need for palliative care, as well as being the compassionate visitor that Darren needed at this time, just two days prior to his death. It was only after Darren's burial that the family verbalized the importance that Darren had placed on his contact with Barbara. This resolved questions that Barbara had had during her work with Darren, a reluctant and seemingly disconnected participant in his own treatment.

Barbara struggled with the treatment plan for Darren in his final months. She made decisions with him and for him based on her experience rather than on the explicit information communicated by him. The work with Darren represented for Barbara

> much of the skill and expertise I have acquired and internalized over the years. The use of self as well as the continuing process of self-reflection often mesh into an ultimately gratifying experience that provides sustenance for this work.

A MODEL OF HOSPITAL AIDS WORK

How do those of us working with AIDS patients navigate the waters of grief and associated turmoil? What is needed to assist and sustain us as we embark on and continue the journey of working with AIDS patients? Even the most accomplished professional cannot withstand the intensity and constancy of the onslaught of powerful feelings that erupt at varying times during the work if there are insufficient supports. Even though our relationship with patients is usually peripheral rather than central, as are family and sig-nificant others, we too can experience "bereavement overload" (Rando, 1984, p. 430), unless the losses are processed. We can, perhaps, draw a par-allel between PWAs who cope more effectively with their condition through the availability of support and professional caregivers whose potential for burnout is minimized by similar assistance (Rando, 1984; Ross, 1993; Win-iarski, 1991).

Webster's New World Dictionary defines support as "help . . . to advocate . . . to maintain with assistance . . . to endure" (1990, p. 593). We postulate that there are different venues of support potentially available to those working with PWAs: departmental, supervisory, collegial, multidisciplinary team, support group, personal therapy, and life-affirming activities. We have found that the combination of any, if not all, of these, provides the possibil-ity of maximizing individuals' capacity and long-term commitment to the work.

Departmental support. Such support emanates from social work admin-istrators in the form of acknowledgment of, respect for, and validation of the differences and difficulty of AIDS work. In contrast, countertransferential reaction toward PWAs, whether on the part of social work or hospital ad-ministrators who consider AIDS patients a low priority, can potentially di-minish or contaminate a necessary avenue for support.

Supervisory support. Although this will be elaborated upon later in this chapter, authors such as Anderson and Wilke (1991), Rando (1984), Rob-bins (1983), and Ross (1993) emphasize the necessity for adequate support and supervision. Adequate supportive supervision is defined as providing the opportunity for assessment and evaluation of the individual's work per-formance, as well as emotional responses to the work. Working with dying patients evokes varying degrees of emotional reactions and investments. It follows that a grief response and/or decathexis is not only essential but must be legitimized and accepted within the supervisory process to ameliorate or prevent some of the potentially damaging effects of the work.

Collegial support. Although it is not necessary that staff be homogenous in terms of race, class, gender, sexual orientation, HIV status, or profes-sional style and capabilities, it is necessary that they respect one another's differences and care about one another. In this way, they not only individu-ally or collectively share in one another's grieving and growth but also are available for professional coverage and assistance.

Multidisciplinary team support. A variety of perspectives applied to a pa-tient's case can serve all involved, reducing the isolation felt by a worker and providing the patient with a better-balanced care plan. Also, loss and subsequent grieving are more likely to be experienced as a group, potentially allowing for both the acceptance of and follow through with, this process.

Support group. The existence of a hospital-based group depends on numerous factors, ranging from the availability of departmental funds to hire an outside facilitator to the willingness of line staff to share their intimate reactions with peers. However, the literature gives credence to the importance of such a group in alleviating the stress of working with PWAs, thus enhancing the capacity of these individuals to continue their work (Anderson and Wilke, 1991; Grossman and Silverstein, 1993).

Each staff member had different examples about the value of such a support group in doing AIDS work. Whether it was a personal crisis, disclosure, threats of layoffs, discussion of professional difficulties with patients, or the grief of constant loss through death, the group helped pull the team together in a way different from that provided by individual supervision. The group has provided a place for mutual safety in which transferences to supervisors could also be clarified.

Personal therapy. Given that AIDS work frequently touches on one's own archaic feelings, the experience of current or previous individual and/or group therapy can facilitate the processing and understanding of those often-felt turbulent reactions.

Life-affirming activities. These can range from spiritual to physical to intellectual to creative to family-oriented pursuits, as long as they expand and enhance the individual's life. For example, Miriam avidly engages in running and rock climbing as a means of regaining her serenity and control. Lorna attends church regularly and is involved in community affairs.

Supervision

The model of social work AIDS case management we present relies significantly on strong supervision that is flexibly concrete, supportive, challenging, therapeutic (intrapsychic), and educational. Kadushin (1985) enumerates three major components of supervision: administrative, educational, and supportive. He further elaborates that

> one of the major functions of the supervisor is to provide certain emotional supports for the worker. She must encourage, strengthen, stimulate and ever comfort-pacify. The supervisor seeks to allay anxiety, fortify flagging faith, affirm and reinforce the worker's assets, replenish depleted self esteem, nourish and enhance ego capacity for adaptation, alleviate psychological pain, restore emotional equilibrium, comfort, bolster and refresh. (p. 229)

In a positive worker-supervisor relationship, the supervisor is never far from participating in these functions on a daily basis. At the same time, the authors contend that it is the depth of the supervisor's clinical expertise that will raise the work with PWAs above the level of complex discharge planning to an understanding of the intricacies of the patient-worker relationship. This knowledge can come through understanding the unconscious mirroring occurring within the supervisory process—patient-worker, worker-supervisor—as well as the nature of the transference.

Successful supervision will encompass any or all of the indications described, while acting as a holding environment or container of the worker's myriad affective reactions. It was on the strength of Lorna's trusting relationship with her supervisor that her issues with the patient in the following case discussion could be crystallized, understood, and worked through. This was Lorna's second social work position. After one and a half years on a medical/surgical unit of another hospital, where she had begun to see AIDS patients as part of her work, she sought to engage in this practice full time.

Lacquana, a thirty-two-year-old African-American woman with full-blown AIDS, was an active crack abuser with a history of noncompliance. She frequently signed out against medical advice (AMA) and sabotaged medical care or discharge plans to which she had previously agreed. During admissions, she usually related to staff on the unit in a demanding, infantile, and impulsive manner. For some time, she induced in Lorna a sense of anger and helplessness, due to her expressed for interventions and then, ultimately, her rejection of them.

In supervision, Lorna reviewed these interactions while gathering further information about Lacquana's life, which had been and currently was saturated with physical abuse and abandonment. AIDS was just another cruel blow for this already emotionally deprived and regressed woman. In understanding Lacquana's repetition of the need for, and particularly the fear of, intimacy as it emerged in the therapeutic interactions, Lorna was ultimately able to provide Lacquana with a different maternal experience than she had known before. The trust in and knowledge from the supervisory relationship was reflected positively in Lorna's work with Lacquana.

Although Lacquana never made any concrete lifestyle changes in the course of her illness, which lasted one year, she was able to internalize Lorna's sense of constancy and dependability. This allowed her to utilize Lorna as her auxiliary ego to discuss her dying process as her respiratory functioning deteriorated. Lacquana initiated the discussion that resulted in her decision not to be intubated and to die with appropriate comfort care. Perhaps for the first time in her life, Lacquana engaged in adult decision making.

Supervision played yet another role as it assisted Mary, after great personal loss, to clarify her relationship to the field of social work. Mary's decision to become a social worker stemmed from the experience of her mother's death. Her family did not verbalize their loss and bereavement, and Mary believed that social work, unlike advertising, her previous career, would offer her such an opportunity.

Mary had done field placement in a hospital neonatal intensive care unit, then she came to AIDS work wanting to expand her skills and intensify her work with terminally ill patients. Within the first months, she experienced several patient deaths and felt sadness for only one whom she had been able to reach as had no other professional provider. Mary felt quite confident not only about her skills in case managing but also in her ability to go through the losses of cognition and physical deterioration experienced by her patients, which she viewed as "part of the package" of working with AIDS patients. This homeostasis was soon interrupted when her father became ill, was admitted to an ICU, and was intubated. Mary continued to work, informing her supervisor of her personal crisis. Not unexpectedly, Mary defended against the emotionality of her AIDS work to remain connected to the myriad feelings of her father's crisis and subsequent death. During that time, her excellence at case management reflected the displacement of her need to remain effective.

When Mary returned to work after her father's burial, she resumed her work by arranging timely discharges and efficiently completing documents and forms. Initially, she addressed the loss of her father in supervision, but eventually this ended. Gradually, Barbara, the supervisor, became aware of a paucity of emotional connectedness in Mary's work with her patients. Due to the sense of a parallel process between the detachment from her patients and Mary's need to protect herself from her own personal loss, Barbara chose not to offer her perception of this impasse. Rather than make a potentially premature and possibly intrusive intervention, Barbara chose to step back and allow Mary to remain in what seemed a protected position, allowing for grieving and healing to occur in Mary's own style. It was a patient situation, however, that jettisoned Mary toward the emotional re-evaluation of self that she had begun months earlier.

The patient, Alonzo, received his AIDS diagnosis simultaneously with the results of his HIV test. Alonzo had denied all risk factors despite a diagnosis of *Pneumocystis carinii* pneumonia (PCP). Mary listened to his fears and provided information aimed at comforting him. Since PCP is now usually resolvable, no one—least of all Mary—expected his quick decline. Alonzo was soon transferred to ICU and intubated. He remained on the respirator for two weeks, with chart notations showing his declining prognosis from poor to dismal. Mary visited him several times, despite his inability to communicate with or recognize anyone. After his death, Barbara and Mary reviewed the process of the work and Mary's reaction, helping Mary to clarify what had occurred. The phrase "life imitates art" had transformed itself into "work imitates life." During her father's death, Mary needed to be the "professional" for herself and her family; with Alonzo, she could be the "person," as she relived her father's death and felt the emotional impact of her loss.

After this, Mary "felt ready" to tackle her continuing involvement and struggles with her patients. With several of them, her work reflected an emotional connection to their myriad needs. However, in general, she experienced a sense of frustration, initially attributed to the substance abusing population with whom she was primarily working. Exploration of countertransferential reactions, education, clinical techniques, and support were offered over the next several months. Ultimately, Mary was confronted with the need to clarify for herself whether her continuing ambivalence was stemming from her work with a substance abusing population, the AIDS population, or a yet unidentified source. Mary remained in direct AIDS patient care until the summer of 1998.

CONCLUSION

Hospital social work/case management with AIDS patients presents a hybrid of psychosocial needs for which staff must be attuned, skilled, and ever ready to respond. These needs can range from the mixture of a person's receiving an HIV and AIDS diagnosis to a patient's rapid deterioration and death. At the same time, hospital social work demands that staff have the capacity and enjoy being able to react quickly to crisis, "shifting gears" as needed. There is no day in a hospital that is predictable.

It is the authors' combined experience that all this, even multiple deaths, can be managed as long as there is the availability of and time for clinical supervision, as well as the presence of the supervisor for brief consultation as needed to meet the ongoing exigencies of our patients. Despite the supervisor's provision of an atmosphere that meets "the basic psychological needs of safety, trust, power, esteem, and intimacy" (McCann and Pearlman, 1990, p. 137), there is an additional need for the other supports that have been described in this chapter. Without these, AIDS social workers may be prone to becoming overwhelmed by the vulnerability and isolation often cited and felt by our patients.

REFERENCES

Anderson, C. and Wilke, P. (1991). *Reflective helping in HIV and AIDS.* Washington, DC: Open University Press.

Grossman, A. and Silverstein, C. (1993). Facilitating support groups for professionals working with people with AIDS. *Social Work 38*(2): 144-151.

Harper, B.C. (1977). *Death: The coping mechanism of the health professional.* Greenville, SC: Southern University Press.

Kadushin, A. (1985). *Supervision in social work,* Second edition. New York: Columbia University Press.

Kübler-Ross, E. (1969). *On death and dying.* New York: Macmillan.

McCann, L. and Pearlman, L. (1990). Vicarious traumatization: A framework for understanding the psychological effects of working with victims. *Journal of Traumatic Stress 3*(1): 131-148.

Rando, T. (1984). *Grief, dying and death: Clinical intervention for care givers.* Champaign, IL: Research Press.

Robbins, J. (1983). *Caring for the dying patient and family.* New York: Harper and Row.

Ross, E. (1993). Preventing burnout among social workers employed in the field of AIDS/HIV. *Social Work in Healthcare 18*(2): 91-108.

Webster's new world dictionary (1990). V. Neufeldt (Ed.). New York: Warner Books.

Winiarski, M. (1991). *AIDS-related psychotherapy.* Needham Heights, MA: Longwood Professional Books.

SECTION IV:
THE DECLINE/THE FUTURE—
WHAT DOES IT LOOK LIKE?

Chapter 20

Social Work, New York State AIDS Centers, and Special Needs Plans

Eli Camhi

Social workers have been on the front line serving the HIV-infected and -affected community since the very beginning of the epidemic. In New York City, from the mid-1980s through the mid-1990s, most AIDS cases were first encountered in hospitals. Hospital social workers, traditionally employed as discharge planners, were among the first to serve these individuals, partnering with nurses, physicians, and other health care providers struggling to overcome the often lethal consequences of untreated opportunistic infections while attempting to restore the patient's social, economic, and psychological support system.

Hospital administrators, medical directors, and social work departments soon learned that to address the complex and multiple needs of newly diagnosed AIDS patients, dedicated multidisciplinary teams were necessary. The AIDS Institute of the New York State Department of Health developed specialized contracts for hospitals willing to create and support such teams. These hospitals were called designated AIDS centers (DACs) and were required to establish a continuum of care that included dedicated inpatient AIDS units linked with outpatient HIV primary care clinics often within departments of infectious diseases. Experienced multidisciplinary teams were created to include physicians, nurses, social workers, counselors, psychiatrists, dieticians, and assorted hospital clerical and administrative staff.

To recruit hospitals to become DACs, the state compensated them with an enhanced outpatient HIV primary care Medicaid rate to offset care team costs. In addition, the state provided the DACs with the ability to select either per diem or DRG (diagnosis-related group) rate of payment. Most DACs chose the per diem rate over the DRG rate because of the unadjusted DRG rate; for example, the standard of care for treatment of *Pneumocystis carinii* pneumonia (PCP) was twenty-one days of IV therapy in contrast to the DRG rate of only sixteen days. The state's fiscal strategies catalyzed rapid change in the care delivery system. Prominent hospitals added specialized staff members quickly, including AIDS center social workers in inpatient and outpatient settings. A fundamental component of the model was aggressive and specialized case management by specialized social workers at various points of care.

In the mid-1990s, breakthroughs in AIDS drug development resulted in the availability of antiretroviral therapies that dramatically reduced the virus's ability to compromise patient immune systems and permit opportunistic infections. This, in turn, resulted in dramatic and significant declines in deaths, hospitalizations, and lengths of stay. In AIDS centers and other hospitals throughout New York State, the total average daily inpatient AIDS census dropped from 2,646 in 1992 to 1,276 in 1998, approximately 52 percent (Chiasson et al., 1998).

These trends required another significant shift in the service delivery model. Prior to 1995, staff resources for AIDS care were concentrated heavily on hospital inpatient units. Some AIDS centers provided one inpatient social worker for every twelve to eighteen hospitalized AIDS patients. In the early days of the epidemic some New York City hospitals averaged a daily inpatient AIDS census of well over sixty patients (Chiasson et al., 1997). With the success of new treatments, outpatient care was now center stage. Clinics began to experience rapid growth as patients sought access to these new therapies. Some hospitals wisely reallocated the now surplus inpatient team of social workers and others to the outpatient setting to meet the increasing demand for service, but many others did not. Pressure on hospitals to decrease costs resulted in a significant reduction of social work staff and, in some cases, the downsizing of hospital social work departments.

When length of stay (LOS) declined, per diem rates in most cases paid less per patient than DRGs; it was then that most DACs abandoned the per diem rate. When LOS declined, clinic cost increased because more patients entered and remained in care. Unfortunately, outpatient AIDS care is not entirely self-sufficient. For many years, AIDS center clinics were subsidized with inpatient dollars as well as by various federal grants. This trend of shifting from a predominately inpatient model to one of predominately outpatient care did not go unnoticed. The AIDS Institute, again, began to plan for a change in reimbursement for the HIV care delivery system.

As early as 1995, the state began to develop a unique and innovative model of reimbursement that would essentially permit the rapid and specific allocation of funds to where the care was needed. HIV special needs plans (SNPs) were proposed to operate as Medicaid-managed care plans exclusively for HIV-infected adults and their dependent children. Through a remarkable collaboration, the state, persons with AIDS, community-based organizations, and health care providers together crafted a model that would preserve the best of the payment structure of the Medicaid fee-for-service plan while supporting opportunities for new and more effective reimbursement strategies. In addition, SNPs would provide a viable alternative to mainstream Medicaid-managed plans as the state moved toward mandatory enrollment of the uninfected Medicaid community.

HIV special needs plans operate using a monthly capitated rate based upon either an HIV or AIDS diagnosis. All standard Medicaid benefits are included and medication is carved out. Patients continue to fill their prescriptions at local pharmacies. Universal case management is required, provided by the SNP or through linkage agreements with grant-supported community-based organizations and designated AIDS center hospitals. Social workers in the community and in the AIDS centers will continue to have the opportunity to fill significant roles in the SNP case management model.

As of January 2003, HIV special needs plans have yet to be licensed. However, in New York City, seven entities are aggressively preparing for the state's licensure. It is expected that at least three SNPs will be operational by the first quarter of 2003 and the remainder by July 2003. If successful, SNPs will become self-sustaining vehicles that finance the continually evolving HIV care delivery system, insuring and protecting our most precious resource: our community.

REFERENCES

Chiasson, M.A., Berenson, L., Li, W., Schwartz, S., Singh, T., Forlenza, S., and Mojica, B. (1997). Accelerating decline in New York City AIDS mortality. Presented at the Fourth Conference on Retroviruses and Opportunistic Infections, Washington, DC, January.

Chiasson, M.A., Berenson, L., Li, W., Schwartz, S., Singh, T., Forlenza, S., and Mojica, B. (1998). Accelerating decline in New York City AIDS mortality. Presented at the Fifth Conference on Retroviruses and Opportunistic Infections, Chicago, IL, February.

Chapter 21

HIV/AIDS and Social Work Practice in Rural North Carolina: A Retrospective Account

Devin L. Griffith

INTRODUCTION

HIV often affects individuals in diverse social and ethnic groups who are perceived as being outside the community's mainstream and the institutional power structure (Smith, 1996). In the southeastern United States, HIV/AIDS has disproportionately affected socially and politically disenfranchised individuals and collective groups (Kayal, 1993). Societal responses and health care reactions in the rural areas of the South have traditionally been fueled by fear, apathy, and confusion. These factors, combined with a societal denial of homosexuality and drug dependence in the rural South, have often supported the notion that AIDS is a disease of "those people" who live a distinctly different lifestyle. These notions often encompass the perspective that AIDS is not a disease of rural America but one that is found in large urban environments such as New York City and San Francisco. Today, this belief system is changing in the rural South as more people have been impacted and touched personally by HIV/AIDS in their communities. Unfortunately, though, these views have contributed to delayed and fragmented responses to HIV/AIDS prevention and care in many rural southern areas.

HIV is devastating the health and wellness of many of our communities. Currently, the southeastern United States reports more new cases of HIV infection than any other region in the country. As a result, the South now has

The author graciously acknowledges the work of Toni Griffith and Marie Allred for their continued commitment, advocacy, and innovative spirit, and for embodying the social work values of social justice and human rights.

the greatest number of people living with the disease when compared to the Northeast, Midwest, and West. Similar to demographic trends in the United States, minority populations continue to be disproportionately affected by the HIV pandemic in the rural Southeast. In North Carolina specifically, women accounted for 35 percent of all new HIV infections, and 74.9 percent of all reported cases were among African Americans between 1996 and 1998 (North Carolina AIDS Advisory Council, 2000).

Since the early 1990s, I have practiced in a rural community in North Carolina as a hospice social worker, HIV/AIDS program manager, and now as a hospital director. Over this time span, I have had the privilege of working individually and in groups with people infected with HIV and their significant others. My HIV/AIDS professional practice has consisted of the provision of community case management services, discharge and long-term planning, hospice social work services, support groups, adult day health services, and, most recently, a satellite infectious disease clinic in a rural hospital. Through my experiences I have learned more than I could have ever initially imagined about the power and courage of the human spirit. I feel blessed to have been taught by the life journeys of so many coping with the diagnosis of AIDS; they have taught me about love, compassion, and the depth of humanity.

COMMUNITY AND HEALTH CARE PROVIDER REACTIONS

Since 1992 as a social worker providing service in the HIV care system, I have had the opportunity to observe a range of community and health system responses to the needs and issues of people infected and affected by HIV. These responses have often stemmed from communities struggling with growth and its accompanying societal changes as well as the multitude of social and health-related issues that HIV presents. Reactions have ranged from being apathetic or persecutory to being compassionate, innovative, and passionately committed to making a positive difference in the fight against HIV and AIDS. The responses from local health care organizations and direct patient care providers have also been varied and, at times, have created additional challenges in providing effective and culturally competent care to people with HIV. Although community and health care system responses have become more compassionate and informed today, many barriers, such as the lack of specialized community resources and medical services, are still present. The lack of infectious disease specialists in rural areas is a significant barrier that compounds access to care challenges. Rural HIV/AIDS patients may not have access to needed routine medical care due to the geographic distances to their infectious disease providers and, as a result, may interface with the local medical system only in emergency situations.

There have been instances when health care providers have expressed personal biases, such as views that patients got what they deserved for living certain lifestyles or making particular life decisions. In some circumstances, nurses who felt that they were providing appropriate care virtually overlooked the needs of a patient's life partner and provided information and support to only an adult parent or relative. In other situations, patients who had a history of chemical dependency were treated in a manner that aimed to strip them of their self-determination. Health care provider responses have historically been characterized by swift actions to monitor compliance and adherence without efforts to understand and incorporate the patient's underlying psychosocial issues into the treatment plan.

These biases can be reinforced and further complicated in a geographic area where there is a high level of cultural homogeneity and where religious institutions are the center of social, cultural, and moral attitudes and norms. Throughout the 1990s, religious institutions in the rural South have many times opened their doors and their hearts and actively supported people with HIV in the community. However, there have been other instances in which an individual's home church was not supportive and inadvertently compounded the client's feelings of shame and guilt.

I have known Zach for nearly eight years. Zach's significant other received hospice services during the last days of his life, and following his partner's death, Zach enrolled with the agency to receive HIV case management services. In addition to bereavement support, Zach was assisted with accessing specialized medical care and obtaining medications for his drug regimen, as well as going through the difficult transition from employment to long-term and Social Security disability. He truly is a resilient soul who has lived with HIV for over fifteen years. Diagnosed with HIV at age eighteen, just three months after graduation from high school, Zach has experienced and seen many of the reactions of rural health care providers.

He remembers vividly the days he spent in a rural, southeastern hospital in the early 1990s and the treatment he received from the physicians, nurses, nursing assistants, housekeeping, and dietary staff. He knew then and he knows now that he was treated differently. Even though he was weak and ill in his hospital bed, he noticed the white masks, latex gloves, disposable aprons, and sterile environment. More than the barriers, however, he remembers the lack of humane treatment. He felt like a "victim" and was treated like an outcast. He recalls the fear on the faces of his medical providers. Zach remembers that instead of the nursing assistant bringing his meals into his room, the dietary staff opened his door just wide enough to put his cardboard tray on the table nearest to the door. He noticed that when he was finished eating the tray was discarded in the trash can in his room. The staff was clearly afraid of him and acted as if simply being present with him in his hospital room would put them at risk of contracting AIDS.

These reactions to people with HIV and AIDS were common in the early 1990s. Zach was lucky enough to have his sister with him who attended to his needs. Often she has been the family advocate for his care needs. He thinks back now and realizes how uninformed and unaware the hospital staff was about HIV and AIDS. What upset him most was the enormity of the fear at this time and that the majority of the staff showed little, if any, interest in learning about and understanding his experience of living with HIV and AIDS. He felt that their only interest was in transferring him to a larger medical center in a metropolitan area. Zach now looks back as a long-term survivor and feels that he has beaten the odds and the prognosis given to him several times by physicians who told him that he had six months or less to live.

PRACTICE ISSUES

Through my experiences, it is evident that people living with HIV/AIDS in rural communities in the South face multiple barriers to receiving effective medical care. Many individuals struggle to consistently access and obtain needed preventative care, medications, and treatments. In many rural areas, the AIDS service agency is not down the street or on the other side of town. Instead, it may be over an hour away in the nearest metropolitan area. In rural areas of North Carolina, transportation needs cannot be met by providing a voucher for a subway, public bus, or a taxi company; these resources simply do not exist. In addition, in my community and in many others, people with HIV and AIDS have to travel great distances, taking from an hour to several hours to access specialized infectious disease care. These situations cause many social workers practicing in both large teaching medical centers and small rural hospitals to provide case management and support services from a distance. Social workers in the large teaching medical centers with infectious disease clinics often collaborate with community case managers in the rural areas to address service barriers and to coordinate resources to address the needs of clients residing in outlying communities.

People living with HIV/AIDS in rural areas are often dealing with the complicated social and economic challenges associated with poverty, chemical dependency, mental disorders, social isolation, and depression. The stigma and stereotypes associated with substance abuse, race, homosexuality, gender, and disabilities create additional service barriers, personal anxiety, and emotional pain. Many studies indicate that rural HIV/AIDS patients tend to be diagnosed in later stages of the disease (University of California San Francisco, AIDS Institute).

I recall working closely with Susan, a forty-five-year-old African-American woman with a history of chemical dependency who was diagnosed in New York

City and moved back to North Carolina to be closer to her family. Susan and I met in 1995 at a support group meeting where I was presenting information about my agency's scope of services. Susan was often frustrated by the medical and mental health care providers' lack of awareness of not only HIV/AIDS but also chemical dependency issues. She routinely shared that medical providers seemed to overlook the significance of her addiction and recovery process in her treatment and care and that mental health workers were noticeably uncomfortable with and uninformed about HIV/AIDS issues. Susan became a spokesperson for HIV/AIDS in the community to raise awareness about the disease and focused many of her efforts toward people coping with substance abuse and chemical dependency issues. She also felt that by speaking as a woman, she dispelled many of the stereotypes that equated HIV with gay men.

As indicated previously, many of our infected patients are diagnosed late in their disease spectrum, resulting in increased difficulty providing both effective discharge planning and clinical intervention. Inpatient social work is often challenging not only because of resource scarcities but also due to circumstances involving a sudden diagnosis. Family members and patients often experience intense feelings of shock, confusion, loss, anger, and sadness when there is a diagnosis of AIDS. On several occasions family members were unable, emotionally and/or physically, to bring their loved ones home from the hospital. This has often resulted in the challenge of the inpatient social worker finding an appropriate alternative facility and available bed for the patient. Specialized facilities for people with advanced AIDS have not been and are not available in rural areas of North Carolina. Nursing home beds are often not available due to a general shortage and a shortage for Medicaid patients in particular. Many nursing facilities also have not yet admitted AIDS patients because of the rationale that they do not have the resources available to adequately care for the patient's medical needs. In many cases, people with advanced AIDS have been transferred to facilities distant from their home communities. This type of displacement is still common for people with AIDS who are in need of placement for skilled nursing care.

This has been a heavy stressor on inpatient social workers challenged with inadequate resources, time limitations associated with cost restraints of Medicare's hospital diagnosis-related groups (DRG) reimbursement system, and the lack of private and public health insurance of many individuals living with AIDS. The DRG reimbursement system has presented a multitude of challenges for hospital social workers because insurers will reimburse only a set amount for a particular medical diagnosis based on a defined case mix. This reimbursement system often creates an institutional financial incentive to discharge patients as early and as quickly as possible in order to reduce the length of hospital stays. Inpatient social workers have often found themselves in the ethical dilemma of being a paid hospital employee versus being the patient advocate. This is merely one example of the effects of a financially strained reimbursement system and the practice implications for inpatient social workers.

While providing social work services with the local hospice and the acting HIV/AIDS service organization, I was often called to intervene with both patients and their significant others as well as with the inpatient social worker and the hospital staff managing patient care. These consultations were mainly to provide information about resource options and ultimately to assist with details of the discharge plan. Many times patients were initially told of their AIDS diagnosis while in the hospital. In a short period of time, this diagnosis was revealed to family members by the patient who was concerned with his or her own immediate care needs. In many circumstances, this resulted in the patient, the adult child, having to return to live with his or her parents. Often these situations were filled with the initial shock and disbelief over the diagnosis followed by anger, guilt, and shame. In addition, the fear of others knowing one's "business" in rural America became the ultimate confidential dilemma.

John was a gay male who grew up in a rural North Carolina town and moved to Atlanta where he thrived both professionally and personally throughout his adulthood. He had interacted little with his parents during these years but was now faced with the situation of returning home to die rather than living his final months in the Atlanta area. His parents did not know about his life and interests as an adult gay man. He had also kept his life a secret from the rural community and especially from his parents' church. My work with him often focused on his guilt and shame associated with family interactions and judgments, as well as end-of-life care. Although I was able to provide supportive counseling, a major gap in John's support system was strikingly evident. Since most of his support system was in Atlanta, his social isolation steadily increased. He often considered going back to Atlanta but felt strongly about his need for the security of being at home with his parents. After several attempts at encouraging him to come to a support group at an adult day health care center, he finally consented. Although his connection to the group developed slowly, he ultimately became an active member of the group and built a new support system of men and women coping with their diagnosis.

PERSPECTIVES ON SUPPORT RESOURCES

Although the provision of hospital-based social work services has often been complicated by the lack of specialized resources, it has also created opportunities for social workers to be involved in the planning and development of innovative services to address the unique needs of people living with HIV and AIDS in their service areas. Social workers committed to the care needs of infected patients have often utilized their community organization and practice skills to facilitate change processes in resource allocation and development. This has often challenged many hospital social workers to broaden their scope of practice and to act on the basic values and tenets of their profession. The philosophy of "making do with what you have" while advocating for increased resources to meet unmet needs has long been a social work practice mantra. Although specialized resources have been developed in large metropolitan areas, HIV/AIDS community organization and development efforts on a smaller scale have often been overlooked in rural settings. Prior to the 1990s, specialized resources were scarce, but many grassroots groups were beginning to form. Informal groups often met at people's homes, and group names were established to legitimize their mission and purpose. Most of these acted as support groups for infected people and their significant others and were a safe place for people to share their concerns, feelings, and issues.

An adult day health center for people with HIV and AIDS is a rare service in a rural area. I was fortunate to have the opportunity to be involved in the development of one in 1994 through the award of specialized grant funds through the HOPWA (Housing Opportunities for People with AIDS) program. The HIV/AIDS adult day center provided health and social services through a team of social workers, nurses, recreational therapists, and nursing assistants who worked in collaboration with an attending physician and the organization's medical director. The focus of the center was to promote quality of life through holistic care that incorporated the patient's physical, social, emotional, and spiritual needs. This service offered patients an opportunity to connect on a consistent basis in a centralized setting and to build support systems, provided respite care for caregivers, and reduced patients' stress levels through an organized program of recreational activities two days a week. Although the program provided a structured setting and a framework for service delivery, the patients who participated in the program literally created a human spirit of care and compassion beyond what was initially imagined in the service design. For many, the "group" became their family of choice that bisected all socioeconomic, racial, ethnic, cultural, sexual orientation, and gender boundaries. What was shared and overarching was that HIV/AIDS was something they all had in common. The group process often facilitated a collective consciousness. It was a unified challenge each time the group convened for a support or educational meeting. I had the privilege of observing the true nature of client empowerment in having patients identify and utilize previously untapped personal strengths.

As the adult day health program grew and endured, the group members faced many internal transitions due to the deaths of fellow participants. As a group, the members coped with multiple losses, survivor's guilt, and complicated bereavement issues. With each death of a group member, concerns about the progression of the illness arose for each member. The group coped with these issues through the creation and use of rituals. An internal memorial service was developed for each person who was no longer with the group in body but was still present in spirit. This memorial service often took a life of its own with each member sharing his or her own belief and faith system in an open and respectful environment. The legacy of each individual was shared during these memorial services and chronicled in the evolving scrapbook of the program and its participants.

The adult day health center underscored the presence of informal support systems that subtly exist in rural areas. These informal support systems have often been the foundation of the caregiving of people with HIV and AIDS in small towns. Many of these individuals are no longer with us, but their legacy of caring and compassion lives on and is a constant reminder of the many long-term survivors of days past. Whether I was the social worker working with the hospital discharge planner or the community-based case manager in the outpatient clinic setting, a major source of practical and emotional support for many patients came from a companion or friend also living with the disease. It could be the manager of the local flower store or the owner of the nearby hair salon. Many times, it was another patient who had taken early retirement and had informally accepted a new vocation of caring for those who were in the advanced stages of the disease. This often involved moving in with dying patients to assist with their end-of-life care needs.

Hospice social workers and interdisciplinary care teams have long recognized the significant role that people living with HIV have filled in caring for dying AIDS patients. Inpatient social workers have also acknowledged the presence of this caregiving and its essential contribution to allowing patients to remain at home and live out their final days in the comfort of familiar surroundings. Effective discharge planning for AIDS patients has often meant the incorporation of informal caregivers with HIV to support the patient's transition to the home and assist in home care arrangements.

PROFESSIONAL AWARENESS
AND FUTURE PRACTICE CONSIDERATIONS

As a provider of HIV/AIDS-related services, I have been touched by the strength and resilience of the patients with whom I have had contact and the colleagues that have been involved in this care provision. I have recognized that doing this work in a rural area can potentially be professionally isolating, as many individuals from other health disciplines and the social work profession do not want to practice in this field. I have watched many of my colleagues leave the profession over the past several years due to the cumulative effects of complex care issues, growing caseloads, and resource shortfalls resulting in compassion fatigue and the need for professional change. For many of us, the development and utilization of an informal support network of professionals has been essential in sustaining ourselves in this work. This informal support network has been instrumental in helping me cope with my professional grief and loss issues from caring for a countless number of people who died from this disease.

Although some of my professional support system exists within the community setting where I practice, it has also been helpful to have a network of social work professionals involved in HIV/AIDS care regionally, statewide, and nationally. In this more extensive network, program-planning strategies are discussed that have facilitated innovative service delivery development. These strategies address new and increasingly complicated issues such as family-centered services for women, children, and youths infected and affected by the disease and treatment adherence services to provide information and support for clients on complex drug regimens.

The epidemic has changed in many ways over the past ten years in the rural South. Unfortunately, our work is increasing due to the growth in the current identified number of people infected with HIV and the projected growth over the next five years. Despite the notion that treatments have lengthened life spans, many of my patients are getting sicker and developing opportunistic infections and new life-threatening complications from years of being on intense and aggressive medication protocols. I find myself often frustrated with the media, which seems to downplay the prevalence of HIV and to present a view that the "cure" is among us with each and every emerging medication. The care of people with HIV and AIDS also has become increasingly complex with overlapping mental health, chemical dependency, poverty, and end-of-life care issues demanding a higher level of service coordination across professional fields and settings.

As I look to the future and the work to be done, I am hopeful for more effective treatments and lower infection rates, but I remain grounded in the reality of my practice setting and current epidemiological trends. I am grateful and feel privileged to have worked with many people with HIV and their significant others through challenging life situations and some of their most intimate moments. Although it is hope that sustains me, it is also the lessons that patients have taught me about living, dying, challenges, individuality, changes, healing, and growth. Each patient has touched me in some special way and inspired me to sustain my commitment to the struggle against HIV and AIDS. When I look to the past, I am reminded of the courage and strength of those individuals who shared their struggle for future improvements in public policy and the delivery of care, treatment, and prevention services. Their legacies live on in the work that many of us as HIV/AIDS social workers do today.

REFERENCES

Kayal, P.M. (1993). *Bearing witness: Gay Men's Health Crisis and the politics of AIDS*. San Francisco: Westview Press.

North Carolina AIDS Advisory Council (2000). *The North Carolina AIDS Index 1999/2000.*

Smith, J.M. (1996). *AIDS and society.* Upper Saddle River, NJ: Prentice Hall.

University of California at San Francisco, AIDS Research Institute. HIV InSite. <http://hivinsite.ucsf.edu>.

THE FACE OF HOSPITAL INPATIENT SOCIAL WORK: THEN AND NOW

Chapter 22

Hospital Social Work with HIV/AIDS Patients to 1995: Death, Dying, Layoffs, and Managed Care

Chris Carlson

In graduate school, hospital social work was generally considered to be a lesser member of the family, perhaps not quite "real" social work. The primary task of the hospital social worker—discharge planning—was initially odious to many an idealistic student. It seemed to go against the social work ideals of developing relationships over time through exploration of client circumstances, then following up with meaningful interventions. The job of the hospital social worker appeared to be little more than catering to medical staff and serving the hospital administration's desire for fast discharges. HIV/AIDS hospital social work proved itself to be much more than what these impressions suggested.

The following is part discussion and part remembrance, about frontline social work with HIV/AIDS-infected patients in a hospital setting before protease inhibitors and highly active antiretroviral therapy (HAART). It was a time of working within a huge epidemic with few options for disease management and certainly no cure. This was also a time when the health care system was being considerably altered by the managed care revolution.

In the late 1980s, the impact of the HIV/AIDS epidemic, combined with activism by gay and medical communities, pushed the state of New York to create the AIDS Institute, which led to the establishment of hospital-based comprehensive AIDS centers, called designated AIDS centers (DACs). As work with this new disease continued, social work became a key component of the multidisciplinary team concept set forth by this plan (Mantell et al., 1989; Nacman, 1991). By the late 1980s, social work case management was formally established to address the multiple concerns of HIV/AIDS patients—concrete and psychosocial—addressing the roles of substance use, mental health, poverty, family dynamics, disease progression, stigmatization, and, in fact, most nonmedical issues, apart from nutrition, in each patient's treatment (Nacman, 1991).

A continuity of care/multidisciplinary team model was established at St. Luke's Hospital. (Each DAC created its own system of care within the guidelines.) Upon first admission to the hospital, patients were assigned to a CSW (a master's degree certified social worker) who followed that patient during the current and subsequent hospitalizations. The patient might also attend the program's outpatient clinic for follow-up. Our patient population in upper Manhattan was, and continues to be, primarily African-American and Hispanic people who were infected with HIV via intravenous drug use or heterosexual sex. Gay male patients have made up no more than 15 percent of our cases. The social work team remained professionally linked to the hospital's social work department and within its cost center, although we worked exclusively with HIV/AIDS-diagnosed patients.

In the early 1990s, our HIV/AIDS adult care team consisted of five inpatient CSWs, one CSW for the outpatient clinic, and a supervising CSW. Each member of the inpatient social work team maintained eight to fourteen cases at a time. A pediatric HIV/AIDS program, the Program for Children and Families (PCF), which involved three CSWs in intensive case management, was a grant-funded program functioning separately from the adult care team. This total of ten CSWs in 1994 was gradually reduced to four by the end of 2001, which included the loss of the supervisor position. By that time we had also been moved from the social work department affiliation to grant-funded status under the HIV/AIDS Program/Center for Comprehensive Care. Our direct manager after the loss of the supervisor position was one of the program administrators, who had neither patient care nor social work experience.

An additional and valuable component of the DAC plan into the mid-1990s was a designated unit within the hospital, a floor solely dedicated to our HIV/AIDS population. It was an asset because the staff was self-selected: all of us wanted to be working with these patients. This made for efficient and multifaceted care on a unit where patient stigmatization was at a minimum and understanding of the epidemic was at a maximum. For instance, when any substance-using patient was admitted, the staff was likely to be familiar with him or her and could help the medical staff differentiate those patients seeking pain medications inappropriately from those who might actually need them. Social workers were often familiar with each patient's psychosocial and medical history, as well as how the patient would handle herself or himself during the admission. This created a better and deeper understanding of our returning patients and provided them with a place where they were known, and likewise allowed the staff to provide greater efficiency in ongoing care.

By 1998 this designated unit had been disbanded to the sorrow of patients and staff; there were no longer enough HIV/AIDS patients in the hospital at any one time to warrant the assignment of an entire unit. Lengths of stay had been shortened significantly; HIV medications were improving care options; and outpatient clinics were gaining prominence. The hospital also wanted greater flexibility in admitting any patient from the emergency room to any available bed. After the disbanding, and continuing into the present, our patients could be admitted to any one of seven different units. We retained our continuity of social work patient assignment but now had to do more traveling and communicate actively with many more staff members every day. This took additional time and energy to follow patients effectively.

The preantiretroviral therapy era was a dire situation for both patients and staff as we fought off death while striving for hope and dignity in the dying process. The work our team did often felt more like constantly throwing on sandbags against an advancing flood that never relented. Our work was as much about death and dying as anything else. A cautious perusal of the units' patient rosters was a morning ritual for each social worker to find out which patients might have died during the night. We confirmed the deaths of 185 of our patients in 1994, 126 in 1995, and 120 in 1996. We lost contact with others and their possible deaths were not confirmed by our team. An HIV or AIDS diagnosis, at that point, usually meant death within two years. This was a grueling situation and was made bearable at our hospital only by good social work supervision, a team support group, and the camaraderie within the social work team and the larger multidisciplinary team. These provided substantial antidotes to burnout.

At this stage, the intensity of the epidemic required that we go beyond our training and experience almost daily. The challenges were of a professional nature but were also very much of a personal nature. The situation called upon us to attend, to witness, to participate, and to lend our humanity. The professional technique—the clinical work, the social work skills—came in keeping these events on the patients' terms, so that they could do the best possible with the remainder of their lives. Together families, friends, and staff attempted to find ways to be with the patients as they experienced their lives moving steadily toward death, as they were challenged to face great difficulties and loss while staying engaged in living. We were there to provide the means to keep the patients engaged in their care while navigating the numerous difficulties involved.

The following three pre-1995 vignettes give some sense of the complexity of the work in which social workers were involved:

Jesus was a Puerto Rican male, employed throughout his adult life, now near death from AIDS. He had a history of intravenous heroin use. His HIV-negative, employed wife, with whom he had stopped having sex when he discovered his diagnosis, was still his supportive companion. The wife, able to maintain her role as primary caretaker, relied heavily on me during this period for emotional support in managing both her role with him and the family dynamics. Their thirteen-year-old daughter, who refused to admit that her father was dying and blamed her mother for her father's illness, was never able to trust any of the hospital staff, presumably because of our association with her father's illness. She had a more discernable reliance on her father's biological family. Jesus' mother, who seemed to relate to her son, family, and the staff more as symbols in her religious construct, responded to his imminent death but not to any of its causes. She viewed his impending death, funeral, and burial in fantastical religious terms that were in distinct conflict with those of his wife. Then there was the patient—man, husband, son, father—trying to fulfill these roles as he grew steadily sicker. He was matter of fact in these efforts. Both his sadness and his love for his family members were obvious as he explained to them how he got to this point in his life, expressing his care for them until he no longer could. It was necessary to work individually with each family member because the family dynamics were such a strain on Jesus. I was also able to meet with the patient, wife, and daughter together in family counseling sessions. Jesus relied on me for support throughout the progression of his illness and until his death.

Stan was a young white man from the Midwest who grew up sixty miles from where I went to grade school. It was easy to imagine him growing up and planning to move to New York City. Designing clothes in New York City had been part of his dream, which he had fulfilled, and now he was dying. During his last two-month hospital stay, friends visited and his family came to New York to be with him. We were able to allow his mother to sleep in his room by providing him a larger, private room. This was one of the ways in which the team showed its flexibility in addressing the challenges our patients presented. Stan had fought long and hard to keep hold of his life but deteriorated steadily to the point of being unresponsive. During this stage, one of his best friends asked me what she could or should say to him. I suggested that she assume he could hear her and that she might acknowledge his brave battle, speaking simply to him, to the person she cared about. He died the next day. His father sat crying with me, both for the loss of his son and because he had never been able to accept his son as a gay man, despite efforts to do so. He asked for my forgiveness and for some way to understand. I held his hand as he continued crying. It was at this point that I started to understand that doing this work also meant being as fully human as possible. The dying process demands an honesty and personal availability that other work may not. The patients are at their most essential and are sensitive to what can be intrusive good deeds that serve the worker's desire to help more than the patient's needs. The dying process forces one to be honest as a clinical worker.

Janina was an African-American woman with AIDS, diagnosed during an admission with tuberculosis (TB). We had known her from previous admissions as being somewhat depressed but good natured, appearing physically healthy and connected to those around her, including her mother and sister. This admission was different: she refused treatment while remaining in TB isolation. She wanted nature to take its course. I worked with the psychiatrist in confirming her mental capacity to make this decision and then presented the situation to the team. It was necessary to determine that she was not in the midst of a clinical depression, other psychiatric illness, or altered mental status that would prevent her from making such a decision without understanding its probable consequence: her death. It was, however, this probable consequence that she sought. Psychiatry, medicine, nursing, and social work all assessed her status regarding this decision because each group had to determine and grapple with its professional and personal stance. In this instance, the nurses were the most resistant but deferred to the HIV/AIDS team's acceptance of Janina's plan. She had the legal right to decline treatment, and the hospital had the mandate to control and contain the spread of TB, in other words, to keep her hospitalized. Ordinarily patients who decline treatment have to leave the hospital, but not in this case. Janina explained her decision, saying that she was facing the inevitable. She did not want to continue fighting a losing battle that could eventually leave her emaciated and helpless. She did not see a purpose in reaching such a point and soon thereafter died under our care. The inevitability of death during this period created a unique legal/ethical/medical environment: troubling, but still demanding our thoughtful participation.

The HIV/AIDS epidemic required seeing difficult situations in different ways. Patients, along with family, friends, and staff, were put in positions to make unique decisions, particularly about life and death. One could not escape the existential component of the work.

It is ironic that the job description for inpatient social work was "discharge planning," given the frequency of cases similar to the ones noted, but there were numerous opportunities to engage in the discharge planning process as well. The clinical work, negotiation, and orchestration inherent in our mandate of establishing safe discharges from the hospital was a complex situation of its own. In that era of HIV/AIDS care, it was easy to feel that the hospital was the epicenter of a patient's life because of the intensity of the work, but the key for the patients was meaningful hospital alliance with the varied governmental and community-based efforts that existed.

A larger public health perspective potentially engaged the patient on many levels. New York City's Division of AIDS Services (DAS), New York State's AIDS Drug Assistance Program (ADAP), home care agencies, nursing intravenous medication services, substance use treatment and methadone maintenance, housing organizations, and supportive and skilled nursing residential facilities were all active participants in the community of care that addressed this epidemic. Numerous organizations and publications emerged to promote access to information and treatment. People With Aids Coalition and Gay Men's Health Crisis were among the better known. Publications, such as *HIV Newsline* and *Body Positive,* put out the messages of "living with HIV" and finding hope, good nutrition, and community in the midst of the stigmatizing and isolating effects of the epidemic. The "Creed" at the beginning of each *Body Positive* issue was titled, "You Are Not Alone." It discusses living with HIV: "For better or worse, your life will always be different now. Some people blame themselves for being HIV+. This kind of guilt and self-hate are very destructive"—while promoting hope, support, and emotional health—"You are not damaged goods. You are still a valuable person, as capable of giving and receiving love as ever" (Lewis and Slocum, 1995, p. 1).

Hospital social work experienced struggles on the systems level as well during this period. In 1995 the state of New York passed a law stating that hospitals were no longer mandated to maintain a social work department—a professional identity; only one CSW was required on site as a supervisor, as needed. Our hospital did not leap to this option, partly because social work here had been such a successful part of its overall public and medical health provision, but cuts in staff were immediate and ongoing. Social work was, along with most participants in health care, challenged in new ways to account for its value, not to patients but to the changing economic realities, particularly at the national level. Legislation severely cut funding for Medicaid and Medicare while the HMO (health maintenance organization) movement was continuing to gain power. (AIDS health care reimbursement was not yet impacted.) The paradox here was that this "revolution" was fueled by claims that physicians and hospitals had abused the system by overusing funds for patient care. HMOs run by businesspeople would now decide on patient care and ultimately reap profits by denying care, sharing those profits with stockholders in the HMO. Health care funds allocated for patient care were now being dispersed to those with no direct involvement in that care and those who would profit most by denying it. This was more than disheartening for many of us in the health care field. It posed a threat to our livelihoods but was also demoralizing as we watched profits take precedence at the expense of patient care.

This coincided with the shift, which had already begun nationally, from an emphasis on inpatient hospital care to outpatient clinic visits. The new medications for those infected with HIV/AIDS supported this shift by moving the epidemic in the direction of being a manageable condition. As protease inhibitors and HAART came into use, options increased, hope increased, and lives were sustained. Confirmed patient deaths in our caseload dropped from 120 in 1996 to sixty in 1997 to twenty-eight in 2001. For a majority of our patients these medications improved their quality of life, allowed for a greater degree of hope, and made living life seem more possible. Now they, and we, had to address the management of difficult medication regimens and their side effects.

Hospital social work, in general, had taken some blows. HIV/AIDS social work had been cut back and was now subject to productivity quotas, responding to economic changes. For frontline workers it was a time characterized by the question, "Why are accountants telling us how to handle patient care?" The emerging corporate style of work was vertical and top-down: executives make decisions and those decisions are passed down to the frontline staff. What had been very effective care, determined by the multidisciplinary team, faced increasing incursions from nonpatient care perspectives. Soon we were told that patients were "consumers." Although the HIV/AIDS team still consisted of infectious disease physicians, CSWs, mental health practitioners, and a nutritionist, the integrity of our health care professionals' decisions and actions was increasingly under external scrutiny.

Soon after 1995, the outpatient clinic, along with other outpatient services, became the focus of policy and funding. We also saw the prevailing use of numbers and productivity to indicate and even dictate patient care. This is not to discount the importance of sound business practice, but sadly, leadership in patient care too often came to be a function of a leader's ability to work with numbers rather than with staff or with patients. As medical management of HIV/AIDS became increasingly successful after 1995, many administrators and policymakers viewed our role differently. Social work's versatility and ability to be in the trenches where there are no clear answers was less visible to these decision makers when they thought they could start relying on the more predictable and measurable use of medications. Hospitals are medical settings, after all, where the prevailing mode of professional training is based on predictable phenomena and where human behavior tends to be seen more as a mathematical equation than the irrational jumble that it often can be (Valdiserri, 1994). The fact remains that patients, their friends, and their families still need what they needed before these changes occurred. Social work is not available to do nice things for patients. It exists, rather, to work with patients in doing that which is difficult—perhaps excruciatingly difficult. And yes, there is still discharge planning to do.

BIBLIOGRAPHY

Abramson, J. S. and Mizrahi, T. (1996). When social workers and physicians collaborate. *Social Work 41*(3): 270-281.

Beckerman, N. and Rock, M. (1996). Themes for the frontlines: Hospital social work with people with AIDS. *Social Work in Health Care 23*(4): 75-89.

Cowles, L. A. and Lefcowitz, M. J. (1995). Interdisciplinary expectations of the medical social worker in the hospital setting: Part 2. *Health and Social Work 20*(4): 279-286.

Fahs, M. C. and Wade, K. (1996). An economic analysis of two models of hospital care for AIDS patients: Implications for hospital discharge planning. *Social Work in Health Care 25*(3): 21-34.

Gebbie, K. M. (1989). The President's Commission on AIDS: What did it do? *American Journal of Public Health 79*(7): 868-873.

Lewis, J. and Slocum, M. (1995). You are not alone. *Body Positive 8*(7): 1-2.

Mantell, J. E., Shulman, L. C., Belmont, M. F., and Spivak, H. B. (1989). Social workers respond to the AIDS epidemic in an acute care hospital. *Health and Social Work 14:* 41-51.

Matorin, S. (2001). Letter of response to effect of a changing health care environment on social leaders. *Social Work 46*(4): 376.

Nacman, M. (1991). *Case Management Training Manual.* New York: New York State Department of Health AIDS Institute.

Rauch, A., Kaufer, S., and Rodriguez, P. (1993). *Views from the Frontline/ The Impact of Health Policy on the Lives of New Yorkers.* New York: New York City Chapter National Association of Social Workers and Society for Social Work Administrators in Health Care Metropolitan New York Chapter, Inc.

Rice, A. and Willinger, B. (1998). AIDS social work glory: A relic of the past. Presentation at the Annual Conference on HIV/AIDS, New Orleans, May 27.

Shilts, R. (1987). *And the Band Played On.* New York: Penguin Books.

Valdiserri, R. O. (1994). *Gardening in Clay; Reflections on AIDS.* Ithaca, NY: Cornell University.

Volland, P. (1996). Social work practice in health care. In M. Mailick and P. Caroff (Eds.), *Social Work Practice in Health Care: Professional Social Work Education and Health Care* (pp. 35-51). Binghamton, NY: The Haworth Press, Inc.

Widman, M., Light, D. W., and Pratt, J. J. (1994). Barriers to out-of-hospital care for AIDS patients. *AIDS Care 6*(1): 59-68.

Chapter 23

Acute Care: Personal Reflections on Providing Social Work Interventions to Patients with HIV/AIDS

Matthew Rofofsky

It was just at the moment I sat down to have what would be an already brief lunch break that my pager sounded: 2733—then again 2733. That was the number to one of the nursing units at St. Luke's Hospital, a full-service community care hospital adjacent to the campus of Columbia University in New York City. My first response to the page was a hearty sigh, a roll of my eyes, and a quiet, quick plea to whichever higher power was listening that this was merely a collegial social call. Next, a cleansing breath, and with a flip to a clean page on my Embassy writing tablet, I hesitantly dialed from the cafeteria house phone. "Yes, this is Matt responding to a page" ("For the ninth time today," I was thinking). The nurse caring for the patient in question took the call and proceeded to flood me with the following:

> I think you need to see this patient by the name of Manny [he is new to our hospital]. He's kneeling on his bed with his hospital gown on backward and he's having a conversation with Jesus in Spanish. He's coming down from a weeklong cocaine and alcohol binge and his LFTs [liver function tests] are off the charts. His aunt and mother are here visiting from the Dominican Republic and he's panicked that they will find out about the "SIDA" [Spanish translation for AIDS]. His aunt is completely frustrated and wants answers. The family speaks only Spanish [of which I speak only *un poquito*]. I tried to page the doctor twice but he hasn't responded. Come quick!

As an inpatient social worker dealing with patients with HIV/AIDS, the scenario with this particular nurse and patient, although it sounds extreme, is one that frequently happens. This is hospital social work and discharge planning today.

As a graduate student, I could not have contemplated such a scenario. For a moment I paused, somewhat overwhelmed by the amount of information I needed to absorb and perplexed over the direction in which I needed to proceed. In moments like this I find myself reaching for the mental energy to do the work. My day had already included participation in a staff meeting, a quality assurance meeting, completion of four initial psychosocial assessments of new patient referrals, facilitation of three discharges and review of two student process recordings for the next day's two-hour supervision meeting. The pause was not so much because I didn't know what to do, but rather the sum of all of the tasks already accomplished that day leaving me overstimulated. To my surprise, the years of social work practice combined with the good fortune of excellent supervision have provided me with the skills to meet the external chaos of my patients and the nature of the work with an inner calm.

I took a few seconds to create a mental picture of the patient. This phenomenon of information gathering or preengagement serves as the foundation for my assessment. I reminded myself to "stay where the client is" as I began to enter his world. Now, having processed the information that was presented, I was ready to meet Manny and his family members. In a manner that is unique to social work, I embarked on a journey with this man and his family through what would be several weeks of intense involvement. The next few weeks required cautious navigation as I engaged and established a relationship with a somewhat volatile man who had an altered mental status. The task at hand was to provide assessment, ongoing intensive bedside counseling, and a tentative discharge plan. All of these must occur while providing support to the family system and being cautious not to disclose HIV status.

As a social work student I learned the academic model for social work practice that included certain steps: preengagement, engagement, exploration, evaluation, termination. It appeared to be a slow and thorough process. Relationships were established over a period of time, and each stage evolved from the one before. Clinical practice in a hospital setting, however, lacks the luxury of time. In these days of managed health care, as was true in the case of Manny, hospital stays are often shockingly brief. In this situation, I was meeting Manny for the first time and was required to make an assessment of his current psychosocial status and to hypothesize his future needs as if he were being discharged the next day. Working within an undetermined time frame challenges the theoretical unfolding of the worker-client relationship. Although Manny stayed in the hospital for a few weeks, it is not uncommon for an inpatient social worker to work with patients who are hospitalized for shorter periods of time—two to three days. In each case the relationship must be established almost immediately so that the social worker can act on the patient's needs.

In order to work with Manny, it was necessary to hone in on his delusional behavior. I had to consider whether it was solely substance induced or was possibly organic in nature. In carefully observing Manny's behavior, choice of words, and body language, I elected to collaborate with our consulting psychiatrist. A psychotropic medication was prescribed for Manny in an attempt to address his psychosis. Two days later, according to his family, Manny was closer to his baseline. I was thus able to engage Manny. In this situation, I now had to work with my secondary clients (his family unit) as well, while being cognizant of the needs of both. This is not atypical. Although Manny seemed more stable, I was still presented with the challenge of language and cognition. Did Manny truly understand the implications of an AIDS diagnosis and the consequences of the disease if left untreated? Those of us doing inpatient work commonly face these questions. Through discussion (much of which required translation) we determined that Manny did in fact understand the nature of his illness. Subsequent conversations addressed Manny's living arrangements and the necessity for posthospital care. Although he initially opposed placement in a skilled nursing facility, Manny later agreed to tour two recommended facilities with his mother and aunt. He eventually decided to accept placement.

As I worked with Manny's family, they continued to voice concerns about his health. Although I attempted to alleviate their anxiety, I could not answer all of their questions due to Manny's desire for strict confidentiality. Since I sensed from their questions that they suspected the extent and nature of his HIV status, I encouraged them to direct their concerns to Manny. However, Manny remained firm in his position not to disclose the extent of his substance abuse or his HIV status to his family. In our simple dialogue, he shared with me the extreme shame he felt. He feared that knowing the information would kill his mother. When the family learned that Manny would be going to a nursing facility, they appeared to be satisfied with the resolution. One wonders what conclusions they came to. Although Manny's discharge plan was not exceptional, nursing facility placement is not universal. Other patients have varying discharge needs, including community hemodialysis placements, nursing care in the home, home infusion therapy, access to housing, adherence strategies for antiretroviral therapy, and outpatient medical follow-up.

Given its complexity, hospital social work sets a standard for social work practice skills because of the need for all stages of the social work process to occur in a brief span of time. Sharp assessment skills must be employed to quickly and effectively facilitate a discharge plan. Patients' individual discharge barriers must be identified, and appropriate measures must be taken to ensure a safe discharge from the hospital. A successful discharge in this brief span is achievable through a collaborative effort. In 1996 Abramson and Mizrahi discussed the social worker in a collaborative role as an integral part of a multidisciplinary team: "In today's climate of cutbacks, managed care, and deprofessionalization, the efficiency of the health care system will increasingly depend on the ability of social workers, physicians, and other health care providers to collaborate effectively in the provision of services to patients."

In the case of Manny, the role of the social worker is apparent in the nurse's initial outreach call. In her perception of a patient presenting with altered mental status and a family unit desiring feedback from staff, it is not unusual that she thought first to call upon the social worker. This is, perhaps, due in part to the loss of the psychiatrist as a predominant figure on our inpatient team. Though once available full-time and on site for collaboration, at present a psychiatrist is generally called upon primarily for consultation purpose, usually for medication management or capacity screenings. Such a consultation often follows a thorough psychosocial assessment completed by the social worker. It is therefore necessary for us to possess knowledge of psychopathology and to be familiar with the psychotropic medications generally offered after a differential diagnoses has been made by the psychiatrist. Inpatient social work today also requires a solid foundation in working with mentally ill chemically addicted (MICA) patients, substance users, and patients with multiple medical diagnoses often associated with HIV/AIDS.

Inpatient social work with people with HIV/AIDS today also requires a social worker to be familiar with the roles and functions of nursing, rehabilitation therapy, substance abuse counseling, diagnostic testing procedures, patient relations, billing, admitting, and outpatient medical treatment options. A common example of the social worker's interdisciplinary competence is in collaborating with a doctor and recommending that a patient scheduled for an MRI be given sedation to calm anxiety engendered by having been told the procedure "is like being inside a coffin." Another example might be to encourage a frightened patient to undergo a lumbar puncture (spinal tap) with the assistance of pain medication. In each situation, the skill in counseling is clearly parallel to a strong familiarity with medical procedures. Since the social worker must function as clinician and facilitator of often complex and multilayered components of a patient's hospital experience, the job can be extremely challenging. A medical analogy to our work might be to say that the inpatient social worker functions much the way the central nervous system works in the human body; this correlation may be understood in terms of systems theory.

Due to managed care, most patients now experience brief hospital stays. Therefore, the social worker is compelled to act as a bridge between inpatient and outpatient care. It is not uncommon for a hospitalized person with HIV/AIDS in deteriorating health to present with multiple issues often including substance abuse, lack of housing, lack of entitlements and/or insufficient or no insurance for medical and prescription coverage, and a compromised ability to manage these and other activities of daily living. Although it may be feasible to address and arrange some of these issues during a given hospitalization, ongoing follow-up is clearly indicated. It is necessary for the inpatient social worker to identify the issues a patient will face when he or she leaves the hospital. Assessment is critical for identification of vital issues to occur. Although intervention is contemplated by the inpatient social worker, given time constraints, these treatment plans are often carried out by the outpatient social worker. In this manner, collaboration and continuity of care are ensured.

Although facilitating a safe and expeditious discharge plan is the inpatient social worker's primary function, it is also necessary for us to be available for patients' emotional reactions to an HIV/AIDS diagnosis. Unlike other mental health professionals, inpatient social work requires finding the balance between concrete service negotiation and provision and meeting the psychological needs of patients in a therapeutic context. It would be difficult and redundant to overstate how rapidly this process must occur, given the time constraints inherent in hospital work today.

Working with the emotional reactions of newly diagnosed people today is similar to what it was before antiretroviral therapy. In my work, I still see emotions ranging from anger and fear to shame, denial, and shock. People struggle with the complicated science of the HIV virus, trying to make sense of its biotechnical and complex nature. It raises issues of identity as clients struggle to own this diagnosis. All too often the virus becomes a defining characteristic of a person and for many leaves a permanent stigma. Unfortunately, ignorance still abounds and people are often defined as "AIDS patients" rather than patients infected with HIV. Social workers help their patients cope with these extraordinary circumstances. The inpatient social worker is often involved in helping patients explore to whom they feel it is necessary to disclose their HIV status, and when and how to say it. Social workers consistently become entrenched in relationship and family work. Despite medical advancements, we continue to assist people by exploring the skills necessary for coping, living, and dying. In these areas, the present work is similar to that of the past.

Social work with persons with AIDS (PWAs) today has changed since the advent of antiretroviral therapy in 1995. Today the work requires helping people to prepare for the future and living with HIV/AIDS. A social worker may have once worked with an individual for several weeks or months before the work terminated because of the patient's death. The work differs today in that we may work with the same patient across multiple admissions. Thus, it becomes our responsibility to provide ongoing continuity of care. The goal and agenda in the worker-client relationship must change accordingly. For some patients this might mean returning to work and negotiating an intricate benefit system so as to not lose medical coverage or supplemental income support with housing.

Medication adherence and the difficulty in managing an HIV medication regimen are issues faced by a great number of individuals. Side effects of the medications can often be debilitating, and the concern of long-term toxicity is a real fear faced by many patients. The decision to start HIV medications can be overwhelming and varies for every individual. People who started highly active antiretroviral therapy (HAART) are developing increased cholesterol, which leads to heart disease and diabetes. It is essential to provide counseling to patients while staying abreast of medical complications. Being HIV infected now includes facing illnesses that noninfected people also contend with on a day-to-day basis.

It is also incumbent for us to review with patients educational materials including safer-sex practices and harm reduction techniques for substance abusers. In addition, it is necessary to inform patients of current laws about HIV partner notification and names reporting. Many of these issues constitute the nature of inpatient social work today. It can be challenging to forge through some of this territory because there is no precedent.

Not long after I began my work at St. Luke's Hospital in 1998, I experienced the deconstruction of a specific HIV/AIDS unit. This new model of HIV/AIDS care created new challenges. What this has meant logistically for staff is a breakdown in communication. Although previously HIV/AIDS patients were treated by a team of professionals including doctors and nurses electing to work with PWAs, this is not the case today. Today the social worker must be prepared to advocate for patients in an environment that might provide less awareness about HIV/AIDS treatment and less interest in working with people infected with the virus. In addition, support has diminished for the inpatient social worker. The position of the renal social worker that once coordinated outpatient hemodialysis placement has been eliminated. Similar is the loss of a certified addiction liaison nurse who once provided substance abuse counseling and referrals. The inpatient HIV/AIDS social worker now must manage these responsibilities. The deconstruction of a specific unit in many ways complicates patient care. The new model has systemic issues because it lacks the consistency and convenience of a unit specifically devoted to PWAs. Where an inpatient social worker was once a part of a specialized HIV/AIDS unit with a core staff, today patients with

HIV/AIDS are admitted to various floors in the hospital. The crux of the work is now working effectively on several nursing units with many non-specialized staff members. In today's milieu, nursing staffs on varied units are unfamiliar with paperwork and related HIV/AIDS social service systems and delivery. The difficulty in accessing patients and the physical complexity of the work environment lead to breakdowns in staff communication and ultimately hold up discharge.

As the focus of HIV/AIDS treatment shifts toward fewer and briefer hospitalizations, I am concerned that the demand for specialty inpatient social work may decrease, especially given the wave of downsizing and reorganization that I have already witnessed. I fear this may lead to new structures causing deprofessionalization, which will ultimately have a negative impact on patient care.

It is difficult to summarize what an average day is like for me as an inpatient social worker. There is nothing average about it. When first assigned a new patient with multiple issues and, perhaps, very poor health, I could be left feeling overwhelmed and wondering how to proceed with the helping process. That is the beauty of social work practice. Social work training prepares us to meet these challenging issues. We draw from previous experience and rely on our clinical instinct. Whether in collaboration with a physician, the patient, a partner, or a family member, we find the words to assist in the healing process, and it is apparent when this helping phenomenon happens. Then I realize again the power of social work and why I am here.

REFERENCE

Abramson, J.S. and Mizrahi, T. (1996). When social workers and physicians collaborate. *Social Work* 41(3): 270-281.

THE INTERFACE OF HOSPITALS AND CLINICS

Chapter 24

Social Work in an Interdisciplinary HIV/AIDS Program

Holly H. Dando
Charles J. Finlon

The Center for Special Studies (CSS) at the Weill Cornell Medical Center of New York Presbyterian Hospital was created by a team of doctors, patients, and volunteers in the late 1980s in response to the growing crisis of the AIDS epidemic. The traditional model using physician and nursing care alone was failing to meet the medical, social, and psychological challenges presented by the disease. Providers sought to create a model that could address the medical needs of a person with HIV or AIDS, as well as problems related to stigma, disability, the psychological effects of impending death, and the recurring need to negotiate complex social entitlement systems. The staff at San Francisco General Hospital had already created a specialized interdisciplinary team model of care in the early days of the epidemic (Jacobs, Damson, and Rogers, 1996) and, because our patient population was demographically similar to theirs, that team model became the basis for our program.

Our model gave a central role to those professional services that are considered "ancillary," or subordinate, to medicine and nursing in mainstream health care settings. In a traditional physician-directed system, an individual doctor makes outside referrals based on his or her assessment of a patient's needs. In our program, services such as social work, nutrition, and chaplainary are integrated into the patient care system, and practitioners from each of those disciplines provide assessment and service directly to the patient. The program's "democratic structure" emphasizes participation by all relevant disciplines in making a plan for patient care (Jacobs, Damson, and Rogers, 1996).

In this model some aspects of patient care are more clearly "owned" by different disciplines than others are. The team's physician will decide which antibiotic to use to treat a patient's infection; the dietician will discuss nutritional supplements; and the social worker will advise patients about insurance and entitlements. More complex questions, however, require the participation of the entire team. Problems such as a patient's difficulty adhering to an antiretroviral regimen or deciding how to approach end-of-life care discussions with struggling family members are discussed and sometimes argued out by the whole team. This emphasis on communication and shared decision making makes CSS a truly *inter*disciplinary program as opposed to a simple *multi*disciplinary one that might provide the same services but in a less coordinated manner.

THE TEAM

Each patient at CSS is assigned a primary care attending physician and a master's level social worker with New York State certification. If psychiatric care is indicated, the patient is also assigned to one of the program's five psychiatrists. This team remains stable over time and serves the patient in both the outpatient clinic and during hospital admissions. This continuity of care differs from standard programs in which a patient may meet with a different provider at each visit or admission. In most programs, a patient who attends an outpatient medical clinic will not see the social worker from that clinic if admitted to the hospital but will be assigned to whichever social worker serves the area he is admitted to (e.g., surgery, fracture, intensive care, etc.). Our social workers, physicians, nutritionists, and chaplains follow our patients no matter where they are admitted in the hospital. This ensures that providers familiar with the patient are, at the very least, consulting with other specialties and disciplines about the patient's treatment.

Such attention can be time consuming but has proven to be worth the effort. Patients express relief at not having to adjust to new staff when they are admitted, and seeing familiar faces can be grounding during a crisis. Working with the same team in both our outpatient clinic and during a hospital admission allows patients and extended family members to build a different kind of long-term relationship with their providers. The trust that develops can give patients the confidence to tackle complex problems in their lives. These issues can then be addressed over time, rather than in the usual single session of crisis counseling. When crisis interventions are needed, the established, ongoing relationship between patient (or family member) and provider increases the intervention's power and likelihood of success.

FUNDING

Our enhanced specialty care center was made possible partly through public funding from the New York State Department of Health's AIDS Institute. The institute permits hospitals identified as designated AIDS centers (DACs) to receive a higher rate of reimbursement for services in exchange for creating enhanced programs to serve the needs of people with HIV and AIDS. These public funds are supplemented by a dedicated group of private fund-raisers through an event called the "Fete de Famille," which was organized by this group in conjunction with the hospital's development department. These additional funds have made many wonderful projects possible, such as purchasing refrigerators for each inpatient room on our designated AIDS unit and the provision of TV and phone service for all patients in our program who become hospitalized. These services are normally provided at considerable cost to the patient. The generosity and commitment of our donors also allow us to provide emergency cash grants for patients in need, as well as supporting research projects and staff education programs.

STAFFING

The center's staff has grown significantly since the program's inception in 1989. Our current charge nurse began at the center that year, working as a home care specialist performing patient assessments and coordinating services between agencies and insurers. She recalls that the program originally held one outpatient clinic per week and was staffed by three part-time physicians, two social workers, several volunteers, and one other outpatient nurse. By 1996, the clinic was holding seven clinics each week and staff had grown to include two home care nurse specialists, eight master's level social workers, a medical director, four full-time general internists, sixteen part-time physicians (including subspecialists such as dermatology and rheumatology), two full-time and four graduate staff psychiatrists, three ambulatory care nurses, twenty-two floor nurses, eleven nurses' aides, a registered dietician, an occupational therapist, a volunteer coordinator, a chaplain, a part-time research coordinator, an emergency medical technician/van operator, and a medical/surgical technician, in addition to a full complement of administrative staff (Jacobs, Damson, and Rogers, 1996). The following year we opened a freestanding clinic in another part of the city and almost doubled our staff. Our current clinical staff now includes nine full-time internists, five psychiatrists, and twenty social workers between the two sites.

Staffing changes over the years have reflected changes in the epidemic. For example, although overall caseloads have remained about the same (about ninety patients per social worker), inpatient caseloads have gotten smaller (between zero and five per social worker at any given time) due to the increasing numbers of patients who avoid hospitalization through improved treatment options. We therefore have fewer floor nurses and, as less time is spent on discharge planning, we have returned to using only one home care specialist to assist our social workers. We have also eliminated some positions such as our occupational therapist and volunteer coordinator because these services became less important as patients' needs changed. We have, conversely, increased our outpatient clinic staff to care for the growing numbers of ambulatory patients we see.

While other AIDS programs in the city have been forced to reduce social work staff due to budget cuts, we have continued to grow due to solid funding and our administration's firm belief in the importance of providing social work service. Social workers, following patients both in and out of the hospital, now make up more than 30 percent of our staff. Each of our MSWs has approximately ninety patients on his or her caseload—relatively reasonable compared to the 250 to 400 patients followed by social workers in some other hospital-based HIV clinics in New York City.

Manageable caseloads maintain morale and reduce the incidence of burnout, but having a large proportion of social workers on staff also has other advantages. Social work's holistic perspective adds balance to the medical model that quite naturally flourishes in hospitals. Our doctors and nurses are able to view problems—and patients—more systemically because of our social workers' influence. It's also less daunting for a social worker to question an unrealistically simplistic interpretation of a patient's behavior when there are others with similar viewpoints sitting in the daily case conference.

COMMUNICATION

Team care without regular and direct communication can lead to fragmentation and duplication of services, so the CSS model incorporates daily patient case conferences. At the end of the clinic session, all providers involved in patient care meet to discuss every patient seen in the outpatient clinic that day. Once a week we also have a full team case conference discussing the inpatients followed by our program. This latter meeting also includes the floor nurses caring for our patients. At both inpatient and out-patient conferences we present and discuss new diagnoses, medications, and social and psychological problems, and care plans are made and agreed upon by team members. There is an enormous benefit to the providers in having their work reviewed by their peers in this way. Helpful suggestions, comments, and questions are integral to this process.

Communication between disciplines is also fostered through weekly meetings to discuss administrative issues, answer current questions, and plan for the future. All staff are also invited to participate in biweekly support groups facilitated by an outside social worker at each site. In these groups team members can share their experiences and gain meaning about this profound and difficult work in an atmosphere of trust and empathy.

The groups began before the introduction of highly active antiretroviral therapy (HAART) when so many of our patients were suffering horrific deaths. Often abandoned by their families, they were wasting away, incontinent, demented from brain infections, and disfigured by Kaposi's sarcoma lesions. Team members clearly suffered the effects of secondary traumatic stress. Now that more of our patients are living longer, it is sometimes easier to deny the effects of job-related stress. Although they present less dramatically, trauma and stress continue to pervade our work. Patients still die isolated from loved ones and supported only by our staff. Our ambulatory patients also present repeatedly with substance abuse relapses, adherence failures, and unremitting social problems, making our work seem futile and increasing our risk for burnout. Having a safe place to vent frustrations and remind one another of past successes is needed as much now as it was in 1994.

In addition to support, social workers receive regular supervision through the hospital's social work department. Each unit meets separately on alternate weeks for group supervision with the director of the department, and several times a year both units meet together for a combined group supervision. New social workers also receive individual supervision during their first year of employment. Working with nineteen other social work colleagues allows many opportunities for informal support and peer supervision as well.

COMMITTEES

Topics such as substance abuse, adherence, and patient education are discussed and explored by staff in a committee format as well. When an area of patient care is identified as particularly complex or compelling, staff is encouraged to form a committee to examine the issues and create a plan of action. An example of the efficacy of this plan is the development of an AIDS education committee. At the outset of the epidemic, our staff members noticed that other departments, often due to staff ignorance or "AIDS phobia," occasionally treated CSS patients differently. We therefore invited other hospital departments who treated AIDS patients, such as pediatrics, the hemophilia clinic, and gynecology, to participate in a committee dedicated to educating the hospital as a whole on AIDS and its attendant issues. Working with managers of all hospital departments, we were able to schedule in-service education seminars. Committee members prepared material appropriate for each audience and, after providing basic HIV/AIDS education, were able to answer questions from staff in areas such as security, nutrition, laundry, escort, laboratory, and registration. Evaluation questionnaires indicated that staff enjoyed and benefited from these meetings. The committee's goal to improve conditions in our hospital by educating our colleagues was met during the many years this committee was in session.

More recently, we have formed a committee to coordinate our developing relationship with an HIV clinic in Sagamu, Nigeria. Staff from many disciplines come together biweekly to sort and pack donated medications for patients at that clinic. We are also developing teaching modules for the Nigerian patients and staff and arranging for reciprocal visits to increase learning opportunities for both programs.

RECENT GROWTH

In the late 1990s, Gay Men's Health Crisis (GMHC), the oldest and largest AIDS service organization in the country, moved to a newly renovated building and decided to lease a part of their ground floor space to an HIV/AIDS care provider. After reviewing submissions from other designated AIDS centers in New York City, they offered the space to our program, and in October 1997 the David E. Rogers Unit of the Center for Special Studies opened at GMHC. Dr. Rogers was an early champion of the cause of AIDS treatment and an inspiration to many of us who worked with him when he was on staff as the Walsh McDermott University Professor of Medicine and Psychiatry at Cornell Medical School. The providers at the Rogers Unit continue to follow their patients both in and out of the hospital, commuting to the main campus as needed. Our original clinic, at the hospital's Sixty-Eighth Street campus, was named for one of our most active donors, Glenn Bernbaum. Between the two units, the Center for Special Studies now cares for over 2,000 patients.

CLINIC STRUCTURE

Each unit holds six clinic sessions per week, during which their care teams see twenty to thirty patients per session. Appointments are scheduled as in a private practice where providers see patients at specific times rather than the typical "clinic" scheduling in which patients are booked for one block of time and seen on a first-come, first-served basis.

All patients receive and sign a care contract at their initial appointment to clarify patients' rights and responsibilities. This document provides for the safety and comfort of patients and staff in our setting by establishing rules for conduct and use of the clinic. We developed this contract in response to some patients' behavioral problems that put clinic staff and patient safety at risk. The contract also addresses chronic lateness and missed appointments. It sets expectations for mutual respect from the first appointment and is a good opportunity for staff to explain to our patients how we work. Patients who are not able to adhere to these rules are given alternate referrals and discharged from care.

SUBSTANCE ABUSE

Drug and alcohol abuse are problems for many of our patients. We intervene with the expertise of many fields, but social workers and psychiatrists become most involved in this area, diagnosing, treating, and referring patients to twelve-step groups, inpatient detoxification, inpatient and outpatient rehabilitation, or methadone maintenance programs. Our staff has run harm reduction, "starting to stop," and "parents in recovery" groups for our outpatient population, and we have made twelve-step meetings available to inpatients. Crises that lead to inpatient admission are sometimes opportunities for patients to reexamine the cost of their substance use. Our continuity of care allows us to continue working with them on solutions to these problems even after discharge.

Before the introduction of HAART in 1996, the combination of AIDS, opportunistic infections, and the risks associated with substance use yielded short lives for many of our substance abusing patients. Now that medication can reduce viral load and allow some immune system reconstitution, we increasingly see a phenomenon in which chronic substance abusers "yo-yo" between periods of abstinence (or at least more controlled use) when they adhere to medication regimens and periods of uncontrolled drug use when they are unable to follow a treatment plan. Such patients are doing the best they can with their current skills, but dealing with multiple relapses can be exhausting for staff. An interdisciplinary team model enables members to "share the load" and support one another in situations that seem hopeless. Social workers can put these repeated relapses or adherence failures into a larger context for both the patient and provider, helping them manage their feelings of futility. When the patient is ready to attempt treatment again, both patient and social worker may have learned something from the previous failure and be able to develop a better treatment plan.

GROUPS

Support groups, such as those mentioned previously, have always been an effective way of caring for our patients. They allow patients to form support networks that often continue well past the group's meeting. Group members can exchange advice and opinions as well as express the range of emotions, from fear and despair to hope and joy, for which they may have no other outlet. They find that they are not alone and can find comfort in this community. Our chaplain also runs several groups focusing on spirituality.

Through the years our social workers have run many different kinds of support groups. As the populations affected by the epidemic have shifted, we have initiated groups to deal with new needs. In early years we ran groups for men who have sex with men, and as need presented itself, we added other groups, including groups for Spanish-speaking women, the newly diagnosed, mothers, people with a diagnosis of AIDS (as opposed to those only HIV positive), young men, and transgender women. When it became clear that combination therapy would fail unless regimens were followed almost perfectly, we also started a treatment support group run by a social worker and a nurse.

Each of our social workers cares for a specific caseload, but those who choose to run groups also end up treating other workers' patients. Information about how the patient functions in a group has often proven helpful to the primary social worker's understanding of that patient. Careful attention to communication between social workers and ongoing clinical exploration of the process with patients has minimized role confusion or boundary transgression.

CONCRETE SERVICES

Most people, correctly or not, associate social workers with public benefits, and the workers in our program do spend a great deal of time assisting patients with these. Housing continues to be a major problem for many HIV-infected individuals, and the combination of longer lives, welfare "reform," and New York City's perennially tight housing market make the current situation even more difficult than it has been in the past. A great deal of our time is spent helping patients who are homeless or living in substandard housing, such as the city's many drug-infested welfare hotels, find resources to access safer, more stable living quarters. This includes time spent advocating with landlords, community-based programs designed to help patients with their housing searches, and the city's HIV/AIDS Services Administration (HASA) (formerly the Division of AIDS Services), which offers rent supplements for qualifying patients. Being a hospital-based program, our social workers cannot go out into the community to assist directly. We therefore increasingly refer patients to intensive case management programs based in the community. These programs have employees who can accompany patients as they make the rounds to welfare and realtors' offices to navigate the city bureaucracy in arranging for rent assistance. The process can be long and frustrating, but this kind of collaboration can benefit patients enormously when it works.

One of the most gratifying indicators of HAART's reduction of HIV morbidity has been the number of our patients returning to work. Historically, people with AIDS became ill, left work, and applied for public and private disability benefits. Social workers helped patients navigate these systems and adjust to their increasing loss of function and to their new, unemployed situation. Lately, we find more patients leaving disability to return to work than patients who want to go on disability. The social worker's basic job remains the same: help the patient navigate the system and adjust to his or her new social role, but it is more gratifying when done in this "reverse" direction, when success feels like victory rather than surrender.

Working with patients hospitalized for acute illness is probably the area of social work that has changed the most at CSS in the past twelve years. In the early years workers' caseloads were about the same as they are now, but acuity (i.e., severity of illness) was naturally higher. A larger number of patients on any given caseload were hospitalized at any given time, and a greater portion of time was spent on labor-intensive inpatient tasks. Many of these hospitalizations ended in death, and a good share of those patients who did survive required home nursing services or transfers to long-term care facilities. Social workers had volumes of paperwork to complete and hours of negotiations with nursing homes and home care agencies, but their primary function was then, as it is now, to help patients and family members make some kind of sense of what was happening to them. This might be dealing with the loss of autonomy that going to a nursing home symbolized or reworking the guilty feelings that they somehow "deserved" what was happening to them. Almost all of the inpatient work was, however, preparing in some way for death. It was exhausting, but the connection with patients, families, and other team members was profound. These days, the levels of acuity for inpatients is much lower, stays are generally brief, and provider caseloads are stable over much longer periods of time.

CELEBRATION

This spirit of community is celebrated during the holiday season at our annual holiday party. What once was held in our clinic space has grown to require a much larger space in the hospital's cafeteria. Staff members from all disciplines serve patients a hot meal. We also have a Santa (a volunteer from a neighborhood restaurant that also donates food) and a tree where children and adults can get a Polaroid of them on Santa's lap. We provide each child with a gift bag, and high spirits abound during the live entertainment and dancing. Patients start asking about the party as early as October of every year. It seems to be an important demonstration that they are cared for in a more personal way by clinic staff.

Our chaplain also organizes an annual memorial ceremony to honor those patients who have died in the previous year. Staff and the deceased patients' loved ones have found this an important way to acknowledge their losses. Even though the list of names seems shorter each year, the depth of emotion felt at the ceremony does not diminish.

THE FUTURE

We have relocated our pediatric AIDS clinic to a space one floor below the adult clinic. We are now treating the HIV-negative children of our adult patients, as well as those infected. Same-day appointment scheduling facilitates adherence to clinic appointments. The new space has playroom facilities for the younger children and computer and Internet access for the older ones.

The staff of both clinics find collaboration enhanced by the physical proximity. Some of our congenitally infected children who are now over twenty-one have also made a successful transition to the adult clinic. In previous years none of us would have thought it possible that these young people, infected at the beginning of the epidemic, would live long enough to become adults. Treatment advances made this possible, and we can hope that future discoveries will lead to other outcomes that we currently consider impossible.

BIBLIOGRAPHY

Germain, C. B. and Gitterman, A. (1996). The Life Model of Social Work Practice: Advances in Theory and Practice. New York: Columbia University Press.
Jacobs, J. L., Damson, L., and Rogers, D. E. (1996). One approach to care for patients infected with human immunodeficiency virus in an academic medical center. *Bulletin of the New York Academy of Medicine 73:* 301-311.

Chapter 25

The Integration of a Permanency Planning Program

Dina Franchi

I first began working with people infected with HIV in the fall of 1991. I remember returning home after the first week and realizing that I was a suburban white woman and had lived such a sheltered life. Not that I hadn't thought that previously—I had worked within the foster care system for several years and at a therapeutic community for substance users for four years. Yet walking into an HIV outpatient clinic at a major medical center on the Lower East Side of Manhattan and looking at my extremely diverse caseload of patients made me realize that I had little experience working with transgender populations, specifically the diversity within the Hispanic and African-American populations. I remember one of my colleagues transferring all of the transgender cases to me and stating "Now let's see what you are made of." I should explain that I had been working at this medical center for only two weeks when my colleague handed me these cases. Years later, he confessed that he did that to show me what was out in the "real world" and to see if I would "rise to the occasion." It was one of the best learning experiences in my life and taught me to be even more understanding and tolerant of people from every walk of life.

My experience with HIV and knowledge about the illness was minimal at that time, but I learned quickly. The disease then was much more physically apparent, and I remember the feelings seeing patients with Kaposi's sarcoma and/or cellulitis evoked in me. These two infections stood out most in my mind as being the most painful and difficult for the patients. There was little way to hide these two infections, and I remember how much more stigmatized these patients often felt about their diagnosis. Patients did not even have to discuss their physical appearance. The way they hid in the corners of the waiting room, came in late for appointments, sat with sunglasses on, or wore clothing they thought would hide their infections spoke volumes about how they felt about themselves. These patients were so concerned about what other people would think of them that they wore makeup to hide the lesions. At times empathy was the only therapeutic tool available to support and comfort these patients. Initially it was difficult for me to remain professional when hearing patients describe the way they felt about their appearance. I remember often wanting to cry with them and becoming angry upon hearing how people stared at them, moved away, or expressed shock at the way they looked. I began holding patients' hands and touching their arms when they became emotional. This was the opposite of what social workers were taught in school, but I realized that we were not always taught the appropriate responses to the gamut of situations and populations that existed in the real world.

Not only was I learning to deal with new situations and emotions in my work, but I was also experiencing different reactions in my personal life. As I mentioned before, I am a white woman from suburbia. There were many people in 1991 who believed that HIV/AIDS did not affect people living on Long Island, and the stigmas around the people who became infected ran deep. I was shocked by the reactions and comments from friends about the population I chose to help. I need to say that my parents, even though I knew they were concerned for me and held some reservations, did not reveal these concerns to me and supported me in my endeavors. Some of my friends, on the other hand, surprised me. I did not expect them to react with such fear for my safety or fail to comprehend why I wanted to work with this population. Initially, many felt that I was just on another one of my crusades. It was not until I educated them about HIV and the number of people it affected that they began to understand my desire and passion to work in this field.

The longer I worked with HIV-infected individuals the more I began to learn and understand about their daily lives. My interest in looking at how HIV affected not just the infected individuals but also their families, friends, colleagues, and support networks grew. There was such a ripple effect with this illness that patients often seemed like salmon swimming against the current. By 1995 there was an increased focus on the orphans of the HIV epidemic; this is where my career took a wonderful turn. I was given the opportunity to start a grant-funded program (through New York State Department of Health's AIDS Institute) focusing on HIV-infected mothers and the need for them to establish permanency plans for their minor children. This program, named Families in Transition (FIT), was unique in that it viewed permanency planning (establishing formalized legal guardianship) as a long-term process and not a process that should be completed when patients were in the end stage of their illness. The staff consisted of a coordinator, me, who also provided all of the direct services, and two outreach workers, each working ten hours a week providing outreach for the program and support to the patients.

Although this opportunity was wonderful, the decision to take on this new program and leave my old position was difficult. I had established many wonderful friends working in the clinic, and I felt that I was assisting patients in making changes in their lives and their self-perceptions. I felt guilty leaving. I felt as if I was abandoning them, a feeling they often experienced with other people in their lives. I was tormented about whether I should transfer. I agonized over whom to transfer certain patients to and experienced many emotions at the thought of having to terminate from patients I had worked with for four years. The termination process was difficult, and during this time I often thought that I could not leave. However, my patients, although sad that I was moving on, were quite supportive about the new program and often gave me encouragement to move on. I also began obtaining a caseload for this new program because many of the women I worked with were mothers and needed this service. Some also did not want to terminate contact with me.

The program allowed parents to understand the different types of guardianship available and assisted them in making the most appropriate choice for their children. For this to occur, I believed that the program needed to link with a legal program to assist these patients. My plan was to allow parents to feel safe and comfortable when making one of the most important decisions in their lives: "Whom do I trust to raise my child when I die?" I attended a permanency planning network meeting and met a lawyer from the Legal Aid Society. She was working on a grant-funded program assisting HIV-infected parents in establishing guardianship plans. We met, brainstormed, and presented to our respective funding sources the benefits of establishing a formal link between our two programs to best meet the needs of the parents we served. My program dealt with the psychosocial aspects of permanency planning, and the legal program dealt with all of the legal issues, including attending any court appearances.

From the beginning there were obstacles. My office was moved to a different building because the administration thought it should be closer to the OB/GYN clinic, which was located three blocks away. The idea of this move was to better identify high-risk women during pregnancy or those mothers who were diagnosed during their pregnancy. The administrators believed that the identified population for HIV-infected mothers would be pregnant women. This turned out to be a disaster. What the administrators did not realize was that women who were pregnant and HIV infected were focusing on birth and life, not planning for their children in the event of their demise. The last person any of these women wanted to deal with was me. These women viewed me as the person who took away their hopes and dreams and kept shoving reality into their faces. Thus, there were few referrals and not much discussion about my program with the staff.

The women who were referred from the HIV outpatient clinic saw my new space as a constant reminder of the changes in their lives and their unwillingness to have more children for fear of perinatal infection. For months I struggled with getting administration to understand the beliefs and feelings of these women and my need to remove my presence from the OB/GYN clinic and return to the HIV outpatient clinic. After several months these changes were made. During this time, I discovered that there were men who were in the same situation as these women: HIV-positive fathers who needed assistance or were part of a couple. The funding source, however, was written only for infected mothers, so I technically could not enroll these infected fathers. Since there were not a large number of fathers, I began seeing them to discuss the clinical aspects of permanency planning and assist them with parenting skills. This role was difficult for most of the fathers since traditionally parenting has been the mother's role. Paralleling this effort was my plea with the funding source to allow the program to become one for infected parents, not just infected mothers. Initially, the funding source wanted to know how I learned about these fathers. I knew if I lied, I would be placing the program and myself in jeopardy. So, I told the truth. I explained that referrals came in for HIV-infected fathers, and I ethically believed that I could not turn them away since there were no other resources available. I apologized for working outside the parameters of the grant (even though I was not really sorry), but I explained that since this was a virtually untouched area, we, as professionals, needed to be open to ensuring the provision of services for unmet needs; the needs of these fathers were unmet. Thankfully, this was met with little resistance. In one site visit and with references from fathers I was working with, the contract manager agreed to my request, and the program was changed to incorporate HIV-infected parents.

Before I knew it, nine of the twelve months of the contract period had passed. There were twenty parents enrolled in the program, and I had barely begun to scratch the surface on permanency planning. What I was beginning to observe was that most parents were no closer now to formalizing a plan for their children's future care and custody than they were when they enrolled. The number of parents enrolled in the program had exceeded the proposed number by twelve, but not one parent had formalized a permanency plan. There were several reasons for this: many had not fully accepted their diagnosis; others had not disclosed to family members or children; many feared abandonment and stigmatization if they disclosed; and most had little idea as to who a potential caregiver for their children would be. Many opted for their own parents, whom they had not yet disclosed to, and many of these parents were elderly, and some were ill themselves. This could be a short-term solution but not a long-term permanency plan; however, the infected parents were not in any emotional position to acknowledge this. I had to re-direct my focus and look at the final outcome, formalizing a permanency plan, as the end result of a long process to assist parents to make the best choice possible. The program had to be revised to first encompass assisting parents in accepting their diagnosis (breaking down denial). Only then could we begin discussing disclosure, reasons to disclose or not, and teaching parents how to disclose to children. Parents also needed education about what children at different developmental stages could comprehend. The next step was to assist parents in identifying a caregiver within their support network and determining who would be a positive role model and provider for their children. All of this was occurring while the parent was dealing with illness, daily life stressors, and other issues such as substance abuse, poverty, legal issues, and school problems for their children. In addition, if a parent was unable to identify a caregiver, then much exploration was involved in finding suitable caregivers without having to potentially place children in the foster care system. During my first year, I learned that what appeared on paper in the grant, a relatively straightforward process, was just the opposite when dealing with real people. I understood this because I was working with these parents on a daily basis, but making others understand this was a much more difficult and frustrating task. Eventually, the process to formalize a permanency plan became clearer and those involved realized that this process is most successful when time is taken to meet the clients' needs and establish a comfort level before discussing issues of mortality and leaving their children.

Finally, the program seemed to be progressing well. However, in building a program situations and aspects that were not accounted for often developed as the program evolved. This occurred as the identified caregivers became involved in the program. As parents died, these newly constituted families were dealing with more than the loss of their loved ones. Often children lost their homes, communities, school districts, and friends. Now these children were living with different family members and learning new rules and structures. This often caused many conflicts with the new family structure, even if the placement was with grandparents. Mourning the loss of a parent was no longer the primary concern. Unfortunately, there were no resources to assist the families through this transition process. Entitlements were also limited, and new caregivers often had to rebudget their finances and reapply for medical benefits for these children. At this time, the Families in Transition Act was not yet even a concept. Our staff was in a quandary as to where to refer these families. The families were quite vocal in not wanting to have to begin with a new staff that did not know what they had endured. Once again, I needed to advocate for the patients and the program to allow the staff to assist and provide supportive counseling for these newly constituted families during this emotionally charged transition period. My contract manager and I were on quite friendly terms because of all the interactions we previously had, and the New York State Department of Health AIDS Institute approved the program's expansion to assist families during this transitional period. However, this added service needed to be conducted without any additional funds to hire more staff. Therefore, my focus had to shift toward finding additional funding while not diminishing the quality of care provided to these families thus far. Grant writing was another foreign concept to me, but I learned quickly. I knew that burnout was a real concern and that if more staff was not provided, the patients' quality of treatment would suffer. I was the only staff member providing direct services to these families, and the issues around mortality, denial, disclosure, and fears of abandonment, in addition to daily life stressors, became overwhelming for me at times. I was lucky enough to have great peer support and sound clinical supervision, but supervision occurred only once a month. There were many times when I felt stressed, overwhelmed, and overworked. Those were the times when I really appreciated having great colleagues to provide support and encouragement.

Four years after the program was initiated, enhanced funding was obtained to meet the larger number of families being seen. At that point, my staff, which now consisted of another social worker besides myself, two outreach workers, and a peer educator, seemed to have a clear direction as to the mission of the project and the steps needed to establish a formalized permanency plan. However, as one aspect of a program comes together, other obstacles often arise. One of these obstacles was the referral base for client recruitment. Almost half of the referrals came from the hospital's outpatient HIV clinic; other referrals came from street outreach, community-based organizations, and methadone clinics. Oddly enough, no referrals were coming in from the HIV pediatric component. This was a major concern for the project directors, and it was often a large source of conflict for me. Believing that the two divisions, the HIV pediatric program and my program, could mutually benefit each other, I hoped for an integration of services. The notion was that as the pediatric unit's children were being cared for, their parents would be able to discuss issues of disclosure for themselves and their children and establish guardianship. I believe part of the reason for the difficulty with integration is that part of the pediatric component was also grant funded. The director of that program might feel that patients would choose one program over the other, as opposed to them having comprehensive services for different issues, thereby viewing the programs as competitive rather than complementary. Unfortunately, that did not occur and still remains a sensitive area today.

What was becoming clear and frustrating to me was that although we had a program that was successful and benefiting many families, many colleagues did not view HIV as a family issue. This innovative program was working with families through the progression of the illness and with the newly constituted families after the parent's demise. Permanency plans that had been established were successful in that the children knew where and with whom they would be living. Parents did not feel that incorporating caregivers into their lives was diminishing their roles. Instead, parents used this time to forge bonds, increase their support networks, and communicate their hopes and dreams for their children. Professionals in other disciplines believed that the focus of treatment was on the individual; they did not understand that everyone in the patient's life is affected by the illness. Much of my time was spent educating colleagues and staff about the need to expand their views regarding how HIV impacts the lives of patients and their families. With this, I became more entrenched in the political arena of a large bureaucracy. As a social worker coming from a clinical perspective, hospital politics was a foreign concept. I had interactions with hospital politics and met with some success previously. However, attempting to change people's paradigms was unbelievably difficult. My frustration, stress, and anger were more intense than I could have imagined. Staff and medical providers needed to understand that family sessions often are longer than individual sessions, that family issues are just as acute as any other part of the patient's life, that family stress can contribute to the poor health of the patient, and that the family needs to be involved in the patient's care and treatment. Most staff finally realized that we could no longer function as if we were working in a vacuum. In the end compromises were reached. Family treatment is now an integral part of our patients' HIV care.

Over the past two decades the face of AIDS has changed, and I have grown as a professional. Yet the underlying issues remain the same. Professionals working in this field still struggle with assisting our clients in overcoming stigma and feelings of being disenfranchised, and in helping them learn to live with a chronic illness. We also deal with the issues in our relationships with colleagues and in our personal life. It continues to boggle my mind that even today people fear this disease, continue to believe the myths about this illness, and alienate people who are infected and affected by HIV. Medical interns continue at times to be indifferent to those hospitalized, confidentiality is not adhered to, and often hurtful statements are made to clients. Social workers also have to deal with the discrimination that occurs because we have chosen to work with this population. Now that people are living longer with HIV, it is no longer on the forefront of the media. People are not as aware of the disease, therefore education and prevention methods have lessened. My fear is that the general public will become complacent about this illness, leading to an increase in the rate of infection. These were concerns ten years ago when I first entered this field, and they remain real concerns today. We struggle daily with assisting our clients in their lives while advocating for tolerance within personal lives and systems. I continue to wait for the day when those infected with HIV will no longer be seen in a negative light. Will that day ever arrive?

Chapter 26

A Personal Journey to Improve Access to HIV-Related Mental Health Services

Nan O'Connor

Mental health care has played an important role in the spectrum of care for individuals living with HIV over the past two decades. Anxiety and mood disorders sometimes result after an individual has been diagnosed with HIV or has contended with opportunistic infections associated with HIV. Primary care providers in hospital-based clinics are often the first to learn of a patient's HIV-related mental health issue such as anxiety or depression. Since patients often feel most comfortable confiding in a medical provider with whom they have a long-standing, trusting relationship, if the patient is amenable, then a referral to mental health treatment can occur. Referrals usually involve the resources, knowledge, and assistance of medical social workers to help patients access these services as expeditiously as possible. This has often proven to be a daunting task.

In my experience working as a medical social worker at the University of California San Francisco (UCSF) Women's Specialty Program for women with HIV in the early to mid-1990s, challenges abounded in trying to access the limited number of available mental health services. The Women's Specialty Program is an outpatient medical clinic designed to provide comprehensive medical care to women living with HIV/AIDS. During my tenure there, I was responsible for providing case management services including referring clients to housing, transportation, and child care services, as well as to agencies that would assist with food, clothing, and emergency funding. For many of the approximately 100 women being served at the clinic, mental health issues were also prevalent. Although I could offer limited individual psychotherapy to some of them, the demand for mental health services clearly exceeded the available resources.

Capacity problems were also an issue at the four outpatient mental health clinics to which I referred patients. Limited staffing at these agencies translated into restricted availability for initial phone screenings and intake assessments. When patients called these agencies, they had difficulty directly reaching the staff who provided the initial screening. Phone recordings at these agencies instructed patients to call back during very specific and often inconvenient times. This was difficult for those marginally housed or homeless who were often without readily available access to a phone. For those who felt they needed the emotional support of their medical social worker to establish contact, the wait seemed to be a frustrating obstacle. Upon completion of the phone screening, clients frequently waited several weeks to two months for their initial intake evaluations, only then to be placed on a waiting list for sometimes a month or two longer. For clients suffering from severe depression or anxiety, this wait was interminable. As the social worker trying to help them gain access to mental health services, I too felt frustrated and somewhat powerless about the waiting period and deeply concerned that patient mental health needs were not being addressed in a timely fashion. This experience instilled in me the desire to advocate for improved access to mental health services for those living with HIV.

STRATEGIES TOWARD IMPROVING MENTAL HEALTH ACCESS

In April 1996, I was invited to apply for a psychiatric social work position at the Center for Special Problems (CSP) by their HIV program coordinator, who was familiar with my work with HIV-infected women and my advocacy for improved access to mental health. I began working there later that month. CSP is an outpatient community mental health clinic with five specialty programs including trauma, domestic violence, gender, sex offenders, and the HIV Mental Health Case Management program to which I was assigned. The HIV program provides individual and group psychotherapy, psychiatric evaluations, medication monitoring, peer support, and case management services as they relate to clients' mental health. I was determined in my new position to see whether I could improve patient access to our services. I was particularly interested in improving access for women at UCSF's Women's Specialty Program and for patients at UCSF's Positive Health Practice located at San Francisco General Hospital's Ward 86. The latter is an outpatient medical clinic designed to provide comprehensive care to those living with HIV/AIDS. At the time I began working at CSP, Ward 86 had a weekly clinic for women, many of whom were uninsured, poor, isolated, and badly in need of mental health services.

ACHIEVING THE GOAL

The first step in achieving the goal of improved mental health access was to solidify my working relationships with the staff at the Women's Specialty Program and to develop and foster new working relationships with the staff at Ward 86, since both make many referrals to our program. In addition, making connections with primary care providers who prefer initiating their own patients' mental health referrals directly was also helpful.

Part of the trust-building process included my initial efforts to help UCSF clients navigate successfully through the intake evaluation. The first part of this process is the phone screening, which our clinic originally conducted Monday through Friday between 9:30 and 11:30 a.m. This limited time slot proved difficult for UCSF clients being seen in afternoon clinics and also for those who needed both practical and emotional support in making the call. For medical social workers, quite often the best time to help clients make calls after a busy morning clinic is in the early afternoon, and our mental health agency did not allow for that. Therefore, I suggested that UCSF staff members call me directly at any time during the day so that, when possible, I could conduct initial phone screenings on demand. This measure, which facilitated patient access, also strengthened my relationships with the UCSF staff. The ease in which this process occurred is in part related to the confluence of the funding stream support for enhanced service delivery to women and to the vision of the coordinator of the HIV program, Dr. Melissa Bloom.

The outgrowth of these relationships was developing a memorandum of understanding (MOU) with both UCSF's Women's Specialty Program and with the Positive Health Practice at Ward 86. An MOU serves as a written document that describes in detail the cross-referral relationship between service providers. In ours we agreed to give each other's clients priority status for receiving services whenever possible. In addition to the already established phone screening, "priority status" included, when clinically appropriate, an intake evaluation within a week or two of the phone screening. Provision of timely access to services when the client is ready and willing to participate improves the course of treatment.

I received a call about fourteen months ago from a medical social worker at Ward 86, requesting individual therapy for her client, Martine, who was a single, thirty-eight-year-old French woman suffering from AIDS-related lymphoma. According to the social worker, Martine's prognosis was poor. In addition, she was suffering from major depression and living a very isolated existence. Martine wanted to decrease her depressive symptoms but was adamantly opposed to being on antidepressants. Due to the severity of both her medical and psychiatric symptoms, I conducted a phone screening with Martine the day she called and completed an intake evaluation later that week. At the completion of the intake, I assigned her a therapist immediately, and she has done very well in individual therapy. She is very motivated and engaged in treatment. She often makes lists of goals she wishes to accomplish and then follows through and achieves them. Moreover, her health has dramatically improved due to her excellent response to combination therapy, and her depressive symptoms have subsided. Throughout the course of treatment, Martine was able to freely process her fear of antidepressants and explore all the obstacles that were interfering with her willingness to try them. As a result, she has been on Prozac for over nine months. Due to her improved health and mood, she is now enrolled in a support group for women with HIV who want to return to work. Her career goal is to become an elementary school teacher.

Certainly many factors contributed to Martine's treatment success. However, her easy access to our services is a factor that should not be overlooked. Ideally, all clients should be able to access mental health services so quickly, but given the frequent capacity issues this is often not the reality.

Another measure that CSP has taken which has resulted in improved access to services from hospital-based clinics is increasing our daily phone screening hours beyond the designated daily 9:30 to 11:30 a.m. time to include afternoon hours from 2:00 to 4:00 p.m., Monday through Friday. This client-centered approach has proven beneficial in that clients are now far more likely to speak with someone directly when they call to request services rather than being asked to call back the following day.

In an effort to improve outreach to HIV-positive women attending hospital-based clinics, I have often used creative strategies to facilitate intake evaluations. One such strategy involves conducting intake evaluations in a location where clients feel both safe and comfortable.

I received a phone call from a medical social worker who had recently seen a flyer advertising the weekly group I facilitate for infected mothers. She described the case management services she was providing to Ines, a thirty-two-year-old Latina woman who was recently diagnosed with HIV and who had only shared her status with select members of her family and her former partner. Although Ines had never before received mental health services or spoken with anyone other than her family or her medical team about her status, she was intrigued by the group. The worker planned to see Ines the next day, and I suggested she have the client call me in her presence so that I could describe the group in detail and conduct a phone screening. It has often proven helpful for clients to sit in the presence of their medical social worker to receive emotional support when reaching out to ask for mental health services for the first time. Although the phone screening went well, Ines was very fearful about entering a mental health agency to complete an intake. In addition to fearing that people would think she was "crazy" if she entered CSP, she was also concerned that if she ran into someone she knew, they would know she had HIV. After hearing Ines' concerns,

I offered to conduct the intake in her home, and she quickly agreed to this plan. This proved to be an instrumental first step in successfully engaging and building trust with her. At the conclusion of the meeting, Ines was willing to come to group. She has been a dedicated group member for the past eighteen months, and she has been working very hard to be more accepting of her HIV diagnosis as well as to become more comfortable with self-disclosure about her HIV status with those she trusts.

Although conducting this intake was successful, staffing limitations, time constraints, and competing demands make such efforts not always possible.

TREATMENT GROUPS

After completing an intake evaluation, a client can sometimes wait two weeks to a month before being assigned a therapist. This presents another capacity challenge at CSP. Because this wait is not optimal, the HIV team has begun to offer clients the opportunity to enroll in time-limited ten-week group therapy sessions as a way to engage in treatment while they are awaiting assignment of an individual therapist. Some of the group topics include coping strategies for living with HIV-related anxiety and depression, spirituality, and midlife issues. Clients who enroll in these groups are asked to complete the entire ten-week group session even if they are assigned an individual therapist before the conclusion of the group. This plan has proven helpful, as the group quite frequently serves as a safe holding environment where a client can begin to explore various mental health issues with peers while awaiting individual treatment. Furthermore, clients who are socially isolated frequently meet others with whom they have issues in common so the group can also serve as a way to enhance an individual's social support network.

PROBLEMS OF THE PSYCHIATRIC PATIENT

Many of the clients referred to us from hospital-based outpatient clinics are dually and triply diagnosed as they are struggling not only with HIV but also with mental health issues and substance abuse. Some of these clients have severe substance abuse problems, which exacerbate preexisting mental health issues and put them at risk for becoming gravely disabled, sometimes requiring psychiatric hospitalization. Still others become actively suicidal, necessitating involuntary hospitalization. Quite frequently, when the client is ready to leave the hospital, outpatient mental health services are included in the discharge plan. Excellent communication and planning is required between the psychiatric social worker and the mental health clinician during this time so that the client's transition into outpatient psychotherapy is seamless. Our practice at CSP is to provide a phone screening to the client while he or she is still psychiatrically hospitalized, followed by a complete intake evaluation within five working days of the discharge.

Recently, I received a call from San Francisco General Hospital's psychiatric ward with a request for services for a client diagnosed with AIDS, paranoid schizophrenia, and cocaine dependence. Joseph had been in the hospital for over three months and needed follow-up psychiatric care including medication management. He had difficulty talking with people over the phone, so I completed the phone evaluation with the inpatient social worker and scheduled him for an intake evaluation the day after he was released. Upon completion of the intake, Joseph was assigned a therapist in two days. Remarkably enough, he engaged in treatment quickly. However, after a few months, Joseph relapsed to renewed cocaine use; the treatment team recommended a residential treatment program designed for triply diagnosed clients, but he refused. However, he did agree to participate in an intensive case management program that provides twenty-four-hour care to high-risk clients, who are too disorganized to benefit from more traditional outpatient care. There, Joseph will receive daily check-ins, referrals, and follow-up with outpatient substance abuse treatment, psychiatric care, and access to a payee for money management.

TREATMENT FOCUS SHIFT

The HIV Mental Health Case Management Program has been providing outpatient mental health services to people living with HIV since 1991. During our program's early days, we saw many more clients who were simply dying. Clinical treatment focused on helping the client cope with the loss of independence and autonomy and the loss of physical mobility secondary to fatigue or wasting. In addition, the treatment process involved exploring the client's fears and concerns regarding issues of mortality. Case management treatment issues included ensuring the client had completed a durable power of attorney for health and a will, and for parents, also ensuring that plans for guardianship had been completed. According to my colleagues who were working at CSP in the early 1990s, length of treatment was not a prominent issue as the therapy quite often continued until the client died.

With the advent of HAART, much of the treatment focus has shifted. Although some of our clients still die of AIDS, many are actually living longer and beginning to face the reality that they do indeed have a future that requires both attention and planning. Goals of treatment for these clients include returning to school to complete GEDs, college, or advanced degrees and returning to work, which frequently involves job and computer training.

For those who have been critically ill and were prepared to die but then rebounded rapidly as a result of the efficacy of their combination therapy, the adjustment to having a future can be quite overwhelming. The myriad mental health issues that accompany this reality include fear, anxiety, panic, issues of low self-esteem, and an immobilizing form of depression. For some clients who spent much time in their twenties and thirties using drugs and engaging in the exchange of sex for drugs, they are confronted with being middle-aged with virtually no marketable skills. For those who have been clean and sober for an extended period of time, the prospect of a return to work can seem overwhelming and may lead to relapse.

As a result of these issues, the clinician needs to work closely with the client and come to a mutual agreement regarding both the most pressing clinical goals as well as an appropriate length of treatment. Operating under an assumption that treatment is lifelong is no longer an option, except for those who are indeed terminally ill. The focus in many ways has now shifted to helping the client best live with a chronic illness and working with the client to take manageable steps toward achieving future goals. Often, engaging in time-limited treatment can serve as a motivating force for clients.

This shift in treatment has been challenging for staff who formerly considered that every client was a candidate for long-term therapy. Shifting the frame to a more time-limited model has proven difficult for the more seasoned clinicians who had espoused the belief that long-term treatment was optimal. Training in brief psychodynamic therapy has proven useful, as has training on termination, which underscores the importance of ending in a way that helps clients to consolidate the gains they have made in treatment. As part of a successful termination process, clients integrate these changes into their daily lives.

For clients who are more characterologically disturbed, long-term therapy continues to be the preferred method of treatment. The focus of this type of treatment includes helping clients with mood stabilization, affect regulation, impulse control, and interpersonal skills. Accomplishing such goals is usually both labor and time intensive. However, for our higher functioning clients, the focus of our more time-limited approach has shifted toward helping them take charge of the future that is now very much their own. Moreover, using a time-limited focus allows us to make treatment slots readily available to those clients newly diagnosed with an HIV-related mental health issue. This type of response is in keeping with our commitment to provide timely and accessible mental health services to those living with HIV/AIDS. Such prompt access can only contribute to a more positive therapeutic outcome.

Chapter 27

Revisiting the "Lazarus Syndrome"

Mary Tucker

HIV/AIDS was still considered a terminal illness, virtually a "death sentence," in 1994, when I began working as an HIV/AIDS social worker in a New York City hospital-based clinic. At that time the standard of care within the medical profession thought to be effective against the virus was AZT, which was observed to have severe side effects at the recommended doses. My primary task then was to help clients understand and accept their illness and face the prospect of many losses, most notably the loss of life's potential and perhaps even the loss of life itself.

In December 1995, protease inhibitors were introduced and eventually combined with certain antiretroviral medications (referred to as the "combination cocktail"). Some people with HIV/AIDS (PWAs) began to show enormous improvements. This combination of medications, commonly referred to as highly active antiretroviral therapy (HAART), began to have a direct and immediate effect by dramatically decreasing morbidity and mortality rates.

With this new promise of a lengthened and improved quality of life for many PWAs, a significant shift in perspective also took place. Dealing with old, but renewed, life issues took on an intensity previously reserved for "death anxiety" in those PWAs who had faced serious illness from AIDS complications. "This phenomenon was dubbed 'the Lazarus Syndrome' describing the biblical figure that Christ raised from the dead, and researchers estimated that tens of thousands of AIDS patients may suffer from it." Many PWAs have regressed to depressive and/or anxiety states. "Some patients have ended long term romantic relationships and others have become suicidal, an odd response to being given a reprieve from death" (France, 1998, Section F, p. 7).

Five years have passed since the term *Lazarus Syndrome* was first used in reference to HIV/AIDS patients, yet many of the same symptoms (i.e., depression, anxiety) and struggles with life issues still persist. This chapter focuses on these ongoing life issues, struggles, and challenges that resulted from improved medications and longer life expectancy. As social workers, we have a responsibility to keep up with the changes in treatment for HIV/AIDS and to help patients develop the skills to cope with these new life issues.

NEW ISSUES AND CHALLENGES

The improved quality of life experienced following HAART presented continuing physiological, psychological, and social challenges for many PWAs.

Learning to live with *all* of the medications that many choose to take is a serious issue, especially as they begin to move on with other areas of their lives. The quantity, timing, food requirements, and often serious side effects (e.g., nausea, vomiting, diarrhea, fatigue, etc.) of HAART are factors patients need to cope with. There is also uncertainty among many patients about how long the positive effects of HAART will last. Fears abound about the possibility of developing resistance to different combination therapies. Resistance, in fact, can occur when a person does not follow the often rigorous medication regimen or receives a resistant strain of HIV from someone else.

Before HAART and the resulting, often dramatic, health improvements, many PWAs felt their lives were "on hold." Now the questions arose: How do I get back to "living"? What does that mean on a very personal/individual level? How do I fill up my time and keep isolation and boredom at a minimum? How do I maintain meaning and connection in my life?

Other patients vacillate between continuing to receive benefits versus returning to work. Many PWAs were forced to leave work and go on disability or public assistance after struggling with serious illness. Anxieties now relate to questions about a return to the workplace: How do I transition back? What are the implications/effects on hard-won benefits such as Social Security Disability (SSD), Supplemental Support Income (SSI), public assistance (PA), Division of Aids Service (DAS), Medicaid, and food stamps? Can benefits be lost for good? Or decreased? Is it better to work part-time or full-time? Do I begin vocational training to regain lost skills or do I develop new skills? How do I maintain rigorous medication regimens while working? Ultimately, what happens if I can't manage working or get sick again? Do I need to start over with the benefit process? Will I be successful in reestablishing my DAS, SSI, etc.?

A third area of concern revolves around social issues such as family and intimate relationships and disclosure. How do I evaluate existing or previous relationships with family, friends, and partners? What are the expectations for future relationships? How do I tell my family, especially my children? How and when do I disclose my HIV-positive status to a potential sexual partner?

These are the conundrums most frequently posed by patients over the past few years.

SOCIAL WORK RESPONSES TO THESE CHALLENGES

Our task as social workers, in addition to recognizing and acknowledging these dilemmas, is to help patients adjust to their new life circumstances.

One way in which we helped address these issues for our clinic population was to develop a time-limited group that provided a forum for PWAs to discuss their views and concerns with respect to a variety of ongoing life issues. The format of the group was originally educational in nature, yet the group moved fairly quickly to a mutual support and self-education format. Brian Armstrong (1999), a social work student at the time, was instrumental in developing and facilitating this group, time limited to eight sessions. Group members bonded personally and strongly connected around common issues. They highlighted their need for self-validation and self-fulfillment, wanting others to help them move forward in their quest for physical, spiritual, and emotional self-caring. The group members viewed their new outlook as being a flexible approach to life.

Although holding a job continues to be important for many, for others it might not be feasible or necessary as a way to feel good about themselves. For those group members who were interested in resuming employment, such issues as balancing job income and government benefits, levels of stress associated with working, possible stigmatization, adhering to medications during the workday, and choosing between full-time and part-time work were all explored. On the other hand, some members still experienced living with HIV as their job, in and of itself. Alternatives to working were also discussed including stipend positions funded by grants, which involve work with other individuals living with HIV/AIDS. The income from these positions need not interfere with government benefits. Volunteer activities can also be meaningful additions or alternatives to jobs. Perhaps the most important aspect of the group was providing a forum whereby patients felt empowered by coming together to discuss, share information, problem solve, and support one another.

Individual therapy sessions were also available to patients and similar "back-to-life" issues also surfaced. Traditional social work interventions that helped patients cope were engagement; empathic listening; understanding "where the client is at"; assessment/identification of problem areas;

partialization and focusing on problem areas; emphasis on client strengths and abilities; validation of the wide variety of feelings that are expressed; and advocacy.

David, a thirty-one-year-old Caribbean man, was working as a home attendant about three years ago when his medical doctor first referred him to me. His physical condition was rapidly deteriorating, and it appeared as though illness and fatigue would necessitate his leaving his job. My task was to help him accept his present physical limitations and explore all of his feelings about *not* working. David needed to examine and resolve his intense feelings about accepting benefits that he had previously perceived as "accepting a handout." Education about the purpose of Social Security taxes as insurance against becoming ill and "reality testing" about the need to survive until he was ready to return to work were the focus of much of our work. Only then could I assist him with the process of obtaining disability. Helping David acknowledge his feelings of anger and sadness about getting sick after years of being healthy also became an important clinical issue. Over a period of two years and with continued therapy, David was able to make the transition back to work after HAART dramatically improved his health. He is currently contemplating a return to school for a nursing degree.

Another clinic response to difficulties faced by PWAs dealing with the physical and psychological impact of complicated medication regimens was the development of a treatment adherence program in May 2001. Adherence to medications remains a vital component to HIV treatment for two different reasons. First, treatment effectiveness is optimal when medications are taken exactly as prescribed. Second, resistance can develop if doses are missed. Either of these factors can seriously limit future treatment options.

Our treatment adherence team consists of a nurse/educator and a social worker who evaluate and help reduce or resolve the barriers—physical, psychological, financial, and social—that prevent patients from complying with their complicated medication regimens. Education, support, and individualized plans and strategies are provided for each patient; thus far, this approach appears to address the changing needs of our clients in dealing with their medications.

Lila, a twenty-eight-year-old African-American single mother with two children, was referred by her medical doctor in 1997. Before testing HIV positive, she had struggled financially. Her AIDS diagnosis came as a shock, resulting in her leaving her job as a security guard because of weakness and fatigue. In addition, her diagnosis left her feeling profoundly depressed. Initially, Lila needed help stabilizing her physical, emotional, and financial situation. Physically, medications helped at first, both antidepressants and HAART, but she began to experience severe side effects and quickly went through a series of different "combination cocktails." She was also hospitalized several times and became convinced she would be one of the "failures" of HAART treatment. Lila became increasingly anxious and depressed. Although disability and DAS benefits helped stabilize her financial situation, her physical and emotional health was still quite fragile. Consistent individual and group supportive therapy helped her cope with her emotional stressors that were identified as her inability to deal with her children and her profound sadness about her loss of life's potential. Over time her symptoms of depression and anxiety abated with the assistance of medication and counseling. Lila recently began our treatment adherence program, which helped stabilize her on her current regimen of HAART and provided her with additional educational and emotional support. Today, she is physically and emotionally stable and is presently looking at options for her future, including training, school, or volunteer activities.

Although many of our clients are responding positively to HAART therapy and beginning to move on with their lives, a number experience greater difficulties with this shift in "life" perspective. In particular, undocumented immigrants continue to have very limited access to benefits and often struggle just to survive.

Joe, a forty-year-old man from Africa, did not have legal resident status and therefore was not eligible for Medicaid or any other benefits with the exception of ADAP/AIDS Drug Assistance Program, a federally funded, state-administered program which pays for clinic treatments and medications. His clinic physician referred him to social work last year because he was struggling financially and feeling overwhelmed. Joe was working sporadically "off the books," living in a substandard room, and having difficulty making ends meet, including feeding himself. I was able to refer Joe to an agency that specifically helped undocumented immigrant PWAs. They provided assistance with services including food pantries and bilingual support groups, but he still needed more in terms of financial support, housing, and legal advocacy specific to his immigration issues. Although these are still unresolved, Joe continues to struggle but is feeling more empowered with the services and support that were provided.

Helping clients such as Joe has become increasingly complicated since the passage of the new immigration laws prohibiting people who entered this country since August 1996 from obtaining benefits, even if they are disabled. This can be terribly frustrating for social workers who are expected, not only by patients but also by medical providers and patients' families, to "fix it."

Active substance users are another group of clients for whom the transition to medication adherence and health maintenance is difficult. Working with addiction issues often necessitates that social workers be familiar with the special resources that are available, such as day treatment, outpatient addiction treatment, and twelve-step programs. In addition, a more recent but controversial philosophy has been added: harm reduction. The harm reduction model includes needle exchange programs, sites where used/dirty needles are exchanged for clean ones, and counseling around decreased substance use rather than immediate abstinence.

Maria, a forty-two-year-old Latina woman, had been fighting serious crack and alcohol addictions when she first came to the clinic in 1995. The initial task of engaging her was complicated by her difficulty in trusting anyone, a typical defense found in substance users. Maria responded to any mention of her substance use as harsh criticism and would disappear for months at a time. Dealing with her ambivalence about her addiction, "gently" cutting through her denial, and consistently being available and accepting of her despite her struggles were important clinical techniques in the work. Over time, a therapeutic alliance formed, trust developed, and Maria was able to face her addiction problems. Like many substance abusers who "bottom out" (the perception that this is their last resort which often results in a readiness for treatment), Maria enrolled in an intensive outpatient substance abuse treatment program for about eighteen months. She has done remarkably well, currently resides in her own apartment, and is regaining old and developing new skills with the help of EPRA (Employment Program for Recovering Alcoholics) and a VESID counselor (Vocational/Educational Services for Individuals with Disabilities) who will help her find and maintain suitable employment. She also continues her recovery with the help of twelve-step programs (AA and NA). Maria is now ready to deal with better adherence to her HAART therapy and demonstrates a new commitment to living well with HIV.

In response to the changing needs of PWAs, many organizations are offering expanded services. Computer training, job readiness programs, job training and placement programs, and general equivalency diploma (GED) programs are proliferating. In addition, seminars are offered by a variety of agencies discussing how returning to work will affect all major benefits.

Although providers and agencies are responding to the changing needs of PWAs, problems still exist. Many issues that appeared at the beginning of the epidemic continue to be problematic even today, such as fear and anxiety about the physical consequences of the virus, a sense of stigmatization, and survivor's guilt. Although many PWAs are experiencing a newfound "healthy" lifestyle, some have not been able to tolerate or have experienced resistance to HAART medications. For them, death anxiety may still be present. There can also be continued uncertainty around long-term efficacy and consequences of these medications.

As social workers, we need to be aware of new treatments for HIV/AIDS and to understand the resulting implications for clients. We need to be flexible, innovative, and sensitive to the changing nature of what it is like for our patients to live with HIV/AIDS in the era of the "Lazarus Syndrome."

REFERENCES

Armstrong, B. (1999). Summary of focus group, May 1999. Unpublished paper for New York University Student Project.

France, D. (1998). Holding AIDS at bay, only to face "Lazarus syndrome." *The New York Times,* October 6, Section F, p. 7.

Chapter 28

A Dialogue About the Changing Face
of Service Delivery and Supervision

Susan C. Rucker
Margaret E. Piazza

The Johns Hopkins University AIDS Service in Baltimore, Maryland, was the vision of Dr. John Bartlett, the chief of infectious disease. In the early 1980s he was working with the Hopkins arm of the Multi-Center AIDS Cohort Study, a research protocol studying the illness in a large co-hort of gay men. As these men became ill, the medical staff of the study felt an obligation to devote time to treating them and volunteered to do so one half-day a week. The Moore Clinic was born in 1984 from this sense of obli-gation. Those patients admitted to the hospital initially received social work services from the general medical social workers assigned to the various ar-eas of the hospital. However, as more and more patients were admitted to the hospital with this new and scary illness, the hospital's department of so-cial work designated this patient population as one that needed the services of an assigned social worker from the medicine unit; Gloria Fairhead be-came the first AIDS social worker at Johns Hopkins. The first inpatient AIDS unit was subsequently opened in 1985 with nine beds. The current unit opened in July 1986 and has capacity for twenty-one patients.

SUSAN: My first AIDS patient was a gay white man who had been admitted to the psychiatry unit where I worked in 1986. I had heard on the nightly

news, like millions had, about this unusual illness that was killing gay
men in San Francisco. Now one of these men was my patient. Oddly
enough, since I was not a gay man, I had no fears of contagion. That
would come later. The patient was suffering from an anxious depression
and was articulate about why he was anxious. For the most part, his issues were reality bound. He was an educated, professional man who was
independent of his parents until his illness cost him his job. He was
forced to return to his parents who loved him but who also clearly did not
understand his "chosen" lifestyle. Instead of supporting his parents
through their declining years to death, he was confronting his own death
too soon with goals unachieved and responsibilities abandoned. As I
talked with him, I saw he had developed a "terrain" of his identity that en-
compassed the history of his achievements, his goals for the future, and
the roles he played. All of this was now turned upside down; all of this
was in question because the act of love had betrayed him. He simply
didn't know who he was anymore, or what he could hope to do or even
hope for. He was articulate and insightful and, although it was painful to
observe, it was also an exhilarating and rich experience for me as a clinician. I was hooked. I transferred to the medicine unit where a program
was being developed to care for this growing population of puzzling patients.

My new colleague, Gloria, explained that we were "hooked on relevance," that is, working with people on issues that are the core of their very
being: sexuality, vocation, mortality. It was being hooked on the depth and
breadth of the issues that played out in a person's life such as medical, economic, and social issues—a cornucopia of issues that twisted, turned,
meshed, and evolved.

PEGGY: In 1987, I decided to take a sharp turn from nursing and go on to social work school. It was a last-minute decision after moving to Maryland,
and I had little choice in my initial field placement. I was assigned to the
nearby military base mental health center where I worked with a diverse
population of active and retired members and their dependents. I began
hearing about an HIV support group that was being facilitated by two of
the civilian social workers. It seemed to be shrouded in a bit of mystery.
The workers would say little about the group to anyone, so the confidentiality and level of protectiveness that surrounded the group was intrigu-
ing to say the least. Even the other mental health providers in the clinic
knew little. I felt that I had to know more about this group and this new
illness called HIV. What could this condition be that the military would
grant someone a medical discharge and guarantee health care for life?
Who was affected by it? What did it mean in terms of social work chal-

lenges? After some time and persistence, the group leaders agreed to ask the members if it might be possible for me to sit in on a session. The little that I learned about HIV and the issues facing these young military members was enough to pull me in completely. These were men and women who were not only stigmatized by their families and friends, they were in the military where, certainly, homosexuality was not condoned and where general discharge was the order of business for someone who was [known to be] gay. Being a military member was an important part of one's identity. And, while they might have some small thought about sacrificing their lives for their country, it seemed a remote possibility in the face of this stigmatizing, deadly disease.

I knew without question where I wanted my second-year field placement, and I put in a request to be assigned to the National Institutes of Health. The university, however, had other plans for me, and I was offered a placement at Johns Hopkins on the inpatient AIDS unit where I subsequently met my field supervisor, Susan Rucker.

Neither of us knew at that time that our partnership in the AIDS service would bring many years of challenge, fulfillment, frustration, joy, and sorrow. We have persevered in the midst of the many evolutions in HIV medical care and funding, which have had enormous impact on delivery of social work services to our patients.

DEVELOPMENT OF AIDS SOCIAL WORK

When the hospital decided to designate two social workers for HIV care, service was provided two afternoons a week in the Moore Clinic and on the inpatient unit, Osler 8. Social work was involved with all social care needs, from concrete to existential, in a comprehensive case management style. A worker might help a patient complete and file an application for financial entitlements, arrange for home nursing, or hold a family meeting. Social workers made rounds with the medical staff and provided illness education to families of origin or families of choice. A true multidisciplinary approach developed because the service included a faculty physician, house staff, nurses, and social workers. Social work staffing allowed for 100 percent screening and service by social work and, because the social worker saw the patient both in the clinic and on the unit, continuity of care was ensured.

Patients felt secure in dealing with fewer staff. Systems were smaller, more intimate, and easier to negotiate. The phone menus of today were then a nightmare of the future. The worker who helped patients apply for a pharmacy program was the same person who heard their fears about disfiguring illness, was the same person who spoke with their parents on the phone, and was the same person at the bedside during admissions. Looking back now, it is clear that although we were busy, volumes were low enough to allow for strong relationship building with the patients and family members who accompanied them to the clinic. This level of personal attention and continuity of care afforded a sense of security to patients during a time when very little else was certain in terms of their treatment. The hospital required all social workers to be master's degree prepared, and the environment afforded us the opportunity to utilize our skills and interventions. It was an extraordinary time in terms of richness of opportunity for mental health interventions and dealing with end-of-life issues.

SUSAN: The strength of the bond between social worker and patient was brought home to me when the fiancée of a patient dissolved into tears upon seeing me with a new, very short haircut. "You should have told me. You should have prepared me for such a big change!" she sobbed. It was sobering to realize I represented such an unimagined stability for this young woman at a time of horrific upheaval. She was dealing with the diagnosis of her partner and the fact that he was already gravely ill and deciding to return to his family in the Southwest, leaving her and her children.

It was not unusual for workers to be reprimanded by patients or family for absences from work for illness or vacation. This sense of abandonment was unexpectedly acute for those patients who developed strong emotional ties to staff.

PEGGY: This became evident while I was seeing a patient for short-term counseling. When I returned after a two-week vacation and met with the patient, I was struck by her coolness and my inability to engage her. At last she became very angry and exploded with, "Where have you been? You're not supposed to be gone." I was taken aback by the vehemence in her voice. It felt like a big burden and took some time for me to put it in perspective in a way that could be used therapeutically with the patient.

During that time, social workers functioned in a strong mental health style. Psychiatric input was minimal, limited to consultations. We completed mental health assessments and were viewed by the medical staff as the first level of intervention. On the inpatient unit, we screened for depression and dementia and conferred with medical staff to obtain psychiatric consultations. The medical staff expected that the social worker would assess the mental state of both the patient and the family in regard to the diagnosis, hope for treatment, and death and dying issues. We frequently maintained counseling clients for short-term therapy, sometimes including a family member or friend. In the outpatient clinic we collaborated with the department of psychiatry and provided mental health screening for all new patients. This assessment included a battery of psychological tests including the Mini-Mental, Trails A and B, the Beck Depression Inventory, and others. The social worker would determine a psychiatric diagnosis when indicated and present the case to the psychiatrist who would confirm the diagnosis and accept the patient into care that day. Most patients were offered psychotropic medications in conjunction with outpatient psychiatric follow-up; when indicated, some were admitted to the inpatient psychiatric unit. This intense screening revealed that approximately 50 percent of new patients presented with an Axis I diagnosis.

SUSAN: This was an exhilarating time, clinically speaking. We had excellent opportunities to use our skills with patients and families. Our diagnostic skills were recognized and valued by the nursing and medical staff.

THE CURRENT CLIMATE

Today the hospital's AIDS service treats approximately 3,000 patients, a far cry from its modest beginnings. Funding for psychiatry has grown significantly, allowing for their daily presence in the clinic. As a result, the mental health role of social work has been diluted. No longer do the social workers do a thorough screening for psychiatric illness. The medical staff looks to the members of the psychiatry team to screen and call upon the psychiatrist as needed. Social work staff is now divided between inpatient and outpatient locations and no longer cross over. The twenty-one bed inpatient unit, with more than 850 admissions a year, is pressured by the managed care organizations and other insurers to move patients to subacute settings quickly. The continuity of care in terms of social work assignments on the inpatient unit remains, but the level of personal attention and mental health care has diminished in the face of complex discharge planning. Our social workers, like many others, are limited in their ability to locate long-term care for patients with multiple medical needs compounded by behavior issues resulting from substance use or psychiatric illness.

Our outpatient clinic has grown from two half-day sessions to five full-day sessions with an average of ninety patients seen on most days and an average of 120 on the day patients are seen by psychiatry. Social work staffing for the clinic has grown to a total of eight providers: one MSW and one

BSW who both spend 80 percent of their time in clinic and 20 percent providing substance treatment groups; one Ryan White case manager (BS degree) with a designated caseload; one Ryan White advocate (high school graduate) who provides specific services; one Social Security eligibility specialist (BS); one managed care case manager (MS) with a designated caseload; and two supervisors (MSWs—Peggy and Susan) who provide cross-coverage and administrative functions. The volume and pace are high because social work staff is available for any patient coming to the clinic that day to see the medical provider or specialist. Since the beginning, work space has been limited and poorly designed for social work interventions and confidentiality. Although our space grew over time, so did the total numbers of staff needing space. The result is that some work is done in public areas. The work is paper heavy, as workers must document for data collection as well as for continuity of care within the clinic and for referral purposes. On the positive side, however, concrete resources such as medications, transportation, and durable medical equipment have increased because of the Ryan White funding acquired through this social work documentation of need and utilization.

SOCIAL WORK RESPONSE TO DEVELOPMENT IN CARE

"Among infectious disease epidemics, there has been no equal in terms of the velocity of scientific discovery and the dramatic changes in outcome resulting from advances in HIV therapy" (Bartlett, 2001, p. 8). The social work staff has been along on this roller-coaster ride since the beginning.

In the early years, we watched as doctors marveled that humans were ill with a disease previously found in birds, *Mycobacterium avium intracellulare.* We were on rounds when a member of the medical staff wondered aloud if cytomegalovirus could infect organs other than the eye; we discovered it could. Today we no longer see deaths from *Pneumocystis carinii* pneumonia except in unusual cases, and we now see great improvements in patients with progressive multifocal leukoencephalopathy and dementia who are able to utilize highly active antiretroviral therapy. With medical advances, we have seen total-care patients return to full functioning. Patients who struggled to get disability payments now present with the problem of boredom and lack of meaning in life because they are not working and feel completely well.

Our practice focus has changed for the most part from helping patients come to terms with death to coming to terms with a new life that includes HIV and other chronic illnesses involving frequent monitoring and complex treatment. Patients have been asked now to play a more active role as providers discuss the benefits and difficulties of medication options. They have incorporated heavy pill burdens into their daily lives and experienced cruel side effects in order to fight HIV. Patients are forced to "ride the HIV roller coaster" of remissions and exacerbations. Once the course was sadly predictable, but predictable to be sure. Today we speak with patients about death and dying as they stand at the precipice when suddenly, with care and a new cocktail, they are scooped up "superman" fashion and rescued from the brink. On the other hand, some patients have been reckless in their compliance with care, assuming that no matter what they do there will be some new medicine to rescue them. Is it any wonder that it becomes ever more difficult to address the end-of-life issues that patients and families come to believe can never happen because there is surely rescue around the corner? Despite this difficulty, we continue to attempt to address end-of-life issues from the beginning of care.

Our social work practice has evolved and expanded hand in hand with the developments in medical care. We have incorporated an understanding of adherence and resistance. We are giving more attention to maintaining pharmacy and insurance coverage. As gatekeepers of Ryan White funds, we are aware of costs and interact more with medical staff as we request substitution of drugs or exert pressure on providers to complete forms needed to apply for benefits and medications. Social work has become valued within the clinical setting for its unique expertise in matters that range from fairly minor interactions to liaison with families and community services, end-of-life issues and care approaches, compliance, and teaching.

PEGGY: We may have lost much of our mental health screening focus to the psychiatric team, but our role has really expanded. We have become a valued part of a true multidisciplinary team. I remember the early days when physicians tended to bypass us and had no real idea what social work could do. Today they recognize us as an important part of the team.

SUSAN: It is gratifying to be so completely integrated into the AIDS service care structure. But when staff are so dependent on us that they panic when we have a staff meeting and they can't find one of us, I know that success has its price.

Our practices regarding usage of medication funds have reflected a total care approach to treating patients. This is a result of our own belief structure and the fact that primary care is provided in our clinic as well as HIV specialty care. The level of funding has for a long time made it possible to purchase any medication prescribed by the provider. Today, suddenly, we are faced with a reduction in funding requiring drastic cuts in the types of medications that we can provide. There will be difficult decisions that must be made that will affect medical practice and patient care.

PEGGY: This makes our position as gatekeepers of the resource very uncomfortable. It feels like we are compromising care because we cannot provide the level of coverage that we have consistently been able to provide. On the other hand, I have to remind myself that despite the cuts, we are still able to provide a level of coverage above and beyond that which is available through most any other area HIV clinic.

FUNDING AND PROGRAM DEVELOPMENT

Evolution of funding streams and program development presents real "chicken-egg" issues. The development of the program has been largely determined by the funding sources available and their criteria. At the same time, the ability to maintain and develop new funding sources is based on success of the program and proper data maintenance and reporting. There are two distinct types of funding, and each has its own level of impact within the clinic setting. One is the type already mentioned: funding for programs. The other is funding specifically for patient care services that include medications, transportation, and durable medical equipment.

SUSAN: Initial funding for HIV social work services was provided by the Johns Hopkins Hospital's Social Work Department. As the AIDS service grew, it became clear to the program administrators that it was advantageous to have social workers who worked solely for the service, without allegiances elsewhere. State funding became available through a grant program called the Diagnostic Evaluation Unit in 1986, which was awarded to Johns Hopkins University Department of Medicine. We were told we were the first social workers to be hired by the university rather than the hospital when we came on in 1988 and 1989. We were MSWs who had experience in the hospital as medical social workers, and we subscribed to the hospital philosophy that "if it isn't documented, it wasn't done." We also subscribed to the belief that a systems approach could address more facets of and result in better patient care. We were able to address the individual patient's problem and identify the system failures that contributed to the problem. I remember when we couldn't get medicines for a patient who was discharged from a nursing home because the institutional medical assistance (a Medicaid type program) had not been converted to community medical assistance.

PEGGY: I discovered that the nursing home had several weeks to complete paperwork notifying the state that the person was no longer institutionalized. This meant that patients were sent to nursing homes for subacute care, were discharged, but then were unable to obtain medications or home care because the form of their medical assistance had not been switched from institutional to community. Unearthing this problem and confronting medical assistance policy officials resulted in a regulation that required nursing homes to act in a timelier manner, thus assuring a patient had access to the means to maintain recovery.

Another change I was able to effect was in the processing of Maryland Pharmacy Assistance applications. It was the practice of the Pharmacy Assistance office to take thirty days to process an application. At the time, this meant that patients who had left the hospital having started HIV medications were not able to continue on these medications after discharge until they received their Pharmacy Assistance. They risked relapse and the development of resistance to HIV medications. I called the director of the Pharmacy Assistance Program and explained the harm to patients caused by this thirty-day lapse in HIV medications. The director was willing to work out a method to process applications in twenty-four to forty-eight hours for those we identified as being in urgent need. Because of this, patients who need to start on HIV medicines will have only a few days delay.

As the AIDS service outpatient clinic grew with increasing numbers of providers and patients, the need for more concrete services increased. Alternative funding was obtained through the Ryan White Care Act to support this growth. As a result, social work staff have become gatekeepers who assess needs, make arrangements for transportation, authorize purchases of medications and durable medical equipment (DME), and negotiate with medical providers over medication costs and substitutions. In addition, social workers maintain data on the use of the resources to support continuing and/or increasing funding needs.

SUSAN: This gatekeeper business is a real mixed bag. Some patients inevitably see us as the people who hand out stuff. At times there is an expectant attitude, as exemplified by the patient who told me he was here for his "annual emergency food voucher." I do try to use the concrete issues as a platform on which to build a more therapeutic relationship with a patient. It has really helped to have something concrete that can demonstrate caring, particularly with very angry or anxious patients.

Ryan White funding continues to support new programs. Of importance to the social work profession is that this funding reflects the federal belief that MSWs should be employed in managerial positions and that direct service can appropriately be provided by persons with less than master's training. This means that the MSW who, due to the nature of social work training, is sensitive to the interplay of individual patient issues (micro) with the larger service delivery system issues (macro) is removed from the arena where these factors intersect. Therefore, the MSW lacks timely opportunities to clearly relate individual problems to wider system failures.

There are now many different grants that exist: grants for new patients without insurance; grants for advocacy for ongoing patients without medical assistance managed care; grants for outreach and assistance with obtaining medical assistance for those who have lost coverage. Delivery of care has become fragmented now that patients have to interact with different staff depending on the insurance or funding source and the service being provided.

THE IMPACT OF MANAGED CARE

Another recent impact on patient care, program development, and practice issues was the introduction of medical assistance managed care in 1997. Simultaneously, the AIDS service inaugurated the first capitated program in Maryland for AIDS-defined patients (Moore Options). Medical assistance managed care quickly proved to be a double-edged sword. On one hand, it prevented much of the "doctor hopping" that was common among patients. These reduced problems such as prescription narcotic abuse and counterproductive care by several physicians with differing approaches. On the other hand, it forced many patients into care with providers they had never seen. In addition, there was a limited enrollment period during which a provider could be chosen, but often patients were auto-assigned to an unknown provider before they were aware of the need to choose one. Patients assumed that they could simply continue to receive care in the clinic they had been associated with for a long period of time. Patients were forced to make difficult choices between, for example, their medical care provider and their substance treatment program when the two providers were not within the same managed care organization.

In terms of program development, our own social work program benefited because a case manager was budgeted in the Moore Options. This added one staff member whose sole responsibility is for the case management of the nearly 300 clients enrolled in the program. The budget also included some transportation money that augmented the Ryan White funds for transportation.

The advent of managed care impacted our practice in other ways. We became responsible for ongoing case management for an additional 200 patients as a result of the agreements between the AIDS service and another managed care organization. This service is provided by the clinic social workers who collaborate with a nurse care coordinator responsible for the medical case management. This adds another layer of management between social work and the resources. The managed care organizations have adopted drug formularies so that the broad drug coverage once provided through medical assistance is a thing of the past. The social worker is now the middleman who negotiates between the provider and the managed care organization's pharmacy to obtain drug substitution or exceptions to the rules.

SUPERVISION

The AIDS Service Social Work and Case Management Program reached its current size in 2000 and is comprised of ten positions.

SUSAN: Peggy and I divide the responsibility of oversight of the staff and program. I function as the program director and handle administrative duties. I also provide direct service to patients and coverage for absent workers. Peggy is the clinical supervisor and provides oversight for all of the staff working with patients; she reviews documentation to assess practice, trends in patient needs, and accuracy of data collection. She is responsible for scheduling and cross coverage. She provides direct service in the clinic and coverage for the inpatient staff. Overall, our program development is largely dictated by funding. Someone else within the AIDS service does the writing of grants and program development. We provide input in terms of what we see is possible as a social work function within the current clinic setting. The social work staff recognizes our individual responsibilities while at the same time understanding that we function as a team.

PEGGY: Historically the inpatient unit has been staffed by two full-time MSWs. This level of staffing is vital as the positions still demand individuals with mental health expertise and the ability to think critically. As a member of the interdisciplinary team, they must be able to function independently, addressing complex discharge planning issues and fragmented family and limited home care and placement resources. They also provide education and direction to interns and residents faced with what may be uncharted waters in their formative professional years.

One of my supervisory challenges evolved from the changes brought on by the insurance and funding sources. I am too frequently the bearer of bad news that impacts workers' autonomy and use of discretionary judgment. For example, with the cuts in funding the list of covered drugs becomes shorter and shorter, leaving little room for negotiations. Also, the increasingly complicated relationships with insurance companies have made discharge planning more difficult. What difference does it make if you have skills in dealing with families if the insurer gives you few options to work with? In the "old days" you could look for the option that was convenient for the family or most appropriate for the patient. Now, sometimes, the most appropriate option for the patient isn't even offered.

SUSAN: These are complex jobs, and we have always looked for MSWs to fill them primarily because *we* are MSWs, but also because that level of training brings with it a common language to describe, discuss, and evaluate patient needs. But as I look back, I think that the level of education had less to do with success in the position than with the personal characteristics of the individuals. The people who stay and thrive on the inpatient unit are those who have a real passion about the work, the setting, and the population. As one of our workers will tell you, he is doing his own soul work every day.

PEGGY: But my fear now is that all of the changes and constraints are bringing such a sense of frustration that this passion and enthusiasm will be dampened. After the intense initial phase of bringing staff up to speed with the job, the policy and procedural environment of the AIDS service and Johns Hopkins settings, supervision with the inpatient workers has become rather informal and less and less dependent on a weekly meeting. Now, staff are likely to contact me for the following: they may hope that I can "magic" a resource unknown to them, or assist in solving a major dilemma the team is facing, such as patient autonomy versus medical paternalism or complicated end-of-life issues.

Supervision in the outpatient setting presents a unique set of challenges. With the diversity of staff in terms of education, experience, and the variety of their roles, supervisory approaches must be tailored to meet the needs of the individual in the particular position. In addition, we have environmental pressures that involve limited space, high patient volumes, a rapid daily pace, and the heavy paperwork demands of documenting our activities and collecting data.

PEGGY: In the clinic setting a large part of supervision takes place on a daily basis with a problem-solving approach rather than a conceptual one. I review all the documentation on two levels: to assess the quality and depth of the interactions and to ensure that all of the data elements are completed and appropriate (this is tedious but vital in reporting to funding agencies and seeking future support).

SUSAN: Peggy's oversight has allowed us to develop practice guidelines so that we have uniformity of approach.

PEGGY: Also challenging is that I am not supervising a group of people who are doing the same job. They are each handling a component of patient care and are working at a variety of levels. This means that I have to work on helping them to integrate the different pieces of our program into a coherent whole. At the same time I am trying to help each one find rewarding activities within the scope of his or her particular job.

Most social work services provided in the clinic happen within a sequential case management format. Various staff members at different times will provide service to a given patient. Therefore, patients must repeat their story and establish some level of relationship with multiple staff members. Each encounter is a discrete intervention that is linked to past and future interventions only by thorough and concise documentation. This ensures that the next worker who sees the patient knows exactly what has been done and what still needs to be done. It also helps prevent staff splitting, which otherwise might be an issue. The patient volume makes for a fast-paced environment that can often allow little time for reflective interventions.

In stark contrast to the sequential case management format is the availability of two funded positions, which allow for ongoing case management service to select clinic patients. These social work case managers have the opportunity to develop relationships over time with the patients they follow, allowing for a more comprehensive view of the patient. Supervision for these workers involves helping them to learn the specific case management requirements of each funding source as well as examining therapeutic relationship building and maintenance. Each has certain data and reporting responsibilities that require periodic monitoring by the supervisors. Both case managers carry heavy caseloads, so helping them to prioritize and focus their efforts efficiently is important. Stress levels are increased because of space limitations. Neither worker has an assigned office in the clinic and often must see patients under less than private, confidential circumstances. As supervisors, we must deal with the frustration experienced by staff as well as by patients who feel that they are receiving service in an inadequate setting.

As the AIDS epidemic has grown and affected more segments of society, the approach to care has evolved and the challenges for social work have multiplied. Focus on concrete needs and shifts in funding for mental health care have impacted our practice. As the number of patients has risen, the greater the pressures have become to acquire funding to support program growth. This, in turn, has put more responsibility on social work to collect and document data to justify the need for this increased funding. This means that there is less time to spend with patients and less time to do insightful work. Supervisors are caught in the dilemma of striving to maintain the quality of interactions in the face of high volume, fragmentation of services, and administrative responsibilities.

SUSAN: We started out being all the staff there was, "doing it all." In the beginning, I had imagined a program to be a phalanx of MSWs "doing it all" with small, intimate caseloads. Ryan White forced me to rethink the types of services to see if they could be subdivided, and they could. Ryan White forced me to think about who delivers the care and whether MSWs were required; they are, but not everywhere. In a year's time we will see two-thirds of the total clinic population and provide over 10,000 individual interventions—big and small. There is a great deal of care to be provided and a great deal of good to be done. We continue to struggle with environmental issues, funding, and dwindling resources; this is AIDS in an inner-city hospital, after all. But we are also blessed with the resource of good-hearted, devoted staff members. Goodness knows what keeps them going some days, but they do. It's hard work even if you *want* to be here. I can't think of any other place I'd rather be.

PEGGY: As the systems change and the challenges to providing quality care in an environment of diminishing health care coverage grow daily, I often lament the "old days." There seemed to be a sense of calling and intensity that brought itself to the work as well as a greater sense of reward amid the highs and lows shared with patients, families, and one another. All this has given way to a more desperate struggle to keep our heads above water while we collect data and do paperwork. Yet there continues to be nothing I would wish to do more than this. I, too, am hooked.

REFERENCE

Bartlett, John G. (2001). HIV: Twenty years in review. *The Hopkins HIV Report* 13(4): 8-9.

Chapter 29

The Challenges of Working with Perinatally Infected Adolescents: Clinical and Concrete Possibilities

Matthew Feldman

One of the greatest triumphs of the AIDS epidemic has been the dramatic decrease in perinatal infections. Between 1992 and 1997, perinatally acquired AIDS cases declined 66 percent in the United States (CDC, 1999), due to the new prenatal medication protocol that HIV-infected mothers could take during pregnancy. However, even as perinatal transmissions continue to decrease, there is still a significant group of infected children and adolescents living with HIV/AIDS. Of the total AIDS cases reported through December 2001, 13,502 are children between birth and nineteen years old (CDC, 2001a). Total deaths of persons reported with AIDS are 467,910, including 462,653 adults and adolescents and 5,257 children under age thirteen (CDC, 2001b). Many of these children were infants infected at birth, before the medical community knew how to significantly decrease the risk of perinatal transmissions. When they were born, there was no effective treatment to control the virus. However, some of these children survived. They were able to live long enough to start antiretroviral treatment and improve medically. There are stories about children who were close to dying and then dramatically improved to the point where they now have high T-cell counts and undetectable viral loads. There is a whole population of children that everyone thought would never reach adolescence. Although they may not be a rising statistic, perinatally infected adolescents are an important, and sometimes forgotten, part of the AIDS epidemic.

PERINATALLY INFECTED ADOLESCENTS

Adolescents who have been infected with HIV since birth face unique challenges that are different from adolescents who contracted the virus from risk-related behaviors. Perinatally infected adolescents experienced the stressors and traumas related to HIV starting at a young age. As children, they may have had multiple hospitalizations, difficult medication regimens with even worse side effects, and countless injections. Many of them watched their parents die and are now being raised by grandparents, aunts and uncles, or older siblings.

At some point in or before their adolescence, a question that is almost inevitably asked of the pediatrician is, "When can I stop taking these pills? I'm so tired of taking them; I've had to all my life. They make me feel worse. I feel fine." Perinatally infected children know only a life with HIV/AIDS. Adults and even adolescents that were infected through risk-related behaviors know a life without HIV, and sometimes this can give them more of a reason to stay healthy. Perinatally infected adolescents do not have this kind of contrast available to them.

ADOLESCENT DEVELOPMENT

The Center for Comprehensive Care at St. Luke's-Roosevelt Hospital Center in New York City treats perinatally infected children and adolescents. As the younger children grow into adolescence, we are encountering an increasing rate of antiretroviral (ARV) nonadherence, despite the adolescents' knowledge of how this could adversely affect their immune systems. There is a range of reasons that nonadherent behavior might emerge at this age. One may be related to normative developmental issues. HIV-infected adolescents, whether or not they have disclosed their diagnosis, have a daily reminder that they are different from their peers. At this time of life, the individual (the adolescent) is increasingly concerned with the peer group's values and codes of behavior. Teenagers also become less interested in their parents' activities and expand their own ideas and values which are sometimes different from those of their families (Rubenstein, 1991). Since adolescence is traditionally marked by movement away from the family and toward the peer group, HIV-infected adolescents may want to stop taking medications as a way to forget about having the virus, as an act of independence, and/or so they can blend in with their peers.

Depression may also be a factor. Given the amount of physical and social changes that take place during adolescence, depression can be a common by-product of this developmental phase. In addition to the anxieties traditionally related to adolescent development, HIV-infected teenagers must contend with additional pressures related to sex and mortality. Although many teenagers with HIV are depressed, we have not worked with any that have any active suicidality or a wish to die. The focus of the depression is more related to the stress of adherence and the desire to be a "normal" adolescent.

FAMILIES WITH PERINATALLY INFECTED ADOLESCENTS

The adolescent's family also plays an important part in maintaining adherence. Brantley, Stabler, and Whitt (1981) noted that the common problems of families with chronically ill children include "lack of money, isolation from the community of the healthy, prejudice, misunderstanding in the schools, loneliness, boredom, and depression" (p. 229). Chronic illness "introduces the external stresses of treatment regimens, separations, hospitalizations, and fears and anxieties which undermine otherwise adequate support systems that reduce dysfunctional families into chaos" ("Pediatric AIDS," 1989, p. 230).

When parents and guardians are not emotionally or physically available, we have found that adolescents are less likely to be adherent. The interaction of family stressors and adolescent development can have serious consequences on adherence. Sometimes parents forget that even though their adolescent appears to want total autonomy, they, the adults, still play an important role in their child's life. As much as adolescents want to be independent, they still need adults on whom they can rely. The penultimate wisdom is the understanding that the adolescent's defensive opposition and withdrawal do not obviate a continuing need for the parental framework during restructuring (Winnicott, 1972).

For adolescents with HIV/AIDS, parents can feel that children are old enough to manage their own medication administration. Parents are often too overwhelmed to monitor adherence carefully, or may not even be involved enough with their child's health to provide the necessary supervision. This could also be due to preexisting family dysfunction, which as suggested, becomes exacerbated by the stresses related to their child's health. On the other hand, this may not be the case. Many parents place unfair and unreasonable responsibilities on their teenagers, holding them to the expectation of following their own complicated medication schedule. The medication regimes tend to be complicated, and adolescents, given varying emotional and cognitive capacities, have different levels of ability in terms of adherence.

CLINICAL CHALLENGES AND NONADHERENCE

Resistance can develop to ARV regimens when adherence is not possible, thereby decreasing the number of remaining ARV combinations. The ARV regimens must be strictly followed. If multiple doses are missed, the regimen could become ineffective and viral resistance could develop. Children and their parents may then be informed that a certain treatment may be their last option. This situation has been discussed many times with the team (medicine, nursing, social work, psychiatry) with whatever interventions possible being made. However, the team is not always successful. When that point is reached, the question we are most often faced with is, "Can this child stay at home or does he or she need to be in a setting where the medications will be administered consistently, so that the responsibility does not rest solely on the child or the support system?" It is important to note that this question emerges in homes both with and without appropriate supervision. Of course, stronger supervision almost always increases the chances of adherence, but that does not ensure complete compliance.

The first intervention tried prior to any separation from the home is to arrange for a visiting nurse and a home health aide to provide more support in the home. This has even included twice a day directly observed medication intake for children who have a significant problem with adherence. However, it has been our experience that if the home is already chaotic, these services are not effective, particularly since parental involvement is required by the nursing agency. The services, however, do succeed in providing support to parents who are involved in their child's health care but are overwhelmed by other responsibilities, such as work or, in some cases, managing their own virus. If the team comes to the conclusion that the child cannot be appropriately medically supervised in the home, the question that follows is, "Where are we going to place this child?"

In New York City there are two skilled nursing facilities that provide services only to children and adolescents with HIV/AIDS. Short stays and a discharge plan either to home or foster care (when family is unavailable) at the time of admission are generally required. A short stay might guarantee that a child takes medication while in the facility. There is constant supervision and encouragement regarding medication adherence. The nursing staffs at these facilities are able to provide the necessary time so that patients take their medication. Some nurses have reported spending up to an hour with an adolescent. However, a short stay may not necessarily give the children time to internalize what they have learned at the facility—especially to the extent that they would be able to continue that level of adherence. When they arrive home, many unfortunately return to the same situation that prompted their original admission.

Short stays, however, can be beneficial in stabilizing an ill child who might require more rehabilitation time after a hospital discharge or as a respite for a family who cannot care for a child for a specific period of time. If a parent remains involved during the stay and really commits to helping the child maintain adherence, then a short stay might potentially be effective. If the parent remains uninvolved, then the stay becomes only a short-lived period of adherence that will not ultimately improve the child's overall immune system in any significant way.

Some children do not have clear discharge plans when they enter these facilities. A clear discharge plan means there is some stable home environment where the child can be placed after their stay at the facility and receive continued support around adherence. If there is no plan and parental supervision is inadequate, child welfare could become involved, and the child might be placed in a foster home. The foster home may or may not be sensitive to the needs of a child or adolescent with HIV/AIDS.

Sarah is a fifteen-year-old girl who was perinatally infected. Her mother died when Sarah was six years old, with her daughter at her bedside. Her father was an alcoholic who, because of his addiction, could not take care of the family. Instead, her twenty-two-year-old brother, Eric, became the primary caretaker, assuming the responsibility for Sarah, their twelve-year-old brother Evan, and Eric's two-year-old son Hal. Two years ago, their father died, and Eric officially became the head of the family and Evan and Sarah's temporary legal guardian. Eric, Evan, Sarah, and Hal lived together in a three-bedroom apartment in the Bronx. Since Sarah had an active public assistance case through the Division of AIDS Services (DAS), the family received rental assistance. In addition, both Sarah and Evan received survivor's benefits and food stamps. Eric had no income of his own. Sarah also had a visiting nurse to help monitor her medications, as well as a home health aide to help her around the house. Throughout the fall of 2000, there were multiple problems with Sarah's DAS case. Eric reported difficulties with the DAS supervisor, indicating the supervisor was abusive and that he was not receiving the rent money on time. His relationship with the landlord was becoming acrimonious, as the amount of back rent he owed increased. There was increasing confusion around who owed whom what monies, and in early 2001, Eric called me repeatedly with complaints that the landlord was harassing him. During this time, Sarah was not taking her ARV medications. In spite of increasing her nursing visits, providing her with more supervision around medication administration was still not enough. Eric was not emotionally or physically available enough to help her, and he was becoming frustrated with his parenting responsibilities, having lost his adolescence and early adult years in the role of father to his two siblings. Eric also began to call and meet with me less frequently, so it became harder to monitor what was happening in the family,

In early February 2001, the family was evicted from their home. Eric and Evan moved to a studio apartment in the Bronx. By this time, Eric's son, Hal, was removed by the Administration for Children's Services (ACS) for medical neglect and returned to his biological mother in Ohio, creating another loss for the family. Sarah went to live with her best friend's family, which was an easy, temporary solution. Although the nursing visits continued, she still was not taking her medications properly. Her pediatrician chose to take her off ARVs, fearing increasing side effects and resistance. This was the scariest time for the treatment team at the clinic, because Sarah began to deteriorate the longer she was off the medications. She developed peripheral neuropathy, lost weight, and her CD4s continued to decrease. The urgency intensified to find her a place where she could stabilize medically and receive her ARVs consistently.

I spent two frustrating months trying to find a place for Sarah to live. I spoke to other social workers who work with terminally ill children but were unaware of any resources for Sarah. I was discovering that there was a dearth of services for terminally ill children, not just those with AIDS, who needed a long-term residence that provided both medical care and a permanent home. For Sarah, there were no other options for a very sick adolescent who needed to be in a skilled nursing facility (SNF) and who had no family to return to. I looked to the adult world of AIDS services, and through my supervisor's relationship with the director of admissions, our first adolescent was admitted to Highbridge Woodycrest Center, an SNF for adults with AIDS and their infected and/or affected children. Many of the current residents are recovering addicts with histories of incarceration, homelessness, and violence.

Given the numbers of adults who are living with AIDS, it is not uncommon to see middle-aged men and women residing in long-term care facilities. People no longer need a place to prepare to die, but rather a place to continue to live with the virus. In New York City, there are currently about fourteen such SNFs. These facilities provide a safe place to stay, along with supportive services, such as primary medical care, nursing, social work, and psychiatric care. Residents who are able often work toward finding an independent living situation.

Although Highbridge Woodycrest was not the "ideal" place for an adolescent girl, our team had confidence in the staff, who made every effort to integrate Sarah into the milieu. The Highbridge staff was aware from the beginning that Sarah would not likely return to live with her brother, even if she became adherent and medically stabilized. Eric was living with Evan, and now Eric's girlfriend had moved in as well. Nothing had changed in Eric's abilities to care for Sarah. Although he loves Sarah, he does not have the skills to care for a sick adolescent. Highbridge would be Sarah's home indefinitely.

Since Sarah has been there, her health has improved dramatically. Her T-cell count has gone from twenty-eight to ninety-eight in the span of ten months. She is on ARVs again, and the regime has been successful. She has gained weight and no longer appears cachectic. She recently started high school again and is enjoying the chance to socialize with peers. During a recent visit with Sarah at Highbridge, it was clear that she is a very popular resident. While she was giving me a tour, practically everyone either acknowledged her, offered help, or stopped to talk with her. In contrast was Sarah's report of her experience: Sarah said to me, "I hate it here, Matt. I want to go to somewhere with kids my own age." It is difficult to tell Sarah that for now there is no other place for her to go. Sarah ideally wants to live with Eric and Evan, but Eric cannot give her the care she needs. Sarah is aware of this on some level, and she often expresses how angry she is at Eric for not taking care of her in the way she needed. As she and I sat in the cafeteria, talking about why she does not like Highbridge, hugs, jokes, and conversations shared with other residents and staff interrupted those thoughts. In spite of Sarah's feelings, it is clear she has made many gains at Highbridge. She has many parental figures, something she has both craved and lacked for most of her life. Her health continues to improve, and for the first time in years she is in an appropriate school setting. Sarah is able to recognize these improvements, but that does not detract from the pain of knowing she cannot be reunited with her family in any real, permanent way. Sarah's stay at Highbridge has been successful so far, mostly due to Sarah's motivation to participate in improving her health. The key issue in her situation was lack of supervision: reminding, encouraging, and supporting her around medication adherence. Her family, unfortunately, could not provide that for her.

In contrast to Sarah is Jamie, a fifteen-year-old adolescent boy, also perinatally infected. His mother died when he was four years old, and his maternal grandmother, Carol, has taken care of him since then. He has an extended family that is also involved in his care and support, primarily his maternal aunt, Mary. Carol loves Jamie very much and will do whatever is necessary in terms of his medical care. However, she is very concrete in her thinking and has difficulty with parenting skills, such as setting and maintaining good limits with Jamie.

Jamie has always presented a challenge to the team. Since his early adolescence Jamie has not taken his medications consistently. Many attempts have been made over the years to try to help him be adherent. When Jamie was eleven years old, he went to a residence and adjusted successfully to his ARV regime. However, soon after his discharge, he regressed. The residence provided him with the structure and encouragement he needed to stay adherent.

When he came to the clinic for appointments, Jamie's presentation and mood seemed depressed. He spoke with a flat affect and appeared to be participating only in areas of his life that he chose. The team thought there could be an underlying depression that could be affecting his noncompliance, but Jamie would not speak with our psychiatrist. Our plan then was to admit him to an inpatient psychiatric adolescent unit for an extended evaluation to determine what, if any, psychiatric treatment might help us treat Jamie more effectively. However, there were no significant psychiatric findings, and he was soon discharged. At fifteen years old, Jamie is intelligent, mentally competent, and wants to live. He does not want to die. In fact, he often talks about his future: he wants to finish high school and buy a car. Unlike Sarah who realized her health was in jeopardy, Jamie clings to the illusion that he is physically doing well.

Over time, my meetings with the family developed a pattern. Carol and Mary would express their frustration that Jamie would not take the medications, and Jamie would repeat that he just does not want to take them. In the summer of 2001, Jamie agreed to go to Highbridge. We had described the facility to him and initially he refused to consider admission. Then one day, he agreed. Given his lack of motivation around his health, Jamie's decision was surprising. He would not tell us why he wanted to go, but the team assumed it related to pressure from his family. While he was there, Jamie's health improved significantly. His ARV regime was successful, and with supervision he was taking all of his medications. However, toward the end of the month, he suddenly became increasingly defiant with the staff: verbally abusive and refusing morning and evening dosages. When Jamie asked to go home for the weekend, this was denied since he had a high fever. He became angry and subsequently destroyed some of the property in his room. Jamie was later hospitalized due to the high fevers and then discharged back home to live with his grandmother as he wished instead of to Highbridge.

The last time the family came into the clinic, the pediatrician decided to give him a medication regime that he could take at home with no toxic side effects. When I met with the family, we had the same conversation that we have had so many times before. Jamie remained quiet and would not answer any questions about his time at Highbridge or what he thought of taking these new medications. Unlike Sarah who needed and responded to supervision and encouragement, Jamie, for some reason, could not. Sarah's family at one time had provided her with the nurturing and love she needed to sustain her health, but Jamie may have never felt that kind of early support. During our meetings Carol is usually quiet, exhausted from trying to convince Jamie to fight to live. It was then that I realized this is what would play out until Jamie dies. I began to see my roles differently. One is to support Jamie's autonomy in making his own decisions as much as possible, while at the same time setting limits so he respects the people involved in his care. The second is to support his family. When Jamie left my office, I looked at Carol, whose eyes had filled with tears. I imagined the pain she was experiencing, having to relive her daughter's death again, but even worse, knowing that her grandson did not have the will to fight as her daughter did. I leaned over, touched her arm, and said, "You have done everything you can for that boy. And you have been wonderful. There is nothing more you could have done." As of this writing, Jamie is still alive but with no change in his behaviors.

A LOOK TOWARD THE FUTURE

Several concrete and clinical issues emerge from some of the issues that this chapter has explored. Given the team's experiences with adolescents, we have intensified our efforts with the families of younger children around adherence issues and focusing on promoting and sustaining adherence throughout the latency and adolescent years. Clinical teams can begin to assess family involvement and patterns and how they impact adherence. Services and counseling could be implemented earlier. The presence of an interested and involved guardian cannot be underestimated, even with an adolescent. Results suggest that caregivers who are unable to describe the medication regimen or who are noncompliant in bringing their children to appointments are unlikely to be able to assist with adherence to a medication regime (Katko et al., 2001). Regardless of age, consistent and caring supervision helps adolescents and children stay adherent to their medications.

Researchers are currently examining the possibility of "drug holidays," or structured treatment interruption (STI). STI may also be useful in patients with multidrug-resistant HIV for whom stopping therapy may allow the emergence of wild-type virus and permit use of recycled ARV drugs to suppress virus replication (Mitsuyasu, 2000).

There is also an interesting strategy we discovered while working with Laura, a fifteen-year-old girl diagnosed with AIDS. She too was not taking her medications regularly, for reasons mostly related to poor supervision and her seeming lack of motivation. In one discussion with her physician, Laura talked about how frustrated she felt being fifteen years old and not having breasts. Also, because of possible medical complications, the pediatrician had advised against manicures and piercings, which also upset her. He explained he was afraid of wound infection given that her immune system was so compromised. He also explained that secondary sex characteristics could sometimes be delayed by a compromised immune system. Part of Laura's motivation to begin her medications became attached to her desire to be a "normal" adolescent. We can use our knowledge of adolescent development to our advantage by integrating and connecting medical issues and information to the struggles that adolescents often experience. As in the case with Laura, when medication adherence became tied to symbols of female adolescence (earrings, breast development), her commitment and interest in adherence increased significantly.

Beyond the clinical work, creative resource planning, interagency collaboration, and advocacy have proved invaluable. Unfortunately, resources are not always available that are tailored to our adolescents' needs. As a profession, we need to continually work creatively with other agencies, both in the public and private sectors, to advocate for more appropriate services for our perinatally infected adolescents. We suggest that an ideal environment would be a residence for adolescents where they could be supervised medically but have the freedom and support to work toward being as independent as possible. They need long-term solutions to complicated issues such as adherence, housing, education, and vocational training. Interdisciplinary involvement is extremely important. The medical and psychosocial systems of a person's life are always interacting; in the case of perinatally infected adolescents, their environment impacts significantly on their ability to remain adherent. We have seen that close collaboration between medical providers and social work staff can improve the quality and depth of treatment plans that are appropriate for the individual patient.

Even though the numbers of new perinatal diagnoses are significantly less than they were in the early 1990s, there is still a population of HIV-infected children who will move into their adolescent years and undoubtedly confront the same issues. We no longer have to be unprepared, now that we have a greater understanding of what needs must be attended to at this age. What we hope for, both on policy and practice levels, are interventions and services that work on a preventive level with the family, so crisis situations do not arise as frequently. In addition, long-term residential treatment facilities are crucial, so these adolescents can have a home when their current living situations are not viable. With these changes, hopefully we will see a shift toward healthier HIV-infected adolescents who are able to look toward a future with infinite possibilities.

BIBLIOGRAPHY

Brantley, H.T., Stabler, B., and Whitt, J.K. (1981). Program considerations in comprehensive care of chronically ill children. *Journal of Pediatric Psychology 6:* 229-238.

Centers for Disease Control and Prevention (2001a). Basic statistics. Summarized from the *HIV/AIDS Surveillance Report.* <http://www.cdc.gov/hiv/stats.htm>.

Centers for Disease Control and Prevention (2001b). Table 21. Total AIDS cases and deaths, by year and age group, through December 2001, United States. *HIV/AIDS Surveillance Report* 13(2). <http://www.cdc.gov/hiv/stats/hasr1302/table21.htm>.

Centers for Disease Control and Prevention, National Center for HIV, STD, and TB Prevention, Division of HIV/AIDS Prevention (1999). Status of perinatal HIV prevention: U.S. declines continue. <http://www.cdc.gov/hiv/pubs/facts/perinatl.htm>.

Katko, E., Johnson, G.M., Fowler, S.L., and Turner, R.B. (2001). Assessment of adherence with medications in human immunodefiency virus-infected children. *Pediatric Infectious Disease Journal 20*(12): 1174-1176.

Mitsuyasu, R. (2000). Immune reconstitution with antiretrovirals, immunotherapy, and after structured treatment interruption. Paper presented at the 2000 Conference on Retroviruses and Opportunistic Infections. <http://www.medscape.com/medscape/cno/2001/RETRO/story.cfm?story_id=2053>.

Pediatric AIDS and human immune deficiency virus infection (1989). *American Psychologist 44*(2): 258-264.

Rubenstein, E. (1991). An overview of adolescent development, behavior, and clinical interventions. *Families in Society 72*(4): 220.

Winnicott, D.W. (1972). Adolescence: Struggling through the doldrums. *Adolescent Psychiatry* 1: 40.

SECTION V:
UNIQUE EXPERIENCES

Chapter 30

The Development of a Custody Planning Program for HIV-Affected Families

Sally Mason

Most of us are aware now, in the early part of the twenty-first century, that women and children as well as men are infected with and affected by HIV. The percentage of women diagnosed with AIDS in the United States tripled between 1985 and 1999 (CDC, 2001). In 1999, one-third of people living with HIV in the United States were women (CDC, 2000). Women of color are especially impacted by HIV/AIDS, with 77 percent of all women diagnosed with AIDS being African American or Hispanic. The vast majority of women with AIDS are also single and have an annual income below $10,000 (NPFHIVRC, 1999). In the early 1990s, however, these trends were just developing and being acknowledged.

At the beginning of the epidemic in the early 1980s, white gay men were the group most impacted by HIV/AIDS. In fact, until the 1993 revision, the Centers for Disease Control definition of AIDS did not include many of the manifestations of HIV that were commonly seen in women, such as cervical cancer and recurrent bacterial pneumonia. Concomitantly, the rising number of children infected perinatally and the "boarder" or abandoned baby phenomenon raised our awareness of the infection rate in women—women who were often single parents and with deteriorating health.

Planning for the children's care became unavoidable for social workers and other medical and social service professionals who worked with HIV-affected families. In child custody cases best interest standards have historically emphasized stability, continuity, and predictability as essential to a child's healthy development (Hall, Pulver, and Cooley, 1996). Though little research had been done on the impact specifically of parental HIV disease on children, the research on parental death and illness, in general, clearly in-

I wish to acknowledge Elizabeth Monk and Cathy Blanford for their contributions to this chapter.

dicated the risk for children's mental health (Garmezy and Rutter, 1988; Rutter, 1979). Chronic stressors common to low-income and minority families also had an impact on children's mental health (Garbarino, 1991; Rutter, 1979). It was, and still is, commonly accepted that the stability of a familiar environment and the continuity of relationships can minimize grief over the loss of a parent. The children's knowledge that there was a plan for them "in case" and then the transition to a warm, nurturing environment at the time of the parent's death meant the children would not be burdened with abrupt changes and would have the support to grieve.

The terms "permanency planning" or "custody planning" are used most often in child welfare and describe the process of finding a permanent home after entering the system for abuse, neglect, or abandonment. The options include adoption or guardianship by a foster parent or the return of the child to the parent's care. Parents with HIV, however, want to plan for the custody of their children because of their potential incapacitation or death. The custody planning literature was surprisingly lacking in the early 1990s, regarding parents with a terminal illness. One group that did have some characteristics in common with HIV-infected mothers was elderly parents of adult children with lifelong disabilities, especially developmental disabilities, who would continue to need daily care after their parent's death. Investigations into the propensity of these parents to plan indicated that most dealt with the decision by not deciding. The topic was avoided because the options were perceived as ugly or painful (Heller and Factor, 1988; Smith and Tobin, 1989).

DEVELOPMENT OF THE PROGRAM—1990 TO 1992

A coalition of service providers to children and families was established in Chicago in the late 1980s by a group of physicians, nurses, and hospital social workers concerned about the medical and psychosocial needs of infected children. Gradually the network's focus expanded to the children *and* their families, affected or infected, incorporating the concerns of HIV-infected women and parents. In the early 1990s, network members became aware of the number of children whose parents were ill or dying of AIDS and for whom no future plans had been made. For example, in one instance a child was taken into the custody of the child welfare system when a mother died in the hospital, since no provision had been made for the child's care.

Attorneys associated with the network were drafting standby guardianship legislation that would expand a parent's legal options for planning. The concept of standby status was fairly new at that point, with only a few states having such legislation. With standby guardianship, parents could designate someone to care for their children contingent on an event, such as death or incapacitating illness. Other options, such as wills or private guardianship, had proved less reliable or less flexible to the needs of the parents and children. Concurrently, a major needs assessment of HIV-infected women in Chicago (Carr, 1990) brought the needs of women and their children into focus and quantified the problem. Chicago was a "second-wave" city for the epidemic; the numbers of infected parents and children, infected and affected, were still relatively low compared to numbers on the East coast. The network's foresight, however, created an opportunity to be proactive and develop a custody planning program before the need became overwhelming.

A network task force was established to stimulate the creation of a custody or permanency planning program. This subgroup of the coalition was a partnership of program administrators, social workers, and attorneys who were associated with HIV services, child welfare services, or health care. The subgroup's task was to develop a planning program that supplemented other HIV social services in Chicago and, at the same time, prevented placement of the children in foster care or involvement with the state child welfare system. At that point, there were no designated custody planning programs in Chicago and only one or two in the United States. Some case managers and hospital social workers had added custody planning to their responsibilities, but they did not always have the expertise or the time. The task force examined issues involved in planning, especially the potential barriers and facilitators at all systems levels; conceptualized the program model; identified an agency to house and develop the project; and identified advocacy work at the larger systems level in support of planning services for HIV-affected families.

About a year into the task force's existence, the group acquired seed money from the state child welfare system. The AIDS project coordinator from the state child welfare system had been actively involved in the coalition and the network task force. Because of the state's overall concern for children and its support for the program's focus on planning without state involvement, the AIDS project coordinator was influential in getting funding from the state to hire a program consultant. This consultant's task was to develop the program ideas, with the product being a proposal template that could be used to seek further funding. The consultant became a member of the task force, interviewed HIV-infected parents, interviewed service providers, and reviewed policy, clinical, and research literature. Fortuitously, two months after the completion of the template proposal, the federal government published a request for proposals for demonstration projects that supported permanency planning for children. The template proposal was quickly turned into a proposal for funding, and the program was funded in the fall of 1992, two years after the inception of the task force.

PROGRAM CONCEPTS AND FEATURES

The major goal of the program was to promote stability and long-term planning for families with an HIV-infected parent. The service approach emphasized family control, specifically over decision making, and empowerment. A major assumption was that children who did not have permanency or custody plans in place at the time of the parent's death or incapacitation might end up being placed in foster care. Although foster care was an alternative, it was generally considered the least desirable option, to be avoided if at all possible.

The newly funded planning program filled a gap in HIV services by providing problem solving, conflict resolution, counseling, and other social service support that families might need when developing and implementing a plan. When a parent identified a potential caregiver and was ready to consider the legal options, then the parent would be referred to the AIDS legal services for the next step in the process. A not-for-profit legal service for people with HIV or AIDS had been established a few years earlier in Chicago. Legal services were provided gratis by attorneys trained in issues relevant to people with HIV/AIDS.

In order to use the program's services, the birth parents had to have legal custody of the children and had to request the services themselves. Although a service provider might make the initial call to the program for information, the parent had to initiate the intake process. The case coordinator's job was to facilitate the planning process by assessing the family's planning needs and providing counseling, education, crisis intervention, and referral as needed. In addition, the case coordinator assisted the parent in a variety of ways: helping the parent talk with children and/or another family member about the parent's HIV status, helping the parent identify a potential caregiver, and participating in discussions with the potential caregiver about their willingness and concerns relating to the potential guardianship. If the birth parent identified a relative or friend as the potential caregiver, then the case coordinator might facilitate discussions between the birth parent and the potential caregiver. In those discussions, the case coordinator might provide education, problem solving, conflict resolution, and reality testing about the viability of the plan and the need for additional support for the potential caregiver if he or she assumed this role.

For the birth parent who had no family or friends available for the children's care, the adoption family worker began the matching process with a potential caregiver. Potential caregivers or adoptive families contacted the agency and expressed an interest in becoming a "second family." After a telephone screening and orientation meeting, the potential adoptive parent completed an eight-session training. Topics in the training included: adoption of older children and sibling groups, HIV/AIDS, grief and loss, birth parent concerns and issues, legal options, and a presentation by a birth parent and an adoptive parent. The potential parent also participated in a home study—a series of meetings to help the adoption worker obtain information that would facilitate the match between birth family and adoptive family. These meetings covered a range of topics from clarification of details, such as ages, numbers of children, and special needs that the adoptive family would consider, to discussion about the potential caregiver's family history, parenting styles, and their understanding of the adoption arrangement.

At the completion of the home study, the potential adoptive parent was licensed as a foster parent for the state. The intent was not, however, for the potential caregiver to become a foster parent. The licensing process gave the birth parent and the agency some security in knowing that the potential caregiver had been thoroughly checked for past abuse or neglect allegations and any criminal charges. At the same time, an assessment was done of the home's physical safety and amount of space to accommodate a child or children. Licensing also left the door open for children to be placed with this family if the parent died after choosing the adoptive family but before a legal plan was in place.

For the match process, the adoptive family made a picture book of their family to be presented to birth families. If a birth family, after viewing the book, indicated an interest in an adoptive family then the potential parent would meet with the case coordinator and the adoption worker to hear about the children and family. If still interested, then the birth parents and adoptive caregivers met. If that meeting was successful, then the potential adoptive caregivers met the children, and the two families began to develop a relationship. At that point, the case coordinator and the adoption worker cooperated to support the ongoing relationship between the birth family and the adoptive family.

Maria, a thirty-three-year-old Latina mother of two uninfected boys, had chosen an adoptive family for her children. As the relationship between the two families developed, the boys stayed with their mother during the week and stayed on the weekend with their new extended family or potential adoptive parents. After one summer when the mother had been very ill, the boys moved at the beginning of the school year to their adoptive parents' home and visited with their mother on the weekends while keeping in contact with her by phone during the week. This relationship supported Maria as her health deteriorated while facilitating the transition for the boys into their new home. The staff helped with these arrangements and mediated if problems arose. The staff also referred Maria to legal services so she could secure her choice with a legal plan.

After a parent's death, staff provided services that helped the caregiver and the children through the transition. The services could include concrete assistance, such as helping the new caregiver get furniture for the children, as well as counseling and grief work as the new family integrated the children into their lives and mourned the parent's loss. New caregivers might also need information and advocacy to access resources and systems that supported a child's special needs, whether medical, emotional, or educational.

The planning services were supplemented with support groups for birth parents, children, and adoptive parents; recreational activities; and legacy work for birth parents, including videotapes, audiotapes, and photo albums. Early in the program, a dedicated case manager was part of the team, but case management seemed to distract from the main focus of the program, using valuable time and resources. The service was also duplicative, as a case management cooperative had been established in the city and every person with HIV was assigned a case manager. Eventually, that case management aspect was phased out and case management was obtained from the assigned community case manager; program staff maintained a close working relationship with the case managers and the cooperative's administration.

FACILITATORS TO IMPLEMENTATION

The task force had successfully developed and launched a respite program for HIV-affected children before attempting this planning program, so they had the experience and commitment to make the new program happen. The members' combined expertise was a great asset in the development and the implementation of the program. Attorneys, child welfare experts, and HIV experts each gave their assistance as needed while the original proposal was being written. During the implementation phase, the network and task force members were also sources for referrals to the program and acted in an advisory capacity.

The private agency that had committed to sponsoring the program had over 100 years of experience in child welfare and was one of the largest social service agencies in the state. The agency also housed one of only two programs in the state, at the time, which provided foster care to HIV-exposed children; the staff was experienced in HIV/AIDS and well educated on the issues of HIV in the family. The agency was also committed to the philosophy of open adoption. Open adoption is the "sharing of information and/or contacts between the adoptive and biological parents of adopted children, before and/or after the placement of the children, and perhaps continuing for the life of the child" (Berry, 1993, p. 125). Open adoption was not, and still is not, a legal arrangement but instead is an informal arrangement that is negotiated between the birth parents and the adoptive parents when it is in the best interests of the child. Open adoption acknowledges the strong ties between birth parents and children, even when they can no longer live together. It also allows for the free sharing of information between the birth parents and adoptive parents in order to make the best choices for the children. Open adoption was and still is a controversial practice, but it is a crucial one for this program in which birth parents and potential caregivers would meet and work together, perhaps even coparenting, until the parent's death.

In the early 1990s, the scholarly and popular press brought the "AIDS orphans" issue into the forefront of the country's consciousness. Michaels and Levine's landmark article on the projected number of "motherless youth" was published in 1992. *The New York Times, Time,* and *Vogue* all ran features about HIV-affected children and parents, or stories of families' struggles with planning. In general, people had sympathy for the children and their loss, so they were able to get past the long-held stigma about the mother or father and focus on the "innocent" children. Finding homes for "AIDS orphans" who did not have a relative or a friend to care for them was an appealing issue. The agency understood the potential for public relations with the program and showcased the program in agency literature and fundraisers. This public relationship increased the external resources available initially to the project, including access to funding and ease in recruitment of adoptive families. The publicity that the program received and the outreach and education that staff provided through an informational toll-free telephone line also raised awareness around the country of the needs of HIV-affected families.

BARRIERS TO IMPLEMENTATION

The task force members and the program staff anticipated that planning would be difficult for some parents for a variety of reasons, including facing one's mortality, keeping sibling groups together, and the day-to-day biopsychosocial challenges for HIV-affected families that take precedence over planning. These barriers were beginning to be documented in the clinical literature and were reported by clinicians who were talking with parents about planning. The largest programmatic barrier, however, other than those which were client based, was maintaining a steady stream of resources, both monetary and human.

As mentioned, initial recruitment of potential adoptive parents was not a problem. One television news story resulted in dozens of phone calls from people who were willing to consider becoming adoptive parents. This was not, however, a traditional adoption program. The birth parents could live a long time, and no one could predict when they would die or become ill enough for the children to move to the new caregiver's home. The potential adoptive parents were making a commitment to become a part of the family's life for an indeterminate period. The potential caregiver could not come to the program looking to adopt children but rather to become a resource to the HIV-affected family or extended family with all of the rewards and challenges that "family" can entail. The AIDS orphan issue that attracted so many, in reality, required a long-term and potentially intense commitment before the children were orphaned.

Recruiting inner-city, minority families was also difficult but important in order for birth families to have a range of choices for adoptive parents for their children. Many of the birth families were African American, and the staff wanted to support the placement of children in families of their own race or culture and perhaps even in the same neighborhood, if that was the parent's wish. The agency had strong ties in middle-class and white communities, and the people who responded initially to recruitment strategies were generally from those communities. In order to widen the diversity of adoptive parents, the staff developed relationships with black churches and broadened publicity campaigns to reach out to families that were demographically and geographically similar to the HIV-affected families. These efforts were somewhat successful, but urban minority families were more likely to have lower incomes. Taking on the care of multiple children, or sometimes even one child, was a financial burden for most families, but even more so for those minority families.

The lack of financial assistance for second families was a great challenge to the recruitment of new caregivers. Subsidies and public medical insurance were not available to the adoptive families, unless the children entered the child welfare system because of neglect, abuse, or abandonment, then were placed in foster care with the potential adoptive parent and eventually adopted by the foster parent/adoptive parent. This scenario, of course, flouted one of the program's original intents: to avoid the children's involvement in the child welfare system. Task force members and the program staff had several meetings with key state-level child welfare administrators to advocate for adoption subsidies to these families. After months of discussion, the state child welfare system decided they could not give subsidies to children other than wards of the state because that change in policy would open the door to many other groups with similar needs.

The program was originally funded for three years through a federal demonstration grant. Initially, other sources of funding were forthcoming because of the program's publicity and the nationwide publicity about the issue. Ongoing funding was much more difficult to obtain to support the program as originally designed. Although the host agency had been supportive of the program initially, it could not make the commitment to financially support the program. The agency was committed to child welfare, but its other programs received reimbursement for services provided from the state child welfare system because the programs were serving wards of the state and contracted with the state to provide those services. The custody planning program, because it sought to keep children out of the system, did not and could not have such an arrangement with the state. In addition, since the services were provided free of charge and served primarily low-income families, the program had no means of self-support.

Unless some other large and long-term funding source was identified, the program could not survive at its original staffing level. Recruitment of potential caregivers was the biggest challenge for the reasons just outlined. Also, birth parents often had family or friends who could provide the future care of the children given some intervention such as education and family conflict resolution. The program narrowed its focus to assisting birth parents in working with extended family, which reduced the need for recruitment of potential caregivers and thus staffing needs. Program staff also sought and received smaller reserves of funding for ancillary services, e.g., groups for affected children and legacy work, such as videotapes and family memory books. These services engaged clients while supplementing the important work of planning.

TEN YEARS LATER

Medical treatment for HIV/AIDS has made great strides since the implementation of the program. As highly active antiretroviral therapy (HAART) improves longevity and quality of life for people with HIV, the need for planning seems less immediate to parents and providers. Despite these developments, the predictions of motherless youth by the year 2000 have indeed come true (Carol Levine, personal communication, 2001). There still is no published research on the impact of custody planning on HIV-infected or -affected children's or adults' mental health or well-being. There are, however, some lessons from the past decade that have been documented, whether through research or the combined clinical experience of social workers and other service providers, that can help us in our practice.

• In the majority of instances, relatives end up caring for the children after the parent's death. In pilot studies, when HIV-infected and HIV-affected children have been placed outside their mother's home, anywhere from 50 to 75 percent of the children were cared for by their relatives (Boxer et al., 1998; Draimin and Levine, 1994). In one Midwest HIV planning program, 81 percent of the potential or current caregivers chosen by infected parents were relatives (Family Options, 2000). Sometimes, of course, extended family members are not willing to care for the children or the parent's past experience indicates that the family members will not be good caregivers. In many families, however, with some discussion and reconciliation, extended family can be educated and conflicts can be resolved so that grandparents or aunts and uncles can take over the care of the children. The recruitment of second families may be necessary in some instances, but in most cases relatives are the best option and one that social workers should explore with parents.

• Several theories or frameworks have impacted program development for HIV planning services—cumulative stress theory, behavioral skills training, and stages of change. Cumulative stress theory acknowledges that HIV families are often low-income, minority, and inner-city families that face daily stresses including crime, violence, poor housing, substance abuse, race and gender discrimination, and now the stigma and uncertainty of HIV. The social worker's job is to help alleviate those emotional or physical barriers to planning (Bauman et al., 2000). The development of behavioral skills—parenting skills, managing illness, and coping with crises—can reduce those stresses while enhancing the parent's ability to plan (Rotheram-Borus and Lightfoot, 2000). The stage process of planning recognizes the steps that parents take to plan—from thinking about the caregiver options to formalizing arrangements legally (Family Options, 2000; Mason, 1998). Movement through that process depends on the issues or stresses that parents and families have to address to pave the way for planning.

• The planning process can be lengthy and labor intensive. In one planning program, birth parents took an average of nine and one half months from intake to securing the legal plan (Family Options, 2000). This nine-and-one-half-month period, however, did not include the amount of time before the parent decided to access the program's services, i.e., the time the parent needed before actively choosing to plan and to seek help doing it. That decision process can take months or years. Planning is a family issue, involving not just the infected person but his or her children, partner, and kin network. The length and intensity of the process depends on the issues or stress that parents and families have to address to pave the way for a plan.

Those issues, to name a few, include disclosure of HIV status to children, relatives, or potential caregivers; resolution of family conflict; grieving past and present losses, such as a child's or partner's death from AIDS or the potential loss of the children to another caregiver; overcoming feelings of guilt or shame about transmission of HIV to a child or loved one; and substance abuse. Social workers must be patiently persistent in helping families move toward their planning goal.

• HIV-infected children represent only a small proportion of the children of infected mothers, and their number is declining, given current screening and treatment of pregnant women. The larger proportion is HIV-*affected* children and/or AIDS orphans. Some studies have documented greater severity of problems among children whose mothers are infected as compared to children whose mothers do not have HIV/AIDS—more depression and aggression and less social and cognitive competence (Forehand et al., 1998; Forsyth et al., 1996). So far, researchers and clinicians can only speculate about the reasons for the differences. Some of the effects of HIV are probably related to the stigma and the uncertainty of the disease process. With this knowledge, planning seems even more significant because it can reduce uncertainty for the parents and children and promote stability.

• Collaboration between social work and legal services is integral to most of the planning programs in the United States. These relationships can be difficult because the two disciplines have different roles and values (Retkin, Stein, and Draimin, 1997). The successful completion of a plan, however, relies on their cooperation. Families often have concrete needs to address or emotional issues to sort through before they are ready for legal assistance. Making legal arrangements secures all of the work that has gone before. Many parents do not plan but instead make informal arrangements with relatives or friends. These arrangements represent important steps for their children's stability. Without a legal plan in place, however, the plan may not hold up after the parent's death, often because of contests by extended family members or biological fathers who have been previously uninvolved.

• The planning process does not stop as soon as the parent dies or becomes incapacitated. New caregivers and their families may need support. Relative caregivers of HIV-affected children are often older with their own health concerns and developmental needs (Joslin, 2000; Mason and Linsk, 2002). As the children move into the new caregiver's home, the family members' roles change and family conflicts can arise. Meanwhile, children and caregivers may be grieving the parent's loss. As noted, HIV-affected children appear to have more emotional and behavioral problems than nonaffected children do, which may put an additional strain on the caregiving family. The newly constituted family and the custody plan may still be vulnerable if case management or therapeutic interventions are not provided through the transition.

• The growing body of neuropsychological research indicates that HIV affects prospective memory and decision making. Prospective memory is "remembering to perform some intended action at a particular point in the future" (McDaniel et al., 1999, p. 103). A study in HIV-positive women showed deficits in this type of memory as compared to HIV-negative women (Harris et al., 2001). In decision making, a person with normal cognitive functioning considers a range of consequences when choosing a course of action. In one study, HIV-positive drug abusers performed more poorly on decision-making tasks than HIV-negative drug abusers, choosing immediate rewards rather than considering future consequences (Reed et al., 2000). These findings do not mean that HIV-infected parents are unable to make future plans for their children. They do suggest that HIV-infected parents may benefit from assistance in making plans and that social workers may need to be more diligent helping parents consider their options and persistent in reminding parents about the completion of tasks.

THE ROLE OF HOSPITAL SOCIAL WORKERS IN CUSTODY PLANNING

Hospital social workers were some of the founding members of the family and child network because they saw the impact of HIV on parents and children in their daily work. Hospital social workers are still positioned to play an important role in helping families plan. First, social workers have a commitment to helping low-income, minority, and/or disenfranchised populations—the populations primarily affected by HIV. Social work education includes information on differences in race, culture, gender, and socioeconomic status and encourages the worker's constant striving for cultural competence in practice.

Second, social workers are knowledgeable about systems, such as families, and the intersection of those systems with health. Social work training emphasizes theories that help us understand how a parent's infection can affect those close to them and the potential impact of stigma on individuals and families. Social workers are trained to see not only the infected person, but also their family, which is a crucial aspect of custody planning.

Third, hospital social workers are at a logical point of intervention for custody planning. Social workers come in contact with family members as they visit the hospital and interact with family members as they make discharge plans. Conversely, social workers may notice the family's absence from the hospital or where the family tensions lie. Through these interactions, hospital social workers can help identify who is available in the support network to be a part of the planning effort and possibly be the future caregiver for the children.

Finally, custody planning is consistent with the introduction of advanced directives, such as living wills, powers of attorney, and health care proxies. Hospital social workers have to talk on a regular basis with people about difficult and taboo subjects, such as death and illness. These are subjects that no one else in the parent's network may be comfortable talking about with him or her. Planning can be a natural extension of the advance directive task; the worker is helping the parent think about what he or she would prefer for the children "in case of" the parent's illness, debilitation, or death. Parents often report that a hospitalization renews their anxiety about their children's future, and they may make a temporary care plan for their children during the hospitalization. Hospitalization can offer an opportunity to explore those options further.

Hospital social workers may not have the opportunity to participate in finalizing a plan; relationships with families are often short term or occur during busy clinic visits. Hospital social workers can, however, help families take the first steps in thinking about planning, reinforce the value of planning whenever possible, and connect families to community-based services that can continue the important work they began.

Finally, as evidenced in the program development process described here, hospital social workers may identify patterns in service needs as they go about their daily work. In those instances where we see needs across families, we must find ways to have our voices heard on behalf of our clients.

REFERENCES

Bauman, L. J., Draimin, B., Levine, C., and Hudis, J. (2000). Who will care for me? Planning the future care and custody of children orphaned by HIV/AIDS. In W. Pequegnat and J. Szapocznik (Eds.), *Working with families in the era of HIV/AIDS* (pp. 155-188). Thousand Oaks, CA: Sage.

Berry, M. (1993). Risk and benefits of open adoption. *Future of Children 3*(1): 125-138.

Boxer, A. M., Burke, J., Cohen, M., Cook, J., Weber, K., Shekarloo, P., and Lubin, H. (1998). Child care arrangements of children whose mothers have died of AIDS. Paper presented at Twelfth World AIDS Conference, Geneva.

Carr, A. (1990). *Summary of research report: The health care and social service needs of HIV-positive women and children in metropolitan Chicago.* Chicago: Visiting Nurse Association of Chicago.

Centers for Disease Control (2001). HIV/AIDS among U.S. women: Minority and young women at continuing risk: Fact Sheet. <http://www.cdc.gov/hiv/pubs/facts/women.htm>.

Draimin, B. H. and Levine, C. (1994). Preliminary analysis of data for *In whose care and custody?*. A joint project of New York City's Division of AIDS Services and The Orphan Project, New York.

Family Options (2000). Final Report. Submitted to Abandoned Infants Assistance Act, U.S. Department of Health and Human Services, Administration for Children and Families.

Forehand, R., Steele, R., Armistead, L., Simon, P., Morese, E., and Clark, L. (1998). The family health project: Psychosocial adjustment of children whose mothers are HIV infected. *Journal of Consulting and Clinical Psychology 77*(3): 513-520.

Forsyth, B. W. C., Damour, L., Nagler, S., and Adnopoz, J. (1996). The psychological effects of parental HIV infection on uninfected children. *Archives of Pediatric and Adolescent Medicine* 150: 1015-1020.

Garbarino, J. (1991). What children can tell us about living in danger. *American Psychologist 46*(4): 376-383.

Garmezy, N. and Rutter, M. (1988). *Stress, coping, and development in children.* Baltimore, MD: Johns Hopkins.

Hall, A. S., Pulver, C. A., and Cooley, M. J. (1996). Psychology of best interest standard: Fifty state statutes and their theoretical antecedents. *American Journal of Family Therapy* 24: 171-180.

Harris, T., Martin, E. M., Reed, R., Carson, V., and Primeau, M. (2001). Prospective memory in HIV-seropositive women. *Journal of the International Neuropsychological Society 7:* 148.

Heller, T. and Factor, A. (1988). Permanency planning among black and white family caregivers of older adults with mental retardation. *Mental Retardation 26:* 203-208.

Joslin, D. (2000). Emotional well being among grandparents raising children affected and orphaned by HIV disease. In B. Hayslip Jr. and R. Goldberg-Glen (Eds.), *Grandparents raising grandchildren: Theoretical, empirical, and clinical perspectives* (pp. 87-105). New York: Springer.

Mason, S. (1998). Custody planning with HIV-affected families: Considerations for child welfare workers. *Child Welfare 77*(2): 161-177.

Mason, S. and Linsk, L. (2002). Relative foster parents of HIV-affected children. *Child Welfare.*

McDaniel, M. A., Glisky, E. L., Rubin, S. R., Guynn, M. J., and Routhieaux, B. C. (1999). Prospective memory: A neuropsychological study. *Neuropsychology 13*(1): 103-110.

Michaels, D. and Levine, C. (1992). Estimates of the number of motherless youth orphaned by AIDS in the United States. *JAMA 268:* 3456-3461.

National Pediatric and Family HIV Resource Center (NPFHIVRC) (1999). Women with HIV: A fact sheet. <http://www.pedhivaids.org/fact/>.

Reed, R. A., Martin, E. M., Pitrak, D. L., Weddington, W., Anderson, D., Carson, V. L., Harris, T., Racenstein, J. M., and Bechara, A. (2000). Decision-making in HIV-seropositive drug abusers: A preliminary study. *Journal of the International Neuropsychological Society 6:* 135.

Retkin, R., Stein, G. L., and Draimin, B. H. (1997). Attorneys and social workers collaborating in HIV care: Breaking new ground. *Fordham Urban Law Journal 24*(3): 533-565.

Rotheram-Borus, M. J. and Lightfoot, M. (2000). Helping adolescents and parents with AIDS to cope effectively in daily life. In W. Pequegnat and J. Szapocznik (Eds.), *Working with families in the era of HIV/AIDS* (pp. 189-211). Thousand Oaks, CA: Sage.

Rutter, M. (1979). Protective factors in children's responses to stress and disadvantage. In M. W. Kent and J. E. Rolf (Eds.), *Primary prevention in psychopathology: Social competency in children* (Volume 3) (pp. 49-74). Hanover, NH: University Press of New England.

Smith, G. C. and Tobin, S. S. (1989). Permanency planning among older parents of adults with lifelong disabilities. *Journal of Gerontological Social Work 14:* 35-59.

Chapter 31

HIV/AIDS Case Management in the ER: A Link to Continuity of Care

Lisa Chapa

INTRODUCTION

The HIV/AIDS program at Parkland Hospital has been in existence since 1986. The HIV emergency room (ER) case management component was instituted in 1993 as a response to the growing need for client advocacy for HIV-infected patients in the emergency services department (ESD). Parkland had seen an increasing number of HIV/AIDS patients utilizing the ESD as their source of primary care. It was decided that ER case management might assist the ESD to achieve client wellness and autonomy through service coordination for every HIV-infected patient seen in the ESD. A registered nurse or a licensed master's level social worker can hold the case management position. The first person, a social worker, to hold the position did so until September 2000, and I have held this position since that time. I worked as the inpatient HIV social worker for three and one-half years before accepting the new women's/teens' advocate position at the Parkland AIDS clinic in January 2000. When the previous HIV ER case manager decided to pursue another career, I applied for and was granted the use of the ESD as primary care for HIV/AIDS patients, and was able to assist the ESD doctors in directing patients to a primary care provider at the Parkland AIDS clinic, Amelia Court, for follow-up care, the overall purpose of HIV/AIDS case management in this position. I have always appreciated the importance of this position as I worked closely with the HIV ER case manager when I was working on the wards and in the clinic.

The HIV ER case manager position is funded by Ryan White Title I, and since September 2000 is supervised by the unit manager of the AIDS clinic, who is a registered nurse. She both understands and embraces the crucial role of social work in health care. She has provided much support and guidance and allows me the autonomy to carry out my tasks as a social work case manager. Prior to September 2000, the social work department supervised the HIV ER case manager but had little or no part in the development of the position. The HIV ER case manager works collaboratively with the patient and the heath care team, including the ESD staff, hospital HIV team, and the AIDS clinic staff, by assessing, planning, implementing, coordinating, monitoring, and evaluating the options and services required to meet the patient's health care and psychosocial needs. The premise is that when an individual reaches the optimal level of wellness and functional capability, everyone benefits: the patients being served, their support systems, the health care delivery system, and the various reimbursement services.

Parkland AIDS Program

Parkland Health & Hospital System is a 900-plus bed hospital that serves as the primary teaching institution for the University of Texas Southwestern Medical School. It is Dallas County's only public hospital and is the largest provider of primary care services for HIV/AIDS patients in the Dallas Eligible Metropolitan Area (EMA). The Dallas EMA includes twelve counties and encompasses more than 4,000 square miles of both urban and rural landscape. Parkland treats over 90 percent of all Ryan White-funded patients in the EMA, is the recipient of Ryan White Titles I, II, III, and IV, and is the site of the regional Texas/Oklahoma AIDS Education & Training Center.

Over 3,500 HIV/AIDS patients were registered at Parkland in 2000. The ethnic breakdown is as follows: 41 percent Caucasian, 42 percent African American, and 17 percent Hispanic. The risk factors of our patients include 65 percent male-to-male transmission, 15 percent male-to-female transmission, 6 percent intravenous drug users, and 14 percent unknown. There were 3,424 visits to the ESD by HIV/AIDS patients that year, which averages 123 visits per month. The ESD, on average, treats 120,000 patients per year.

The hospital HIV team consists of two inpatient HIV RN case managers, two HIV social workers, and the HIV ER case manager. One of the HIV social workers sees only females and the other sees only males. The AIDS clinic, called Amelia Court, is located across the street from the hospital and treats an average of 100 patients per day. The clinic provides primary medical care, HIV specialized treatment, and various ancillary services including social work by two licensed master's-level social workers and home care case management by three registered nurses. There are two other Parkland clinic sites, and approximately 150 HIV patients are registered in each. One clinic has a physician and an HIV/AIDS social worker, and the other has two nurse practitioners and an HIV/AIDS social worker. Historically, these clinics treat patients who are relatively well with regard to their HIV/AIDS diagnosis; therefore, there has not been sufficient need for full-time home care case managers. Weekly continuity-of-care meetings are held in order to discuss the progress and discharge plans for the HIV/AIDS patients hospitalized at that time. The meeting is attended by the hospital HIV team and several staff members of the AIDS clinic, including the pharmacist, social workers, women's/teens' advocate, home care case managers, assistant unit manager, and the clinic providers. The social workers and the providers from the other two clinics are invited to these meetings but often are unable to attend due to the distance and travel time between the clinics and the hospital.

CASE FINDING IN THE ESD

My day begins at 9:00 a.m. with a review of the names of those HIV-infected patients admitted the previous day or weekend. One of the inpatient HIV social workers calls me daily to inform me of the admissions she finds on the floor as of that morning. With this information, I formulate the list of HIV-infected inpatients. This list is e-mailed to the hospital HIV team and the clinic staff. Once that is completed, I can focus on checking the ESD computer system to locate any patients with an HIV diagnosis. The system indicates the patients' names, time of arrival, chief complaints, location in the ESD, and other pertinent information. Most of the time the HIV-infected patients are entered in the computer as IDP (infectious disease protocol). This is often how I identify my patients, but not always. Sometimes the patients' names are familiar to me or the complaints lead me to suspect HIV. For instance, if a thirty-two-year-old presents to the ESD with complaints of nausea, vomiting, and diarrhea, which are often associated with antiretroviral therapy side effects, I will review the triage note in the computer system to ascertain more information about the patient's medical history. Once I find that I have patients in the ESD, I refer to any assessments I may have done during previous visits. I look for their most recent CD4s and viral loads as well as their recent clinic attendance. I am then ready to reassess the patient's current situation.

The number of patients per day varies. On the busiest days I may have ten or eleven patients, and on the slowest days I may have one. The ESD staff will often find or page me to let me know they are working with an HIV-infected patient. There is no second shift HIV ER case manager, so when patients come in at night or over the weekend they are unattended. I do, however, review all of the ESD discharge summaries to identify all HIV-infected patients who come through the ESD monthly. When I find patients who have not been given clinic follow-up, I call them to inquire about their plans for primary care and arrange appointments if necessary.

The overall role and subsequent tasks of the HIV ER case manager can be conceptualized into four roles: liaison, clinician, advocate, and empowerment agent. These roles overlap and require critical thinking and extensive knowledge about HIV/AIDS and the disease process.

HIV ER CASE MANAGER ROLES

Liaison

The liaison role includes interhospital collaboration as well as community-wide collaboration. Many outside agencies, including the county jail, the county health department, and various AIDS service organizations, contact me to both obtain and provide medical information regarding HIV/AIDS patients visiting the ESD. Since patients with HIV/AIDS often have significant medical histories and take numerous medications, it is extremely helpful to the ESD staff when they are provided with this information early in the patient's ESD visit. I often gather important and pertinent medical information about the patient from the provider and/or staff at the AIDS clinic in order to facilitate the assessment and care plan in the ESD. Conversely, I provide information regarding the patient's ESD visit to the clinic providers and staff. They also will call to inquire about a patient's recent ESD visit and the outcome of that visit. Clinic providers will also inform me when one of their patients is coming to the ESD. This collaborative relationship facilitates patient care and treatment.

It is not only the Parkland staff who inform me of patients who are en route to the ESD, but also the AIDS service organizations (ASOs), the Dallas County Health Department, and even patients or their loved ones. Mutual collaboration occurs after securing written and/or verbal consent from the patient in order to facilitate continuity of care. One can imagine how helpful it is to have one point of contact in the ESD for individuals both inside and outside the Parkland system. The role of the HIV ER case manager has proven to be a critical link to continuity of care, especially in light of the fact that there is no other "constant" in the ESD with whom the patients can relate; the nurses rotate in different areas of the ESD and the residents rotate in and out of the ESD altogether.

The wait time in the ESD can range from three to more than eighteen hours depending on how busy the ESD is and the patient's condition. HIV patients often need encouragement to stay in order to receive necessary treatment. My explanations about the reality of the ESD as well as personalizing their presence in the ESD often mitigates against their leaving. If the patient's symptoms are not very serious and they feel they can wait until the next day, I present the option of returning in the morning when it is likely to be far less busy.

As a liaison I, along with other members of the HIV team, represent Parkland at the weekly AIDS Arms network meetings at which five cases are presented. AIDS Arms, which has been in existence for ten years, is an AIDS service organization that provides case management services to persons with HIV/AIDS in the Dallas EMA, including many of Parkland's patients. They host weekly meetings for providers from various Dallas area AIDS service organizations and medical providers for the purpose of case presentations to enhance coordination, mutual problem solving, and anticipation of future needs of the clients.

Clinician

The stigmatization and shame that comes with an HIV/AIDS diagnosis often leaves our patients isolated and estranged from their families and/or friends. Unfortunately, sometimes the ESD visit is the first time the patient faces his or her illness, recognizing that HIV will not simply go away. The ESD visit can be frightening, especially when the patient is experiencing the first HIV-related illness. I have sat with many patients and their loved ones and counseled them regarding the disease.

It is extremely important for someone who is knowledgeable about the diagnosis and the psychosocial issues attached to it to be able to actively listen to the patients and their loved ones discuss their fears and hopes regarding the disease. The ESD visit often provides the opportunity to diffuse and replace anxiety with understanding and compassion. Patients and their loved ones often have many questions about the disease, its treatment, and the lifestyle change that results. I am there to help talk through these concerns in the hopes of making the ESD visit less overwhelming and more productive.

End-of-life care certainly comes up in the ESD. When appropriate, patients and their loved ones receive counseling and information regarding options for end-of-life care. Several patients have been placed in hospice facilities or nursing homes directly from the ESD rather than admitted to the inpatient unit.

Patients also come to the ESD with HIV-related symptoms and may admit to risk factors for HIV. In those instances, I have been asked to do the pretest counseling for these patients and to provide the information they need in order to follow up with the results. I have also been asked to do the posttest counseling for patients who were tested somewhere in the Parkland system but had not followed up for the results. Of all the tasks that I do, this one is the most difficult. The ESD physicians don't usually have time to discuss the new HIV diagnosis with the patient and, frankly, they would rather leave that to someone else. Even after five years of posttest counseling experience, I still get a little nervous before walking into a newly diagnosed patient's room. I will not forget the patient who threatened suicide and banged on the windows, crying out that she did not want HIV. The patients who are stoic, however, are more worrisome to me because I can't get a feel for what they're thinking or how they're really coping with the news. I try to convey the vast improvements in research, the promise of even better medicines, and the good quality of life many people living with HIV are now experiencing. All the while I know they are wondering when the disease will take their lives and how they're going to tell their loved ones. One never gets accustomed to informing someone of an HIV diagnosis. It is especially difficult in the ESD setting because the patient is obviously in a medical crisis and to be informed of an HIV test result exacerbates the anxiety.

Advocate

Some patients I see are unable to clearly articulate their complaints or concerns. As an advocate, I help them express their medical needs to the ESD staff in order to minimize confusion and use their time and the staff's time more efficiently. I often advocate for the patient to have certain lab work done in the ESD that will facilitate their next clinic visit, as well as keep them from making another trip to Parkland to have the lab work done later. If after interviewing the patient in the triage area or the waiting room I feel that he or she is really in need of something such as intravenous fluids, I may stop one of the residents to ask that an order be written for the fluids to be started. I do this sparingly so as not to lose credibility with the doctors and nurses who are actually very receptive to such requests because of their respect for my expertise and knowledge.

The information I learn from assessing the patient in the ESD often expedites social service delivery for the patient. With illness comes some extent of psychosocial stress or crisis, especially when the illness is debilitating for any length of time.

If the patient is to be admitted, I will inform the inpatient HIV team of any pressing needs that require immediate intervention, particularly for those patients who present with altered mental status and difficulty ambulating. Usually, though, with this type of patient I attempt to locate family or friends if no one accompanies the patient, in order to ascertain how the patient was caring for himself or herself and the extent of the available support network. I might assist the family/friends in thinking through scenarios and options for the patient's future living arrangements. I may also make referrals to AIDS service organizations and arrange for them to see the patient during the hospital stay. All of this information would be gathered in the ESD and provided to the inpatient HIV team in order to facilitate discharge planning. In essence, the HIV ER case manager is a pivotal role, one whose function may also encompass initiating the discharge planning, which benefits patients, their support networks, and the hospital.

If the patient is to be discharged from the ESD, I ensure that he or she has either a follow-up appointment or the phone number to the clinic. If the patient needs transportation services to and from the clinic, I arrange for that service through another agency. In essence, I make sure that the patient leaves the ESD with all the information necessary to access services as needed.

Some medical professionals in the ESD who do not work specifically with HIV/AIDS patients have argued that the HIV patients are being "enabled" by having someone designated to assist them with the process. However, patients are told that their diagnosis does not mean that their complaints are more urgent than any other patient waiting to be seen.

Given my varied information about and contact with patients, I can inform the ESD staff about patients who I know have abused various social services or Parkland services in the past so that they are fully informed about the patients and how that history may relate to the current ESD visit. I encourage doctors to do toxicology screens on patients who I know have histories of drug use and whose symptoms appear related to drug use. Although there is often a fine line between advocating and enabling, social work continuity, expertise, and longevity often help us distinguish between the two.

Empowerment Agent

Empowerment—isn't that the goal of social work? Autonomy and self-determination are key, particularly for such a stigmatized and often victimized population. When patients are empowered with information on how best to care for themselves physically, emotionally, and psychosocially, they are able to demonstrate autonomy and self-determination in a way that will improve their well-being. Patients diagnosed with HIV learn more than they ever wanted to know about the disease and its treatment. I see the ESD visit as an opportunity to explain to patients where they are in the disease process (i.e., their CD4 counts and viral loads) and how their adherence or difficulty with adherence is affecting the progression of the disease. I explain to them what procedures the doctors need to do and why, what the results mean, and the importance of taking the medications as prescribed.

I try to empower not only by educating them about their disease but also by explaining how best to utilize the Parkland system and how to apply for various entitlements, such as Social Security benefits, food stamps, and the Parkland's subsidized insurance program.

Tom, a forty-one-year-old, had visited the ESD three times in the last month when I was not there. On his fourth visit we spoke about why he had been coming to the ESD so frequently. He informed me that he was living with different friends because he had no money to pay rent. He had lost his job due to constant illness, and he didn't know where else to get medical attention. I was able to refer him for stable housing, for Social Security benefits, and to the clinic for ongoing medical treatment. The patient has since begun receiving his Social Security benefits and is compliant with medical appointments. Sometimes all patients need is a little boost to help them become more independent and self-sufficient.

At times patients will come into the ESD with the same crisis—no benefits, homelessness, no transportation, or needing drug treatment even though I had previously intervened. There will always be patients who are not ready to be invested in their care and who abuse the ESD. For any patients actively using drugs, I recommend treatment. However, I have found that the outcome is more successful when the patient makes this decision out of readiness as opposed to feeling pressured by me or anyone else. Patients who are not yet ready for treatment but remain frequent ESD users subsequently receive less attention from me. The message I constantly reinforce is that if they really want services then they need to make a commitment to help me help them.

CONCLUSION

The role of the HIV ER case manager as liaison, clinician, advocate, and empowerment agent is beneficial not only to the patients and their loved ones but also to the Parkland staff and the Dallas area HIV community. Some patients will choose to use the ESD as their primary care, but that number has significantly decreased since the start of HIV case management in the ESD. Currently, most of the patients that come through the ESD already have primary care providers but need emergent treatment for particular complaints. Some of the patients come for procedures such as lumbar punctures, CT scans, and EKGs.

Now that many patients are living longer with the disease, HIV is becoming known as a chronic illness more than a terminal one. Although patients continue to present to the ESD with the symptoms of the disease, they now come with adverse side effects from the HIV medications they are taking. Visits to the ESD by HIV/AIDS patients have steadily increased at Parkland over the last four years by an average of 500 visits per year, and Dallas County is still seeing a rise in the numbers of new HIV diagnoses. These trends suggest that the future role of HIV ER case management will continue to be vital to the continuity of care for the HIV/AIDS patients at Parkland Health & Hospital System.

Chapter 32

The Evolution of HIV Case Management Standards for Sonoma County

Kevin Farrell

In 1998, the HIV Planning Council of Sonoma County identified a significant series of challenges for the case management system already in place. A system of care for people with HIV/AIDS had evolved beginning in the early 1980s; although highly professional and medically responsive to client needs, the system was somewhat fragmented, especially in the area of case management. This chapter addresses the process of change in moving to a more systematized delivery of service.

HISTORICAL BACKGROUND

Not long after AIDS was identified in the urban gay centers in 1981, the impact was felt in Sonoma County, an area approximately sixty miles from San Francisco. Since the mid-1960s, the town of Guerneville on the Russian River had been a summer retreat for gay men from San Francisco and its environs. Over time, many of these men had purchased second homes in the area, refurbished fishing cottages for year-round living, or moved to the area because of its attractive climate and reputation for tolerance. The Russian River Health Center, located in Guerneville, treated its first AIDS patient in 1982.

Although many of the men received nonemergency medical care in San Francisco, several hospitals in the Russian River area provided more direct HIV/AIDS care: a 250-bed Kaiser Permanente hospital, a local Catholic hospital (Santa Rosa Memorial), and the county's own hospital, which has since been leased to a private nonprofit. Outpatient, specialized HIV medical care was available at the county's Health Services Clinic Department located in Santa Rosa beginning in 1986. In 1990, the state of California began funding the clinic as an early intervention center. After the federal government funded the Ryan White Care Act, the county became a Title II recipient and, in 1994, a Title I-designated Eligible Metropolitan Area (EMA). Ryan White Title III funds, which are used strictly for medical services, followed in 1997; Title IV funding, providing care for women and children, was obtained in 2001.

Medical care was provided by seven family practice physicians or nurse practitioners at the county clinic, and the Russian River Health Center had two physicians with extensive HIV experience; last, there were three other doctors who had a large gay clientele and practiced within the county. Because Sonoma County covers such a large area geographically, medical care and case management services were dispersed along similar lines.

The community of Sonoma County responded to AIDS with the creation of various AIDS service organizations, the first being Face to Face, started by a group of volunteers in 1984. It eventually operated out of two offices, one on the Russian River and another in Santa Rosa, the county seat. By 1998, each office case managed about 200 HIV/AIDS clients, a mix of people with varying degrees of acuity as well as medical and psychosocial needs. Sunburst Projects, which focused on women and children, provided additional community case management services, and both Title III clinics provided case management services in addition to medical care.

Community-based case management was financed by a combination of community fund-raising and county, state, and federal dollars. Sonoma County, because of the high incidence of AIDS, became a Ryan White Title I EMA in 1994, enabling it to obtain a large share of federal dollars. By 1998, the local planning council was responsible for disbursement of about $1.5 million each year, and almost 15 percent was spent on various forms of case management. In addition, California provided about $130,000 to Face to Face to case manage some of the highest-need clients under its Case Management Program and the Medi-Cal Waiver Program. Both use a nurse/social worker model to provide health care and psychosocial support designed to enable clients to remain in their homes and, ideally, out of emergency rooms and hospital beds.

This system of care worked very well because of the small number of physicians and good communication lines between care providers. But in terms of case management, by 1998 systemic problems became apparent. Many clients were now living longer and having fewer opportunistic infections because of the triple therapy combinations; the sense of emergency had somewhat dissipated. Concomitantly, overall HIV/AIDS financial resources were declining. In fact, under the new Ryan White distribution formulas it was possible that Sonoma County might lose its designation as a Title I EMA, which would then significantly further reduce resources. Clients of the care system began advocating to take a hard look at case management spending that they felt was excessive: they felt less service was needed because of their improved health status. Juxtaposed was the perception of health care providers who were detecting an increase in new clients who were often coming late to care and who presented multiple psychosocial challenges including drug and alcohol abuse and chronic mental health difficulties. The picture of the HIV/AIDS epidemic was rapidly evolving, and the system was not perfectly designed to change with it.

THE BEGINNING OF CHANGE

By 1998, there were approximately 550 people with HIV/AIDS in the care system and over 900 had died since 1981. The Sonoma County AIDS Commission (which had taken over both roles as Title I planning council and Title II consortium) identified a number of challenges to the existing case management system for people with HIV/AIDS in the county, including the following:

- Case management was not well understood and some clients questioned its value.
- Many clients reported having multiple case managers and were unaware of their separate functions.
- Time and energy was being wasted as case managers duplicated one another's work.
- Qualifications for case managers varied widely without a uniformly recognized standard.
- Providers did not consistently assess the level of client acuity.
- Communication among providers was sometimes lacking.
- Client outcomes could not be adequately measured or compared consistently across agencies or providers.

Providers and clients were invited to an initial community meeting at which clients clearly voiced their concerns about duplication of resources within the system as providers explained what they saw as their roles in providing case management to people with HIV/AIDS. It became apparent that there were serious differences between what some clients wanted from the case management system and what they felt they were actually getting.

In addition, clients complained about the duplication of paperwork they were expected to provide to each agency when seeking services. They felt that they went through identical processes at each agency when they applied for various services (i.e., medical care, food bank, emergency financial assistance, each of which was operated by a different provider) and that the system could be streamlined and made more user friendly. At the first communitywide meeting of providers and clients, it became clear that there were significant differences in how each viewed the needs and roles of the other.

In response to these concerns, the AIDS Commission created a Case Management Task Force whose job would be to standardize HIV case management within the county. It would have authority to make recommendations to the AIDS Commission that would define case management, determine who it should serve, set educational and experiential requirements for case managers, create a set of client rights and responsibilities, and establish a way of accurately measuring client acuity, which was a critical component in attempting to standardize care within a system of care that had become fragmented. Stakeholders came to the table in mid-1999 to begin this process, which was funded by a technical assistance grant from the Health Resources and Services Administration (HRSA).

The group initially met with a consultant and established a set of operating principles and values. The value statement's top priority was that providers would take a client-centered approach to case management and work together with clients to maximize positive health outcomes while respecting each client's dignity and worth. It further stated that the goal of the case management system would be to provide a seamless continuum of quality care that would be designed to be culturally appropriate, cost effective, efficient, and accessible to all people with HIV/AIDS in Sonoma County. These were heady goals, but the group believed that they were realistic and attainable.

Ten meetings over a period of eight months were held for the full committee, and subcommittees were established as needed. Particularly thorny questions were predictably passed on to these subcommittees, and the issue with the greatest probability of causing controversy within the larger group was reserved for the end of the process.

This question concerned how each client's need for various services would be assessed and what amount of case management a given client would require in light of his or her needs. This was critically important to many providers because the number of clients an agency served would ultimately determine its share of the case management dollars from the AIDS Commission.

The determination of a given client's acuity level would decide if he or she were eligible for case management services and, if so, what level of care the client would then be assigned. Under the existing system, only people with a diagnosis of AIDS or "symptomatic HIV" were eligible for case management services; attainment of this eligibility standard opened the "gate" for various other services which included financial assistance for rent, utilities, and other needs, generally up to about $1,500 per client per year in Ryan White Title II and HOPWA (Housing Opportunities for Persons with AIDS) funds for housing-related emergencies.

The clients' physician made the determination of "symptomatic HIV" or AIDS, and the criteria used to make these designations varied from provider to provider. Some physicians in the community operated with a stricter definition of what constituted "symptomatic" than others, leading to inequities in terms of who received services and who did not. In addition, community physicians felt that they were being placed in a difficult situation in their relationships with their patients by having to make determinations that impacted not only case management services but also, in effect, emergency financial services, housing, and the availability of psychosocial counseling—all of which were services available only to consumers who could pass the initial HIV/AIDS screen by the physician.

The welcome arrival of effective combination therapy further complicated decision making in this regard. Providers had found decisions of this nature easier to arrive at prior to the reduction in opportunistic infections, morbidity, and mortality. Previously, patients could be expected to follow a fairly predictable course from diagnosis through disease and onto death, generally within two to three years. Because each person with HIV was believed to have a relatively predictable terminal disease, the entire range of resources was made available to all. This system was no longer realistic given reduced morbidity and mortality and the demographic changes in the clients coming into the care system.

Although anyone in any stage of HIV disease could receive Title III medical care in Sonoma County, the two community-based organizations (Face to Face and Sunburst) relied on physicians' letters of diagnosis in order to initiate case management services. Both agencies provided a somewhat different range of services, with Sunburst's geared more toward women and families, but there was some overlap between these two providers in terms of caseload.

Increasingly, from about 1997 on, case managers at these agencies saw consumers who appeared to be in need of services due to their economic or psychosocial challenges but who were unable to obtain the required physician's letter determining medical need. Over time, as more people with HIV presented with a combination of economic, emotional, and social issues, but not necessarily with medical qualifications that would provide them with the necessary diagnosis, the system became murkier and less responsive to people in need. At the same time, some consumers who had responded very favorably to the new medication regimens were clearly doing much better and were no longer in need of intensive services; however, they were still technically eligible and could receive the full range of ancillary services provided by case managers because these consumers had an AIDS diagnosis at one time.

The result of this confluence of factors was that inequities were built into the system of case management so that some people no longer requiring case management and ancillary services were in fact receiving them while others who would benefit from case management were unable to access the system.

NEW INNOVATIONS

Sonoma County, of course, was not alone in facing these questions. Numerous HIV/AIDS providers (as well as other Title I and II grantees) across the country needed to adapt to the new world of HIV/AIDS case management in which they found themselves when effective therapies became available. In Sonoma County, it became increasingly clear that solving this interlocking set of challenges would require a thorough rethinking of the way a consumer entered—and remained in—the case management system.

The determination was made to abandon the "medical model" of case management based on the physician's certification of medical need and replace it with a new system that more accurately reflected the realities of living with HIV in the late 1990s. The solution to these problems was the development of a new acuity scale that would assess clients on four different scales (see Table 32.1):

1. HIV impact on the activities of daily living
2. General health
3. Personal/economic resources
4. Psychosocial issues

Assessment of these four critical areas results in the determination of an "index" or score for each client as determined by the case manager at intake as well as in subsequent follow-up visits (see Figure 32.1). The index determines whether a client is eligible for services and at which level of case management.

The acuity level of the client also determines the educational and experiential requirements of the individual case manager, the regularity with which clients are visited by their case managers, and the number of clients at this level that a case manager can appropriately manage (see Figure 32.2).

For example, a client with relatively minimal needs (as determined by the index achieved on the acuity scale) would be placed in Level I case manage-

TABLE 32.1. Criteria for Assessment of Client Acuity Scale Index

I. HIV IMPACT ON ADLs			
A	B	C	D
Asymptomatic HIV; no ADLs impact	Symptomatic HIV disease; without significant ADLs impact	Symptomatic HIV disease; moderate impact on ADLs	HIV disease with: health failure, life-threatening opportunistic infections; complex health challenges; ADLs severely impacted

II. HEALTH (Score Range: 0-56)				
FACTORS	0	1	3	7
HIV Medical Needs	HIV/AIDS medical needs are monitored and under control	Some HIV related health needs not under control	Has acute or untreated HIV medical conditions	HIV related life-threatening health emergency or situation
Non-HIV Medical Needs (injury, pregnancy, diabetes, etc.)	No non-HIV/AIDS medical needs	Some non-HIV medical needs that are monitored and under control	Emerging or untreated non-HIV medical conditions	Non-HIV related life-threatening health emergency or situation
HIV Medication Side Effects	No side effects or has not started	Minimal side effects	Moderate side effects affecting some ADLs	Severe side effects affecting many ADLs
HIV Medical Care	Has consistent, coordinated HIV speciality care	Has medical care but no HIV speciality care	Inconsistent or intermittent HIV care	Not currently receiving medical care
Activities of Daily Living (ADLs)	Able to perform ADLs without assistance	Needs some assistance with ADLs	Needs 10-15 hours/week in-home support for ADLs	Needs > 15 hours/week support for ADLs
Ability to Adhere to Medications	Client reports ability or willingness to adhere to medications	No level for this factor	Client reports inconsistent ability to adhere to medications	Inability or unwillingness to adhere to medications
Mental Health	Stable; no current mental illness or history of mental illness	Mild symptoms or disorders	Moderate symptoms or disorders	Severe symptoms or disorders; danger to self or others
Drug/Alcohol Use	No current substance abuse or history of substance abuse	Some problems with substance use	Numerous life problems related to substance use	Chaotic life due to substance use

TABLE 32.1 *(continued)*

III. PERSONAL/ECONOMIC RESOURCES (Score Range: 0-20)

FACTORS	0	1	3	5
Housing	Stable, clean housing	Requires short-term assistance with rent/utilities to maintain housing	Eviction imminent or home barely habitable or temporary shelter with family or friends	Homeless on streets or shelter resident or living in car
Financial Situation	Steady, adequate source of income	Income source in jeopardy or requires some assistance for critical needs	Income is inconsistent or too low to meet primary needs	No income or in financial crises
Basic Needs (food, clothing, warmth)	Basic needs met successfully	Primary needs met usually; occasionally needs assistance	Often lacking food or clothing or utilities	Basic needs consistently not met
Benefits/ Insurance	All applicable benefits in place or has private resources	Requires some assistance to obtain some benefits	Requires ongoing assistance to obtain needed benefits	No applicable benefits in place or not eligible

IV. PSYCHOSOCIAL ISSUES (Score Range: 0-63)

FACTORS	0	1	3	5
Behavior	Functions appropriately in most settings	No Level 1 for this factor	Repeated incidents of inappropriate behavior, "acting out," etc.	Abuse or threats to others; lack of impulse control
Social Support System	Dependable network of friends/family/ partner	Existing support system with gaps; friends/family/ partner periodically available	Moderate support mostly provided by professional caregivers	No stable support system other than professionals
Family Functioning	Stable, supportive, relationship with partners and/or children or living independently	Some functional difficulties	Significant multiple difficulties	Family in crisis
Domestic Violence (to or by client)	No history of abuse or domestic violence	History, but no recent episode	Current or recent episode within the past 18 months	Recent pattern of domestic violence or abuse
Dependents	Stable; dependents cared for, or no dependents; no planning necessary for future care	Dependents' needs are mostly met	Permanency or other planning required	Dependents' needs are frequently unmet; crisis needs evident

Criminal Justice System Involvement	No history of CJS involvement	Recent history of CJS involvement or misdeameanor arrest; outstanding warrants	Recent felony arrest; incarcerated pending trial or sentencing	Evading CJS; danger of incarceration
Legal Issues	All documents in order; no current legal problems	Requires assistance with legal documents (i.e., DPOA, W&T, guardianship, adoption)	Involvement in civil justice matters; may require assistance with documents	Bankruptcy or civil action pending with severe impact on the individual
Immigration	Has legal status	In process of obtaining legal status	Having difficulty sustaining status or may lose status	Undocumented
Language Skills (ability to understand English, follow instructions, and communicate in an office setting)	Can speak, read, write, and understand English at an adult level, can fill out forms and follow procedures and instructions	No Level 1 for this factor	Some difficulties with speaking, reading, writing, and understanding English at an adult level, and/or requires assistance in following procedures and instructions and filling out forms	Not able to represent self in English
Cultural/System Issues	Minimal cultural or system barriers	Requires some assistance accessing the system	Unable to access systems without ongoing assistance	Chooses not to access needed services due to fear or distrust of system
Knowledge of HIV Disease	Has been informed and verbalizes understanding about the disease	Some understanding of disease	Little or incorrect understanding of disease	No understanding of HIV disease progression
Risk Reduction (HIV/STDs)	Abstaining from high-risk transmission behavior	Isolated incidents of high-risk behavior	Occasional incidents of high-risk behavior	Ongoing engagement in high-risk behavior
Transportation	Has access to dependable transportation	Occasional transportation problems or access to public transportation only	Requires ongoing assistance for transportation to doctors, etc.	No Level 5 for this factor

ment that is provided by a BSW or MSW-level provider who would see the client in person every 120 days. These case managers could have client loads of up to 100. A client with a medium level of need as determined by the acuity index would be seen by a licensed clinical social worker (LCSW) or an MSW-level case manager every sixty days. These case managers

Case Management Agency: _____

Client: _____	Assessed by:	Client Acuity Scores				Assigned to:
Client ID #: _____		I. (A-D)	II. (0-56)	III. (0-20)	IV. (0-63)	
Date of Assessment / /						

Viral Load/ Date [   ]   CD4/Date [   ]   Multiple Diagnosis? Mental Health ☐   Substance ☐

I. HIV Impact on ADLs (Range A-D)		III. Personal/Economic Resources (Range 0-5)		IV. Psychosocial Issues (Range 0-5)	
A. Asymptomatic HIV		Housing		Behavior	
B. HIV: no significant impact		Financial Situation		Social Support System	
C. HIV: moderate impact					
D. HIV: severe impact		Basic Needs		Family Functioning	
I. SCORE (A-D)		Benefits/Insurance		Domestic Violence	
II. Health (Range 0-7)		III. TOTAL (0-20)		Dependents	
HIV Medical Needs				Criminal Justice Involvement	
Non-HIV Medical Needs				Civil/Legal Issues	
HIV Medication Side Effects				Immigration	
HIV Medical Care				Language Skills	
Activities of Daily Living				Cultural/System Barriers	
Ability to Adhere to Medications				Knowledge of HIV Disease	
Mental Health				Risk Reduction	
Drug/Alcohol Use				Transportation *(No level 5)*	
II. TOTAL (0-56)				IV. TOTAL (0-63)	

NOTES
_____
_____
_____
_____
_____

FIGURE 32.1. HIV Case Management Client Psychosocial Acuity Scale

CLIENT PLACEMENT

Screening, Intake, Assessment
Provided by: Level II or III Case Manager or Supervisor
- On-call client advocate for information and referral
- New client intake/screening/assessment—referrals to level I, II, or III case management
- Comprehensive analysis of needs and resources available to meet needs

Case Management Referrals
Provided by: Case Manager or Supervisor
to Level I, II, or III, depending on severity of need (medical, psychological, and/or social)

	LEVELS OF CASE MANAGEMENT SERVICES			
	case mgmt not required	Level I	Level II	Level III
Acuity (Based on the client's highest acuity scale score on any of these factors)	I. A II. 0 III. 0 IV. 0	I. A-B II. 1-10 III. 1-5 IV. 1-12	I. A-C II. 11-21 III. 6-10 IV. 13-20	I. B-D II. 22+ III. 11+ IV. 21+
Contact—Minimum	Not applicable	1x/120 days	1x/60 days	1x/30 days
Maximum Caseloads	Not applicable	120	40	15
Qualifications (Prioritized)	Not applicable	1. MSW 2. BSW 3. Grantee waiver	HIV experience preferred and: 1. LCSW 2. MSW or MFT 3. MA in counseling/psychology or related field with grantee waiver	HIV experience and medical case management experience required 1. LCSW 2. MSW 3. MFT

FIGURE 32.2. Levels of Case Management Services for Client Placement

would have caseloads ranging up to forty. Clients with the greatest needs as measured by the acuity index would be seen monthly by teams consisting of a registered nurse and an LCSW or MSW whose caseloads would be limited to twenty people.

Clients would move between levels as their health and psychosocial needs required. It was hoped that each agency providing case management would enable clients to maintain case managers even as clients move between levels, so that continuity of care could be maintained with the minimum of disruption to each client's routine.

The new standards of case management and the revised system of acuity measurement was adopted by the Sonoma County AIDS Commission in mid-2000, but implementation of the standards, and in particular the use of the acuity scale, was delayed for a variety of reasons. Although adopted unanimously by the AIDS Commission, the new measures of acuity would radically alter the system if implemented all at once, so a period of gradual implementation was designed.

The new standards required that a subcommittee of the AIDS Commission be established to provide oversight and technical assistance in case management. That group, which had effective consumer representation, decided to produce a consumer guide to case management and a standardized intake tool as its initial tasks. At the same time, the initial acuity scale was tested at various sites where case management was provided, and it was discovered that some clients who were assessed by their medical case managers were viewed much differently than they were by their community-based case management teams. These kinds of realizations necessitated changes in the acuity scale as it had been developed, and increased attention was paid to clients designated by case managers as "multiply diagnosed," meaning that they had a history of or current drug/alcohol abuse and a mental health diagnosis in addition to HIV. These more complex clients, whose numbers were increasing in the system of care, were requiring more resources and coordination among agencies for effective case management.

As these issues were being addressed, an intensive eight-hour training program was designed for case managers to introduce them to the new acuity system. This was conducted in early 2001, and the new acuity system was generally in place throughout the Sonoma County HIV/AIDS case management system by the end of the year.

The results of the new standards and use of the new acuity scale are not yet fully clear. Implementation of the standards has improved the quality and delivery of case management services throughout the system of care, and the county health department, as well as the AIDS Commission, has a clearer and more accurate picture of the clients with HIV/AIDS being served using its combination of local, state, and federal resources. The system of care is on its way to being more responsive to clients. People with HIV who formerly did not fit into the rigid definitions that would allow them to access certain services now find themselves eligible for case management and other forms of assistance. At the same time, a concurrent increase in the number of relatively healthy clients who may no longer need services and leave the system of case management has not been observed. Once significant resources of this nature are offered to consumers, it is difficult to withdraw them, and some case managers have understandably resisted their new roles as service "gatekeepers."

Other challenges remain for Sonoma County. Although it continues to be designated as a Title I EMA, the 2000 census revealed that its population fell just under the 500,000-person mark that would guarantee a Title I designation, and the number of people with AIDS in the county is now about 630. As with other health jurisdictions in California, Sonoma will be required to adopt HIV reporting by 2005, and funding decisions will be based on reported HIV cases, not the number of people with AIDS. As with many local health jurisdictions, Sonoma County continues to witness an increase in multiply diagnosed clients with HIV/AIDS and people who come late to care or return to care only when they are critically ill. This is a complicated picture that will require a system of medical care, case management, and ancillary services that is highly responsive to medical and demographic changes. The case management standards, and in particular the acuity scale adopted to more realistically measure the day-to-day realities of living with HIV in the third decade of AIDS, have played a critical role in building this kind of care system.

Chapter 33

Telling the Social Work Story for Survival

Darrell P. Wheeler

Social workers have been part of the HIV/AIDS care and treatment milieu since the beginning of this epidemic in the United States. We have served on the front lines, and we have served in the back wards. We have been there for individuals, families, and communities. We have provided concrete services, and we have cried with clients. We have made a difference in this epidemic! Having made a difference, then, why do we find ourselves, as a profession, faced with so many serious threats to our survival? What can and should we do to deal with these threats, and how can we position ourselves to survive?

The matter of survival is as real for social workers in this field as it is for our patients and clients. Addressing the onslaught of attacks within our practice settings is a very real agenda for many social workers today. This situation is not just present for those in HIV/AIDS care. In fact, hospital and medical social work departments and units across the country are faced with many of these same dilemmas (Globerman and Bogo, 2002).

Over the past ten years, I have had many opportunities to work alongside social workers in community-based, medical, and health care settings as they provided HIV/AIDS-related services. I have been privileged to collaborate in works that examined what we do, the ways in which we present our work to others, and the ways in which we document the efficacy of our work. This chapter discusses many of the factors identified and confronted during these collaborations. I discuss factors that have likely contributed to our current professional situation, ways in which we have tried to respond to these factors, and things we will need to do to survive in this work. Sharing these narrative experiences is important as we look to our future in HIV/AIDS care and service delivery.

Many of the working collaborations that will be discussed were born out of an urgent need for providers to document the effect and benefits of social work services in response to funding and resource demands. At other times the work grew out of an interest by providers to advance the knowledge of social work interventions in HIV/AIDS care. Regardless of the origin of these collaborations, one constant element was and is always present: the unwavering commitment and compassion demonstrated by social workers to do this work and to make a difference for our clients. Commitment and compassion are essential attributes for doing this work. They are rarely, however, sufficient for keeping programs afloat.

Throughout this discussion I will refer to "storytelling." It is important to note that I am not talking about fictional storytelling, but rather using the narrative process as a mechanism for presenting the work we have done, currently do, and will continue to do in the arena of HIV/AIDS care and services. Another point that needs to be clarified here is that telling the story is just the beginning of the process. It is my hope that readers of this essay will be inspired and challenged to engage in other efforts that promote the work we do with and for our clients. Although it is essential that we celebrate our past successes and lament the losses, it is equally important for us to critically assess our professional strengths and weaknesses.

WHEN COMPASSION AND COMMITMENT ARE NOT ENOUGH: THE DILEMMA OF HIV/AIDS SOCIAL WORK SERVICES

Social workers have tirelessly provided care and services throughout the HIV/AIDS epidemic. We have worked with and for our clients in so many ways. Our efforts have been valiant at times, and they have undoubtedly aided clients and their families in innumerable ways (Claiborne and Vandenburgh, 2001). Along the path of service to clients, we seemingly forgot service to our own survival in these care settings.

Today health care service delivery is not predicated on the need for care as much as it is on the ability to cover the costs for care (Mizrahi and Berger, 2001; Kahn et al., 2001). This holds true for accessing services and providing the vehicles for service delivery. The availability and adequacy of health care in the United States is inextricably linked to market and economic forces. The United States is one of the most, if not the most, technologically rich countries in the world, yet a substantial proportion of our citizens are without adequate medical care (Hackey, 1998). The ability to pay for these services is key to accessing services. Further, the ability to mobilize the resources to provide these services places varying units in the health care industry in better or worse positions for practice. Stated another way, if a unit or profession can get the money and resources to cover the costs for delivering its services, then the group has power within the health care industry. The inability to generate these funds puts groups at the mercy of those who do generate the resources. Striving to attain and retain these resources becomes one of the important tasks for social work in health care settings—including those doing HIV/AIDS care and treatment (Mizrahi and Berger, 2001).

Historically, social work has been a profession committed to work with and on behalf of oppressed, disenfranchised, and marginalized groups. Our roots in health care are linked to our ability to understand and address environmental forces that cause and/or exacerbate medical problems (Bracht, 1978b). In many contemporary medical care settings, this environmental emphasis has been replaced—possibly to our own detriment—by specialization of services and greater emphasis on patient introspection and pharmacological interventions. Our work with patients on individual and psychological adjustments contributes greatly to their well-being. However, what has become increasingly unclear is how our current professional functions and identity are delineated from those of other providers in the health care industry (Bracht, 1978a). Although we may believe fervently in the need for the interventions we deliver, if we cannot substantiate their utility, their benefits, and the continued need for such services, then we are forced to have others define our future within health settings. Further, if we cannot articulate how our services translate into resource generation, and not just resource depletion, then our roles and viability within medical settings become even more tenuous.

THE NEED TO TELL OUR STORIES: DOCUMENTING FOR SURVIVAL

The social work profession has a rich history of advocacy on behalf of various constituencies. Our work has transcended the decades and produced untold benefits for countless groups. As a profession, we have been astute observers of political and social processes. We understand the need for social action and for being change agents for our clients (Mattaini, Meyer, and Lowery, 1999). Somewhere in developing strong advocacy for our clients we have not consistently advocated for ourselves and our professional standing with the same zeal. Developing an agenda for professional advocacy has, in contemporary health care arenas, become an imperative for social workers.

Advocating for the professional presence of social work in HIV/AIDS care requires us to be reflective and self-critical. It calls us to revisit the work we have done. It requires us to evaluate our successes and learn from our mistakes. Ultimately, this professional advocacy demands that we mobilize toward strengthening our professional position in care settings and advancing our professional interventions. Telling our stories, the narratives describing what we do, becomes one way of letting others know about the power, value, and importance of our work. In addition, these narratives should serve as a reminder to other social workers that we are professionals with knowledge, skills, and values that truly make a difference for the clients we serve and the larger society. Before discussing the content of these narratives and stories of our work, it is important to examine the building blocks that give our professional identities life.

TELLING OUR STORIES IS MORE THAN "STORYTELLING": THE THREE Ws

Recently I was asked to present the grand rounds at a large teaching hospital. The social work department sponsored this event and requested that I address three main points: (1) discuss the importance of social work services in the health care milieu; (2) promote the idea that social workers should and could contribute more to the professional health services literature; and (3) make the discussion lively and interesting. (The first two points seemed clear to me but the third required a bit of work.)

In preparing for this discussion, I came across an interesting commentary about barriers to social workers' writing for the professional literature. In this commentary, Mel Gray (1999) writes that many social workers believe what they have to say is uninteresting, which he finds "ironic because social workers often spend more time than other professionals keeping records and writing. Unless this writing is translated into an accessible form, valuable case studies and other impressions may be lost" (p. 305). Translating this valuable material before it is lost is precisely the reason for social workers to tell their stories.

The many ways in which we can tell others about our work are certainly too varied to attempt to address here. What I can offer is a template for structuring an approach to this endeavor. I have used this template many times in classrooms and consultations. This approach, the three Ws, asks the narrator to answer three questions: What is being done? Why is it being done? and What difference does it make?

The first W: What do we do? Here the social worker is being asked to describe the intervention. In this description the worker wants to provide enough information about the intervention or service so that it literally comes to life for the person hearing or reading the narrative. As can happen in professional arenas, jargon is used, assumptions about levels of understanding are made, and shortcuts in describing the work are taken. In exchanges with colleagues familiar with our work, these practices may be acceptable and warranted. However, when it comes to letting others know about the work we do, fleshing out the details is essential.

This is a tricky point, because it is possible to provide so much detail that both the presenter and the receiver of the information get lost. However, enough information must be presented so that the complexities of the work done stand out. Oversimplification of the work can lead to at least two negative outcomes: (1) belief that professional status is not required to accomplish the tasks; and (2) fewer resources can be expended to accomplish the task. Both of these issues have manifested in powerful ways in the area of social work services for HIV/AIDS in health care settings. Namely, there has been an increased reliance on other professionals and/or paraprofessionals to accomplish "social work" duties (also called downgrading) and significant budget cuts (Citrome, 1997). Clearly, many factors contribute to budget cuts. I have listened to colleagues describe (narrate) the details and complexities of their work. When asked to show where and how these activities are linked to budget requests and expenditures, the dollar-to-task correlations were not clear.

Consistency and precision in the narrative are other key elements. Key decision makers who may be less familiar with the intrinsic benefits of establishing rapport with clients may need to be convinced of this. Telling the story can be useful in this endeavor. Another factor that probably contributes to the difficulties we have in telling others what we do is that many, if not most, of the tools we use are intangible. We engage clients in processes that involve dialogue: we talk to clients. We often record information on specific forms, but as a profession we do not have instruments and tools that are readily defined by those outside of social work as social work tools. Take, for example, stethoscopes, syringes, and thermometers. These implements are probably easily identified by the average American as being associated with health care workers. Not having such universally identified symbols of practice, the narratives of what we do, our stories, become critical to our professional survival.

The story should provide a clear and concise description of the steps used to engage the client and how this engagement can result in benefits for the client, the medical/unit service, and the organization. A running commentary among social workers (how we can process everything) cautions us to avoid getting lost in the storytelling process and yet to succinctly convey in sufficient fullness the description of what we are doing with and for the client.

Finally, the concept of telling others what we do is consistent with our professional training. Social workers spend many hours in field and class-room settings developing and mastering practice skills. Often we rehearse and demonstrate our skills in mock and supervised sessions. We are chal-lenged in our training to think about the successive steps needed to imple-ment particular interventions or skills. Repeatedly we conceptualize the pathways needed to demonstrate that we have mastered assessing, explor-ing, intervening, and concluding skills (Cournoyer, 1996). Describing to others these practices should be a common aspect of our professional reper-toire. In a competitive market, such as HIV/AIDS in medical settings, our ability to articulate what we do, in oral and written communications, and to do it concisely and succinctly may be as vital to social work survival as per-forming the skill itself.

The second W: Why do we do it? Having and demonstrating a profes-sional knowledge base is critical not just as an academic exercise. More-over, it is a defining feature of a profession (Baker, 1994). Much like the ability to articulate what we do, being able to defend and justify why we do our interventions is an essential resource in defending the profession's posi-tion in HIV/AIDS care services. Social work services are often character-ized, by the uninitiated, as simply "helping people," and doing so without a specific method, purpose, or theory. Our ability to justify or provide a "grounded" rationale for our services moves the position of the social worker from that of a "do-gooder" to that of a professional equal whose acts are purposive and directed toward targeted change.

For some social work professionals, articulating the theory and concepts that guide their practice is second nature while for others this is a daunting and nearly incomprehensible task. Such diversity in responses speaks to a level of unevenness within our professional ranks. Over the years I have heard and witnessed many interesting responses by social workers to the question "Why do you do the practice/intervention you do?" At times the re-sponses are cogent and passionate articulations of purpose, pathways, and process. In other instances workers present concrete responses, although they are often repetitions of the organizational policy and procedure man-ual. The latter responses do not do justice to the training of and public sanc-tion for professional social work.

Professional social workers are expected to deliver interventions that are appropriate to the situation at hand. A significant aspect of selecting the ap-propriate intervention is having an understanding of various theories, frame-works, models, and concepts that predict and describe human behavior and social interactions. Mattaini (1999) points to two reasons that the profes-sional should have these tools: (1) "to communicate with other profession-als who may be operating from a different conceptual framework" and

(2) "because no theory is adequate to explain all phenomena at all levels of practice, social workers may sometimes need to turn to theories other than the ones from which they usually operate" (p. 111).

The discussion of theories in practice is sometimes elevated, or devalued, to a discussion exclusively for researchers and academicians. This perspective is detrimental to professional social work practice. By distancing practice from the theoretical and conceptual knowledge base, social work and social workers risk two unfortunate outcomes: (1) having their practice blindly guided or perceived as such; and (2) constantly "recreating the wheel" because the worker is unfamiliar with theory that would allow selection of appropriate techniques for intervention(s). The utility of theory in social work practice is arguably only as good as the application. Thus, theories are used to guide the worker in selecting the interventions and not to be the end result of the process. As Turner (1996) notes,

> When theory becomes overly cerebral and mechanistic, stressing labeling and classifying rather than on the individuality of each client and situation, it can become an end in itself. Then the ability to predict, explain and even control becomes the goal, rather than the optimizing of human potential and facilitating growth. (p. 13)

In my own work, and in collaborations with other HIV/AIDS care providers, I often require a drawing of the conceptual practice model. This rendering is used as a tool to flesh out the elements of the underlying theories and concepts employed in the intervention. I have found this process to be particularly beneficial when I am having difficulty articulating the underpinnings of my work or the work of colleagues. The following example illustrates this point.

An HIV/AIDS prevention intervention for adolescents incorporates work with parents and teens to reduce the risk of pregnancy, sexually transmitted infections (STIs), and substance abuse. In discussing the model for the intervention, the staff initially identified stages of change (Prochaska, Redding, and Evers, 1997) as the only guiding force behind their intervention. As we explored and completed drawings of the model of practice, it became apparent that the intervention also contained elements from communications theory and social and community development frameworks (Payne, 1997). This was an important realization for the organization. Because they realized that their intervention was influenced by more than one framework, the administrator examined more carefully the skill sets needed to implement the program successfully. This examination by the administrator led to seeking and obtaining additional funding for staff training and other resources. Success in this process was partially attributed to the ability to articulate to superiors the complexities of the intervention, which had produced favorable outcomes in the past. These complexities were supported based on practice experience with the client group, theories and models of practice, and the documented benefits of the programs.

The third W: What difference does it make? For a great many social work providers, including those in HIV/AIDS care and services, this has become the big question. Increasingly, funders, administrators, and the general public want to know how the billions of dollars spent on HIV/AIDS have made a difference.* This question is being asked in many ways and with a sense of urgency. In my work over the past six years, the role of documenting and evaluating the outcomes and impacts of HIV/AIDS interventions has skyrocketed. Along with the emphasis on evaluation has come an anxiousness among providers and provider systems that is at times palpable. This anxiety is not lost on social work professionals.

The word *evaluation* evokes visions of criticism; using the assessment to edge a person or program out; or just being mean. In sum, evaluation is often viewed as a negative. Evaluation is infused with thoughts of numerical assessments that reduce the human element to its least common denominator or take it completely out of the picture. Undoubtedly, evaluations have been used for these purposes. Social workers in HIV/AIDS care, especially those in medical and hospital care settings, are probably too familiar with the ways in which evaluations have been used to justify downsizing and "outsizing." These, however, are not the only ways in which evaluation should and can be used. Given the prominence of evaluation in HIV/AIDS services today, social workers will need to think strategically and tactically about ways of turning a burden into a benefit.

Professional social workers are familiar with the concepts of evaluation. We are taught in our training that assessing one's practice is an important and essential part of being a professional social worker. Most of us waded through one, two, or possibly three research and/or statistics courses and completed at least one research project or report, and this is where many of us wanted research and evaluation to end. As noted in the discussion of theory and practice, separating the assessment and evaluation of practice from the knowledge and skills base of evaluation methods does not do justice to our professional training. In the competitive HIV/AIDS arena we must, in fact, do a better job of bridging the two worlds. A complete review of evalu-

---

*For example, the Government Performance and Results Act of 1993 has among its stated goals: "Improve the confidence of the American people in the capability of the Federal Government, by systematically holding Federal agencies accountable for achieving program results; and improve Federal program effectiveness and public accountability by promoting a new focus on results, service quality, and customer satisfaction."

ation skills is not possible in this chapter. In this section, I want to highlight a few key points and underscore ways in which evaluation can be used to support the presence and roles of professional social workers in HIV/AIDS services.

Social workers engaged in HIV/AIDS care and services must be able to evaluate practice on at least two levels, process and outcome. Both are important in providing a complete description of the benefits of our interventions. Process evaluation may be intuitively more conducive to social work practice interventions. Since most social workers can recall (or still utilize) process recordings, the learning curve is often less steep than with other types of evaluation. In process evaluation we examine the components of our interventions with a goal of documenting reliable and replicable applications of the intervention steps. If the social worker has delineated the steps and/or stages of the intervention (first W), which are guided by a particular framework or theory (second W), assessing the fidelity and consistency of the process should flow naturally. Certainly, of necessity, interventions with "real" clients will vary. Such variance, however, should not be so dramatic from client to client that the same intervention is not recognizable. Empirical support for the intervention's implementation comes in many formats. One of the most common in social work practice is our case and/or chart notes. These documents become the proof that we have done a specific intervention. These documents, as will be discussed later, also become the mechanism for demonstrating the efficacy of our interventions.

In collaborations and consultations what I have encountered is that intervention processes are described, but often without constant articulation of the core elements. In some instances the absence of the core elements' identification is related to poorly understood and defined concepts, theories, and/or frameworks for practice. Social workers who are clear about the framework for practice are in a far better position to identify the core (essential) elements of the practice. This can be done in a concise manner and still accommodate idiosyncratic elements of the specific client interaction. The constant identification of the core elements of one's practice can be helpful in reinforcing the purposive nature of social work. This may be especially useful to those unfamiliar with professional social work practice.

Another important aspect of evaluation for social workers to address is identifying and documenting outcomes. In this regard, social workers must be able to envision the goals they have established with and for their clients and to translate these visions into observable and measurable terms. Creating observable and measurable means of evaluating practice interventions can create tensions for workers. For some social workers, the client's well-being and success is not something regarded in quantifiable terms. Nevertheless, the ability to translate clinical successes into observable and measurable terms is a skill needed by social workers in competitive markets. In countless consultations I have heard workers say that quantifying a client's situation is artificial and reduces the client to something less than a person. Inasmuch as numbers cannot show the entire picture of a client's situation and/or progress, I concur with this assessment. However, the ability to track client movement and progress by using markers that are both observable and quantifiable can benefit the social worker and often the client as well.

One of the primary benefits is our ability to quickly convey to others the "amount" of movement that a client has made over a period of time. Here both the magnitude and the duration of the change can have important implications for the social worker's articulation of the need for continued services or alterations in the current treatment intervention. Conveying information about clinical interactions in quantifiable terms is not synonymous with turning our backs on the qualitative and idiosyncratic aspects of our clients' situations. In fact, it can serve quite the opposite purpose by demonstrating the degree to which our interventions have a documented impact on clients. Further, it provides evidence for the need to continue such interventions, and hopefully justify why a social worker in particular should deliver the services. With the growing emphasis by funders, administrators, and others on service outcome and impacts, it is essential that social work professionals in HIV/AIDS support their rich clinical work with rigorous evaluations of both the process and outcome of their practice. These evaluations should blend both qualitative (narrative) descriptions of the work done with and for clients and the outcomes of this work. These descriptions, although important, are not sufficient to convey, to an often skeptical audience, that what we do or did really makes a difference and warrants continued support.

I have presented here a framework for telling a story. The story to be told is a story of how social work has, does, and will continue to make meaningful contributions to the lives of clients impacted by HIV/AIDS. One reason for taking the storytelling approach is that it embodies much of what social workers already do in their daily work when they write and speak to one another about the services they provide. Telling the story is a familiar metaphor for most of us, and it can invoke a sense of calm in approach to a sometimes awkward task.

As has been pointed out, telling a story is not just an exercise in futility. Rather, it is presented as one means we have to combat the many forces that have eroded the role of social work in HIV/AIDS. The specific framework presented is simple in its presentation but potentially very powerful in its impact. The cornerstones of this narrative sharing are three points: telling what we do (our intervention and service descriptions); telling why we do it (our theoretical and conceptual frameworks for taking such interventions); and telling what difference our work has made. These three elements are presented as a foundation for conveying to others (social workers and other professions) the importance of social work in HIV/AIDS care. The following example is presented to highlight this. The example is drawn from my experiences as a provider, colleague, collaborator, and consultant with many HIV/AIDS social workers over the past ten years.

CASE EXAMPLE

A local hospital's HIV/AIDS unit that provides both inpatient and outpatient care experienced five to seven years of significant growth. The growth resulted in the addition of twenty full-time staff members. Staff represented multiple disciplines: nursing, nutrition, psychology, social work, art therapy, and dental hygiene. In addition to the growth in number and diversity of staff, there was an accompanying growth in the number of unit patients from an average monthly census of 100 to 300 registered clients. The team of professionals on the unit interacted well with one another and provided many useful services to the clients.

Approximately eighteen months ago two events seemed to converge and change the milieu of the unit. First, a new administrator was assigned to this unit. The incumbent was a social worker with more than ten years of clinical experience and another twelve years as a hospital administrator. Second, immediately preceding the arrival of the administrator there was a precipitous decline in the monthly client census. Staff on the unit speculated about the impact that the census decline and the new administrator would have on their positions.

One of the first things the new administrator did was to meet each of the staff members to get an idea of the person's prior experiences on and vision for the unit. Unknown to the staff, the administrator had been informed that the unit was not fiscally sound and that the budget was being adjusted to reflect declines in census and growing demands elsewhere in the medical corporation. The administrator was faced with two critical tasks: (1) meeting client needs and (2) restructuring the unit given its fiscal standing.

After meeting with the staff individually, the administrator convened a meeting of the entire professional team and shared the news regarding the fiscal standing of the unit and the need to address the corporation's concerns. In addition, she shared with the staff members a vision of the unit that was actually a composite of the stories they had relayed during their individual meetings. The composite told of a unit that grew in response to significant community needs, flourished, and never looked back. The composite was void of critical programmatic analyses or reflections of the work being done, how to sustain it, or how to alter it. Although the composite picture was rich with reflections by staff members about what they had done and wanted to do, it lacked a coordinating and consolidating base for these reflections. The team was impressed by the administrator's attentiveness to their reflections and even more so by the concise and comprehensive story presented. Instead of being demoralized, the team was energized as they reflected on their work, but nonetheless daunted by finding ways to move forward. The administrator recommended that the team think about these issues and reconvene the following week.

Before the next meeting the administrator gave the team members three items to read. One was a newspaper report about their unit. This report was five years old and had been found by the administrator while cleaning her new office. The article was about the "new" unit and three clients that were returning to work as a result of their experiences with this unit. The article included pictures of staff, many of whom were still there, working with clients. The second item she gave the team to read was an article from a professional journal. This article was written by a social worker and focused on family and community as important resources for creating and sustaining client social supports and community stability. The third item distributed was the annual report from the medical corporation. The report, a high gloss and impressive document, was full of statistics about their fiscal, community, and professional standings. There were pictures of and quotes from patients, families, administrators, medical personnel, financial supporters, and elected officials. As might be expected, each of these persons gave brief accounts of why and how the corporation was important to them and to the viability of the surrounding community.

At the next meeting of the professional team, the administrator asked the staff to reflect on and respond to the readings. After a moment of awkward silence the staff began to talk about the readings. Staff recalled fondly and with passion the early days of the unit, including the struggles they had setting up the unit and working out the relationships with community and other staff. They discussed the ways in which the many disciplines had to learn to work in tandem. The team also discussed the ways in which clients informed the development of the unit. Other team members commented on the way the corporation focused on financial outputs and questioned if the clients were truly important at all. The administrator listened attentively and took notes. After about thirty minutes the administrator presented the staff with three drawings she had made during their discussion.

The first drawing depicted the many tasks workers did to support and assist their clients' development. The second depiction was of the many linkages needed to move clients from a starting point to a desired goal. The final drawing was a picture of a client smiling with lines drawn to connect this picture to the other two pictures. Staff asked the administrator to explain this strange collage. In her response she pointed out that the client in the third drawing was a client "successfully" served by the unit team. The lines to the other drawings represented pathways and relationships that assisted the client to get to this point. The second drawing depicted the many systems the team identified as needing to be impacted in working toward client goals. Further, the second drawing underscored philosophical, theoretical, and conceptual frameworks of the team (i.e., emphasis on family and social networks, systems orientation, and cognitive skills). The first drawing not only represented the work staff actually did with clients, but it also linked to the second drawing in that the models and concepts employed by staff related to the activities of their work. At first the staff were surprised and questioned the validity of this exercise, especially since significant changes were looming.

The administrator took time to explain that based on her review of the existing records, individual discussions with staff, and the two staff meetings, she was convinced the unit staff members were not getting full credit for the work they were doing. This included the absence of (1) client satisfaction assessments; (2) documentation of cumulative client outcomes; and (3) any dissemination of their work beyond the unit. She summed up by saying that she realized changes had to occur given the fiscal situation, but she believed part of the dilemma lay in the lack of detail in the narration of the scope and impact of the team's work. The administrator concluded by asking the team to join in a critical examination of the work of the unit, the purpose of that work, and its outcome. The team agreed since, at the very least, it bought time for their positions.

Over the next several months the team mined old records for information, critically and rigorously examined their work with clients, and evaluated the products of their work. The team met regularly, with and without the administrator, to review and record their efforts and progress. At the end of several months the team had not only evaluated their practices, but they had also created a framework that was identified by the corporation as exemplary. The clinical successes of the team were presented during hospital meetings, grand rounds, and during community and professional gatherings. At the end of a year, the team members looked back with amazement at the amount of work they had accomplished. They attributed much of the success to the administrator. The administrator pointed out that she may have been a catalyst for the work, but that it was the team members who had designed and implemented the work. In the end, the financial difficulties faced on this unit were not fully avoided, but they were significantly less than originally projected.

This example is a composite of many experiences, and the linear trajectory was, in practice, not always so linear. The work described here is, however, representative of an approach that has worked for other social workers in practice. Faced with an ever-growing threat to our professional survival in HIV/AIDS care, professional social workers must pick up the mantle and be willing to advocate on their own behalf. This example highlights one method for approaching this work.

CONCLUSION

It may seem that much of the discussion in this chapter has been about the stability of the social work profession and the social worker. This is a correct characterization. I make no claims that the schema I am presenting will result in any significant change in the course of a single client's care and/or treatment. I do posit that with more attention by social work professionals to the definition and articulation of what we do, why we do it, and what difference it makes, we can position ourselves to be more competitive, viable, and visible in service to our clients. By extension, I have suggested that inattentiveness to these issues will allow others to continue to define our position in HIV/AIDS care and usurp our roles. As one, if not the only, profession defined by its commitment to work with and for disenfranchised and oppressed client systems, I sincerely believe it would be a loss to all clients if HIV/AIDS care were devoid of a significant social work presence.

In this struggle we are challenged to develop and deploy mechanisms that, first and foremost, meet the goals of service provision for our clients. In addition, we must work actively to address the need for professional viability and survival. The model presented in this essay will not change the world of social work. What it can do is provide a framework for social workers in HIV/AIDS care to use in assessing their work, advocating for themselves, and assuring a place at the table to advocate for and serve clients. By telling what we do, why we do it, and what difference it makes—in written and oral forms—we increase the likelihood that we will be heard and that we will be there. Our silence at this time may mean more than lost opportunities for our clients later.

REFERENCES

Baker, R.L. (1994). *The Social Work Dictionary,* Second Edition. Washington, DC: NASW.

Bracht, N.F. (1978a). Contributions to comprehensive health care: Basic premises. In N.F. Bracht (Ed.), *Social Work in Health Care: A Guide to Professional Practice* (pp. 19-33). Binghamton, NY: The Haworth Press.

Bracht, N.F. (1978b). The scope and historical development of social work, 1900-1975. In N.F. Bracht (Ed.), *Social Work in Health Care: A Guide to Professional Practice* (pp. 3-18). Binghamton, NY: The Haworth Press.

Citrome, L. (1997). Layoffs, reductions-in-force, downsizing, rightsizing: The case of a state psychiatric hospital. *Administration and Policy in Mental Health* 24(6): 523-533.

Claiborne, N. and Vandenburgh, H. (2001). Social workers' role in disease management. *Health and Social Work* 26(4): 217-225.

Cournoyer, B. (1996). *The Social Work Skills Workbook,* Second Edition. New York: Brooks/Cole Publishing.

Globerman, J. and Bogo, M. (2002). The impact of hospital restructuring on social work field education. *Health and Social Work* 27(1): 7-16.

Gray, M. (1999). Writing for a journal: Blood, sweat, and tears. *Families in Society* 80(3): 305-308.

Hackey, R.B. (1998). *Rethinking Health Care Policy: The New Politics of State Regulation.* Washington, DC: Georgetown University Press.

Kahn, J.G., Haile, B., Rates, J., and Chang, S. (2001). Health and federal budgetary effects of increasing access to antiretroviral medications for HIV by expanding Medicaid. *American Journal of Public Health* 91(9): 1464-1473.

Mattaini, M.A. (1999). Knowledge for practice. In M.A. Mattaini, C.T. Lowery, and C.H. Meyer (Eds.), *The Foundations of Social Work Practice: A Graduate Text,* Second Edition (pp. 87-116). Washington, DC: NASW.

Mattaini, M.A., Meyer, C.H., and Lowery, C.T. (1999). Introduction. In M.A. Mattaini, C.T. Lowery, and C.H. Meyer (Eds.), *The Foundations of Social Work Practice: A Graduate Text,* Second Edition (pp. xiii-xxx). Washington, DC: NASW.

Mizrahi, T. and Berger, C.S. (2001). Effect of a changing health care environment on social work leaders: Obstacles and opportunities in hospital social work. *Social Work* 46(2): 170-182.

Payne, M. (1997). *Modern Social Work Theory,* Second Edition. Chicago, IL: Lyceum.

Prochaska, J.O., Redding, C.A., and Evers, K.E. (1997). The transtheoretical model and stages of change. In K. Glanz, F.M. Lewis, and B.K. Rimer (Eds.), *Health Behavioral and Health Education: Theory, Research and Practice,* Second Edition (pp. 60-84). San Francisco, CA: Jossey Bass.

Turner, F. (1996). *Social work treatment,* Fourth Edition. New York: Free Press.

Afterword

Barbara Willinger

The chapters in this book have taken you through the AIDS epidemic, from its early days of being known as GRID to today when the disease carries the well-known name AIDS—twenty-plus years of a new and deadly epidemic that some people originally likened to the plague. Although once this disease robbed men, women, and children of their lives within two years of being diagnosed with AIDS, those dealing with AIDS now have the possibility of life due to HAART.

Hospital social workers were there from the beginning—on the cutting edge of the work. We were there as an extension of our role within hospitals, but some of us also came out of a personal commitment to confront a powerfully driven disease, as you have seen reflected in the chapters. For other social workers, it was an extension or expansion of social work values of working with people who are considered disenfranchised by society at large. From the beginning and continuing to the present, social work has striven to infuse clients and affected communities with a sense of empowerment.

We can be proud of our many and varied contributions to develop, implement, and extend services to persons with AIDS: from initiating early responses to developing ongoing case management standards, to identifying system impediments to patients' access to care, to the recognition of the need for child care planning mechanisms, to the ongoing daily work of providing services to people with complex needs who are often in devastating medical or psychosocial situations. Across the country we sat on city, state, and local task forces that brainstormed, developed, and implemented services necessitated by our patients' physical, emotional, and economic needs.

In time, more and more of the other helping professions entered into working with HIV/AIDS clients. We now share our work with many other disciplines, such as mental health, complementary therapies, and peer education. So although our work may no longer be heavily focused on ongoing supportive counseling and mental health assessments, our therapeutic exchanges with patients do not have to cease so long as we maintain a clinical understanding of patient dynamics within the context and framework of delivery of concrete services or in the assumption of the case management role.

Today's climate of HIV/AIDS and the interjection of managed care has resulted in a shift of emphasis from inpatient to outpatient care. Several of the chapters have raised questions about the direction and role of hospital-based social work. Will our specialized role be diluted (and will we become generalists) in this new climate? What new paradigms will we need to accept? Will non-master's-level-trained social workers or perhaps nurses undertake the case manager role? Will social work participation veer more toward community-based organizations or in New York to the newly developing special needs plans? These are questions yet to be answered.

It appears that after twenty years we are entering a new era, just as we did when HIV/AIDS appeared on the scene. A change has occurred from patients dying from AIDS to living with HIV. We must now work within different fiscally driven service delivery models. But some of the issues remain the same for our clients: shock, despair, loss, adherence, and shame. On the broad canvas of service delivery, there are many social workers now in the field who have no historical perspective of HIV/AIDS work and enter it with few if any preconceived ideas of what the work was; they are aware only of what it now is. For them and the social workers to come, this book provides a framework of understanding care delivery and what the "fight" was all about.

Many of us who have been in the field for ten years or more heralded the introduction of protease inhibitors and HAART with somewhat less enthusiasm than others. We had experienced other "breakthroughs," such as AZT, that although beneficial also brought ultimate feelings of disappointment and disillusionment for many patients. Today's treatments do offer a respite for many in their struggle with AIDS, a time in which the virus may be undetectable but not gone. We must openly acknowledge, however, that HAART does not work for all and, even when effective, sometimes has difficult side effects or creates other medical complications such as high cholesterol and liver or cardiac disease.

Similar, however, to our initial need to know about AIDS opportunistic infections, we must now educate ourselves about HAART so that we can effectively assist clients in their struggles with adherence. But adherence is only one small part of the larger picture. As several chapters have indicated, we must engage clients in finding ways to manage their time now that it is no longer always focused on their health. This raises questions for us to ponder for the future. As libido returns, will people engage in safer sex practices? Will we need to renew our efforts to educate and remind patients of the risks? Will we be able to assist our clients in their transitions to the workforce? Will there be enough job training programs, let alone employment opportunities, available for HIV clients? Will clients be able to give up their benefits or will they need support from us to reach that decision? Those clients who successfully functioned in the world prior to infection will most likely have the ego capacity and skills to be able to return unless medically depleted. However, even for those who may continue to do well for an indefinite period of time it is also "clear that most people will not be able to stay on treatment for the rest of their lives. Between cumulative drug resistance, long-term side effects and simple weariness with the demands of the various regimens, it is almost naïve to expect people to be able to succeed for periods of 20 to 50 years or more. But that's what it will take to allow people to live a normal life despite HIV" (Project Inform, 2001, p. 2). Finally, there is and will always continue to be an entire group of clients who are well known to social work—those from socially and economically disadvantaged environments, those with substance use or mental illness, or those with a combination of these factors who will continue to struggle with their lives, with HIV being just another blow.

Whereas once AIDS was an illness that devastated adults in their peak productive years (twenties to forties) or attacked neonates robbing them of normal development, if not life itself, today we are seeing our clients living into their sixties and seventies, with some even being newly diagnosed at that age. Will their issues be any different from those we have already confronted? What about perinatally infected children who have survived, many only to be suffering from severe behavioral problems and mental illness? Perhaps these will be the next frontiers of social work.

So although our place in history may be over, our work as social workers and clinicians is not. We are just in another phase—as is the AIDS epidemic.

REFERENCE

Project Inform (2001). Past_Present_and_Future@20Years. *Perspective* 33: 1-4.

Index

Page numbers followed by the letter "f" indicate figures; those followed by the letter "t" indicate tables.

St. Claire's Hospital, NYC, 28, 78
St. Luke's Hospital, NYC, 214, 221, 226
St. Luke's-Roosevelt Hospital Center, NYC, 155, 278
St. Mary's Medical Center, SF, 35, 37, 39
St. Vincent's Hospital, NYC, 28
Staff support, 111. *See also* Collegial support; Professional peer support
  DAS, 75
  group, 164
  groups, MSKCC, 151-152
Stage of change, and custody planning, 298
Standby guardianship legislation, 290
Stigma
  AIDS social workers, 37
  continuing, 245, 309
  early HIV, 7, 43, 106
Structured treatment interruption (STI), 284
Suffering and dependency, Atlanta support group, 137-138
Sunburst, Sonoma County, 319
Supervision
  case management, 171-172, 173-174
  CSS Weill Cornell, 233
  Moore Clinic, Baltimore, 273-276
  one-on-one, 164
  PWAs work, 191-194
Supervisory support systems, 180
Supplemental Support Income (SSI), 256
Support groups. *See also* Collegial support; Patient support group; Professional peer support; Staff support
  bereavement, 151, 174
  chronic disease, 152
  couples, partners, caretakers, 150-151
  family, NYC, 128-130
  patients, Atlanta, 133-134
  PWAs work, 191

Support groups *(continued)*
  recommended rules, 140
  staff, 151-152
  time-limited, 251, 257
Survivor's guilt, 260
"Symptomatic HIV," case management eligibility, 318-319

Team building, 38
Team care, 54-55
Terminal illness, 146-147
Terminally ill work, 184
Theory articulation, social work narrative, 334-336
Therapeutic relationship, dying person, 153
Thompson, Bruce, 85
Three Ws of social work narrative, 332-339
Time-limited group therapy, 251
  life continuance issues, 257
Toxoplasmosis, *xxx*, 6, 144
Transferential "good mother," 188
Transitional care center, 15
Transmission misinformation, 126
Triply diagnosed clients, 251
Tuberculosis (TB), 6, 8, 157
  multidrug resistant, 97
Tulane University School of Social Work, 87, 90
"Twinship," 175

Union College, Schenectady, 64
University of California
  UCSF Center for AIDS Prevention, 166
  UCSF Positive Health Practice, 248
  UCSF Women's Specialty Program, 247
  UCSF-AIDS Health Project, 164
Urban, Susan, 72

Velez, Dennis, 73
Vertical infection, 14